THE PHYSICIAN AS MANAGER

John J. Aluise

THE PHYSICIAN AS MANAGER

Second Edition

With 100 Illustrations

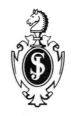

Springer-Verlag
New York Berlin Heidelberg
London Paris Tokyo

John J. Aluise, Ph.D.
Department of Family Medicine
University of North Carolina
Chapel Hill, NC 27514
U.S.A.

Library of Congress Cataloging in Publication Data
Aluise, John J.
    The physician as manager.
    Includes bibliographies and index.
    1. Medicine—Practice.   2. Medical offices—
Management.   I. Title. [DNLM: 1. Practice
Management, Medical. W 80 A471p]
    R728.A4   1986   610′.68   86-21980

The first edition of this book was published by the Charles Press Publishers, Division of the Robert J. Brady Co.,
Bowie, Maryland, in 1980.

Typeset by BiComp, Inc., York, Pennsylvania.
Printed and bound by Quinn-Woodbine Inc., Woodbine, New Jersey.
Printed in the United States of America.

9 8 7 6 5 4 3 2 1

ISBN 0-387-96381-2 Springer-Verlag New York Berlin Heidelberg
ISBN 3-540-96381-2 Springer-Verlag Berlin Heidelberg New York

This book, as well as all my personal and professional accomplishments, are a result of the love and support I have received from my parents, Vanda and Joseph; my wife, Barbara, who has been a partner in my life's work; and my children, Joseph, Edward and Gina, who provide us with a continuing sense of pride and satisfaction.

Foreword to the Second Edition

Physicians generally finish their residencies well trained to manage the medical problems they will face, but poorly prepared to function in the many other roles required. Physicians will have to manage not only their patients, but also their time, personnel, patient scheduling, practice structure and office systems, billing and collecting, as well as practice and personal finances. Although each of these areas has tremendous impact on the quality of their personal and professional lives, physicians usually enter practice without the training and skills needed to manage effectively.

Good management of a medical practice has always been important, but in today's rapidly changing health care environment it is critical. Increased competition and external pressures to contain costs make it mandatory that practices meet the needs of the population served in a cost-efficient manner. An understanding of how and why people choose their physician is required if patients are to be attracted and kept. The physician must provide the leadership necessary to create a therapeutic environment that is mutually satisfying for patients and physician.

The development of alternative practice structures such as health maintenance organizations, independent practice associations, and preferred provider organizations, as well as alterations in reimbursement such as capitation plans, mandate that a physician be knowledgeable in these areas. The practice must be flexible and efficient if access to an adequate patient population is to be retained. Computerization will be required to meet these goals.

The Physician as Manager is the single best source I have found for the information required to manage a successful medical practice. Not only has John Aluise served as a practice management educator, he also has assisted many residents with the development of their practices and has followed them over time. These experiences have given him unique insight into the needs of a physician manager. The result is a textbook that is both comprehensive and practical. Its expansion to include chapters on the economic environment of health care, marketing health services, and the computer-ization of medical practices is most appropriate and timely. *The Physician as Manager* should be required reading for anyone who is involved in medical practice with any management re-sponsibilities. Following the principles outlined will result in a more satisfying personal and pro-fessional life.

THOMAS L. SPEROS, M.D.

Washington Family Medicine Center, Washington, D.C.

Clinical Instructor, Department of Family Medicine, University of North Carolina School of Medicine

Clinical Assistant Professor, Department of Family Practice, East Carolina University School of Medicine

Foreword to the First Edition

Physicians enter the world of practice with a zeal and idealism that is very seldom equalled. Their many years of training have provided them with the knowledge and skills to care for the many problems that patients will present. They have also promised themselves that their continuing education will not be given low priority and they will not make the same errors as the older physicians whom they have observed.

The first year of practice usually equals their expectations. They are able to practice at an enjoyable pace, attend continuing education conferences, and enjoy what they are doing. As the second year begins, they find their practice growing, hours becoming longer, and usually, they have fired the first nurse and receptionist they hired.

At this time, the physician also discovers the accounts receivable has grown to such a large amount his accountant is suggesting firmer collection policies. This suggestion evokes some anger, but mostly guilt, and the physician usually compensates by a further increase in patient load to increase the cash flow. The physician also finds that continuing education hours and time spent with the family are decreasing, whereas the time necessary for the practice increases. The practice is now beginning to control the physician.

By the time the third year begins, the physician finds it necessary to add personnel in order to increase efficiency. The new personnel clash with the older personnel, and instead of decreasing problems, another is added. At this time, complaints about staff treatment of patients begin to increase. Frustration, depression, and anger are some of the feelings that dominate the physician's daily life at this point. Control of time is no longer the physician's. Patient and staff demands, coupled with a rising accounts receivable and inadequate cash flow, make the world of idealism a bit unrealistic.

By this time, continuing education has decreased to the required quarterly staff meetings and the physician's growing family is unhappy about their phantom father/mother. (The physician's spouse thought everything would be better once they went into practice!)

It is now five years into practice and several different things can happen—a change in location, change in specialty, entering a group, taking on a partner, divorce, alcoholism, etc. The physician, being independent and self-sufficient, finds it difficult to admit that he or she was not properly prepared for practice. Seven to eight years of medical school and residency should have been sufficient. Some of the professors said that practice management was something which would come easily and they would learn that when they went out into practice. Could it be that they might have been wrong?

Some physicians will overcome the above deficit by profiting from their mistakes. They may obtain consultation at a very large price and learn how to regain control of their practice and staff. Proper collection emphasis, motivating personnel, improving efficiency, and regaining control of the practice may come about by the seventh or eighth year.

But what will have been lost in those seven years? Reestablishing contacts with patients will produce patient dissatisfaction. The personnel that have been hired and fired usually do not lose their memory of the bad experience. Medical knowledge has a half-life of seven years and the physician now finds a need for a large refresher course, to say nothing of how the lack of recent knowledge may have harmed the patients. The most tragic part of these seven years is with the doctor's family. No matter how stable, they have paid some price for the past seven years.

Managing your practice in a scientific, reasonable manner, so that you can control your life, is what this book is all about. Use of the principles espoused by John Aluise may allow you to get home earlier, spend more time in continuing education, and perhaps, be a healthier person in a healthy family.

EDWARD J. SHAHADY, M.D.
Professor, Department of
Family Medicine,
University of North
Carolina

Acknowledgments

During the more than nine years I have been associated with the University of North Carolina (UNC) Department of Family Medicine, several people were instrumental in the educational and scholarly work that I accomplished. They are Drs David Citron, Lewis Sigmon, George Wolff, Richard Walton, Thomas Cable, Harry Summerlin, Peter Rizzolo, Donald Whitenack, Robert Gwyther, Richard Olson, and, especially, Edward Shahady. These residency program directors were committed to teaching residents the practical aspects of medical practice. Another group deserving recognition are the practice management education colleagues with whom I have worked over the years: Thomas Lee, Scott Pierson, David Gurley, David Michaels, Gary Smith, Stephen Scott, Michael Huppert, Stephen Bogdewic, and Vernon Rolf.

My special thanks go to my secretary, Marcia Hawks, who was an extremely capable and loyal assistant during the past four years.

Several people contributed directly to the second edition of *The Physician as Manager.* Samuel W. Warburton, MD, vice president of medical affairs for Health America, and Charles Kiskaden, health plan manager of Kaiser Foundation of North Carolina, reviewed the chapter on economic environment. Betty Cogswell, PhD, sociologist in the Department of Family Medicine at UNC, and Barnett Parker, PhD, marketing professor in the Department of Health Administration at UNC, reviewed the marketing chapter. Lee Ann Rotherberger, MA, director of research for the Moses Cone Family Practice Residency Program in Greensboro, NC, and Alan Gold, president of Global Health Systems, Rockville, Maryland, made important contributions to the computerization chapter. Others who reviewed various parts of the first edition and who offered suggestions for the revision were Regis Lyons and Thomas Pate, E. F. Hutton; Edward E. Hollowell, LLD, health care lawyer in Raleigh, NC; and William Zelman, PhD, CPA, finance professor in the Department of Health Administration at UNC. Patricia Barron, MPH, Paul Dunn, M.A. family nurse practitioner, and Ron Kellogg,

MD, who contributed patient education handouts included in the marketing appendix.

Finally, the staff and residents of the Family Practice Center of the University of North Carolina and the Family Practice Center of Akron City Hospital, Akron, Ohio, deserve very special recognition for allowing me to work with and learn from them in more ways than I could mention.

I would also like to acknowledge those staff members of the Department of Family Medicine at UNC who assisted in various aspects of the book. Carol Peterson, Patti Wilkerson, Ruth Williams, and Stephanie Kelly contributed directly to the preparation of the manuscript. Leslie Purcell and Linda Houseman provided invaluable editorial suggestions. Mary Beth Shenton, the audiovisual specialist in our department, designed the exhibits for Chapter 1.

Contents

Appendices

Index

Introduction

THE PHYSICIAN AS MANAGER OFFERS PHYSICIANS AND OTHER HEALTH PROFESSIONALS A PRACTICAL GUIDEBOOK TO UNDERSTAND THE ECONOMIC AND MANAGEMENT CONCEPTS RELEVANT TO MEDICAL PRACTICE.

The changing patterns of medical practice have brought with them the need for physicians to have a basic understanding of management principles and their applications to medical practice and the health care field. As insurance companies, health maintenance organizations, government agencies, and industry become major influences on the delivery and financing of medical care, the once exclusive doctor–patient relationship is being modified by contractual agreements with third-party payers. Physicians are no longer the sole authority in their field. Whether they work in a small practice or in a large corporate organization, physicians perform their professional responsibilities in a complex system that requires current knowledge of finance, personnel, communications, medical–legal affairs, automated systems, and public relations.

In the past, physicians relied on their clinical competence and professional reputation to build and maintain their practices. Although these attributes are still necessary, other issues such as accessibility, quality assurance, cost containment, and health maintenance are growing in importance. Although many traditionalists in medicine resist the pressure to become competitive, physicians and other health professionals now have the opportunity to design an innovative health care system. Industry and government want to join forces with the medical field to resolve the problem of unprecedented rising health care costs. If physicians are to function at an *executive* level, they will need to expand their professional competency to include a working knowledge of medical economics and practice management. Health care organizations, of every size and type, need leadership from physicians qualified to perform the full range of personnel, finance, and other managerial responsibilities.

The first edition of this book was written to provide medical students, residents, and practicing physicians with a basic understanding of the business aspects of medical practice. This revision updates the management concepts and applications from the earlier writing and provides a current picture of the economic environment that is influencing the medical care system. It also presents the strategies that physicians may employ to secure their leadership role as health care professionals. The three new chapters, Economic Environment, Marketing Health Services, and Computerization, discuss the leading external and internal influences on the field of medicine. For example, government and industry are now major participants in the planning and decision making of health care and medical services. In addition the lucrative health care market has attracted large corporate competitors, most of whom are sophisticated in designing and promoting high quality, cost-effective medical services. Automation has tremendous potential for enhancing the quality of care and improving the efficiency of office management.

The remaining chapters of the book can be considered the latest edition of the medical management survival kit. The subjects are planning the entrance into practice, personnel supervision, financial management, leadership skills, professional relations, office systems, and communications. Revisions of the initial text were made to reflect the organizational and managerial changes which a physician must be aware of to function as a physician-manager. The appendices provide additional information and references to support the content of the chapters.

1

Economic Environment

- How will changes in life style affect the delivery of health services?
- How will the various cost containment programs influence physicians' practice patterns?
- What are the implications of prospective payment and peer review?
- How will the emergence of large corporate organizations affect health care professionals and community practices?
- What are the distinguishing factors of the various types of health maintenance organizations?
- What impact have health care coalitions had on a community health care systems?

The health care market is in the midst of changes that will revolutionize how medical care will be provided and financed. Emphasis is shifting from high quality at any price to sufficient medical services in a cost-conscious market. High technology and high finance may be tempered by the involvement of government and industry in the health care decision-making process. The doctor-patient relationship is being modified by contractual agreements with third party payers. The changes in the economic and political environment affecting health care have been traced to the rising cost of medical services.

Paul Starr's *The Social Transformation of American Medicine* (1982) provides many insights into the quandary facing the health care profession. According to Starr:

Federal policymaking has been piecemeal, with most of the governmental solutions creating more problems than they solved. Examples included the disproportionate investments in biomedical research and medical center technology, doubling the output of medical schools in less than twenty years, and overpopulating medical and surgical specialists. Financial incentives for physicians and hospitals have encouraged utilization of services and expensive medical facilities. Insurance plans paid the bills while physicians and consumers reaped the benefits, at least in the short run. Research and development subsidies produced such advancements as CAT scans, radiation treatment, heart surgery and many other complex procedures, however the questions remain, who pays for the use of these high-cost treatments and how are decisions made about who receives them.

Starr does not offer a definitive answer, but he and many others who are researching the health-cost-containment dilemma point to several changes that may keep health services and expenditures at appropriate levels. The reimbursement emphasis will have to shift from illness to prevention. It may be that the highest quality of life will come from good diet, no smoking, less drinking, more exercise, and health maintenance activities, *not* heart transplants and massive doses of chemotherapy. Health services research should receive greater

1

funding and, with the increased resources, meet the challenge of dealing with the health and social problems of the wider population. Finally, as the health budget reaches the $400 billion level, physicians should realize that their clinical training and research orientation does not equip them to deal with the economic and political complexities of their field. Just as other industries have grown up from the small, one-owner shop, so has medicine. A corporate environment should not be opposed but welcomed as the organizational system most appropriate to manage and deliver the health care that will best serve 230 million Americans.

The magnitude of the health cost issue from government and industry perspectives was reported in a report published by the Health Care Financing Administration in the Spring 1984 issue of *Health Care Financial Review*. Figures 1.1 and 1.2 present the major categories of health expenditures and sources of funding in the United States. As can be seen, the driving force of health costs has been hospital care. Hospital care as a percentage of total health costs increased from 35% in 1952 to 47% in 1982, and in the past ten years it has grown at an annual rate of 15%. Physician services have a much greater impact than is indicated by the 22% of total cost, since physicians control a substantial proportion of the decision process for health costs. Cost of physician services increased nearly 14% per year from 1972 to 1982. Thus the two largest segments of health pay-

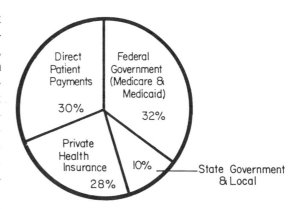

Figure 1.2 Health Care Payments 1990 Projections

ments, hospital care and physician services, will undoubtedly be the focus of attention for legislative and industrial actions. Analysis of the payment side of the health cost equation reveals why government and industry have become active in health care financing. Health care outlays are becoming a larger portion of the federal budget. In 1982 health costs were 12% of total government spending, up from 4% in 1965 (before Medicare and Medicaid). The private sector's portion of the health bill has grown at an average annual rate of 10%, which is of particular concern to business firms who have had to absorb these costs as their profitability declines.

The health cost problem is now a national issue. Medicare and Medicaid expenditures have reached such large amounts that government spending for health care is now a political topic. The medical profession failed at controlling costs, if in fact it made any effort to do so. Health care reimbursement programs provided little or no incentive for hospitals or physicians to keep expenses down. On the contrary, third-party payers may have contributed to the high cost of health care for two reasons. First, when a third party pays for a service, patients are usually not involved in payment and very often are unaware of the total cost. Health care is perhaps the only service that separates consumers from the responsibility to directly pay for a majority of the costs of the services they receive. Second, most third-party reimbursement is cost-based or retrospective, with the insurer making payments based on costs incurred. Thus providers are less inclined to be cost conscious.

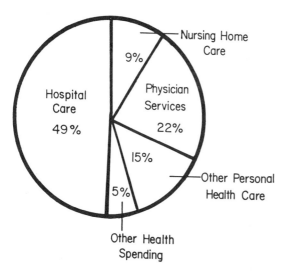

Figure 1.1 Health Care Expenditures 1990 Projections

Health care professionals must be aware of both societal trends influencing their market and the alternative financing systems, if they are to play a major role in shaping the economic changes in their profession. The emphasis on prospective reimbursement and contractual prepayment will alter the financial management system significantly. Fee-for-service and cost-based reimbursement will become less a factor in hospital and physician payments.

A study of expert opinions sponsored by the American College of Hospital Administrations and Arthur Anderson and Company entitled *Health Care in the 1990's: Trends and Strategies* (1984) offered three sets of conclusions.

1. **Cost of Care** Consumers will be more prudent in making health care purchasing decisions. There will be significant competition among physicians, hospitals, and other types of health-care providers. Consumers will increasingly obtain health care services from preferred-providers organizations, health maintenance organizations, and similar systems, all of which will slow the increases in health-care costs. Medical premiums, deductibles, and stop-loss amounts are increasing. Medicare will limit benefits for the chronically ill and the aged.
2. **Access to Care** Access to health care may decline for the medically indigent and those dependent on Medicare and Medicaid. Additional extended-care facilities will be needed because of an aging population and shorter hospital stays. Congress will increasingly work to define life and death to determine when life supports may be withdrawn in cases of terminal illness. The qualifying age for receiving Medicare benefits will be raised. A means test will be implemented for Medicare. Medicare will expand coverage for home care, hospice, outpatient services, rehabilitations, and skill and nursing.
3. **Quality of Care** National standards of health care and treatment may be established. An individual's ability to pay may dictate the extent of the services provided. Consumers will depend more on self-diagnosis and self-treatment. Patients will more often question and reject a physician's recommendations. Second opinions will be the norm. Increased competition among health care organizations

and providers will have a negative impact on quality at least from physicians' perspectives.

Regardless of how many of these predictions become realities, health professionals must be ready to adapt to the changing societal and economical trends. The following discussion of social changes, cost containment, prospective payment, competition, alternative health systems, and health care coalitions offers a more detailed explanation of how these changes will affect health-care organizations and the practice of medicine.

SOCIAL CHANGES

The traditional US family has changed. In the 1950s, 70% of US family households consisted of a wage-earning dad, a stay-at-home mom, and two or three children. As we approach the 1990s, such family units account for only 7% of all US households. Along with the change in family composition, Americans are altering their living patterns, more women are working, and the population is aging.

Living Arrangements

As can be seen in Table 1.1 living arrangements have changed dramatically. Even though the

Table 1.1 Social Trends Affecting Health Care

	1970	1980	%\nChange
	(000)	(000)	
Divorces Granted	708	1,170	+65.3%
Unmarried Couples	532	1,346	+157.4%
Married Couples\nwith Child	25,541	24,625	−3.6%
Married Couples\nwithout Children	19.187	23,037	+20.1%
Persons Living Alone	10,851	17,202	+58.5%
Children Living with\nOne Parent	8,230	11,528	+40.1%
Families with Both\nSpouses Working	20,327	24,253	+19.3%
Percent of Women in\nWorkforce	43%	52%	

Source: Department of Commerce, U.S. Government

number of marriages performed increased, the number of divorces granted and unmarried couples living together increased markedly. Families with both husband and wife working increased nearly 20% in ten years.

Working Women

The percentage of women in the labor force increased steadily in the past decade. In 1980, 42% of the employed workers were women, with projections for a higher percentage in the future. Women are branching out in all fields, including traditionally male occupations such as law, medicine, dentistry, accounting, and engineering. Another phenomenon of the women-at-work situation is the number of working mothers. Single women and working mothers are much more conscious of time constraints and prefer convenient consumer services. Nearly every retail business in the United States has adapted to meet the changing needs and demands of this "new society." Service industries are offering multiple locations, longer hours, more days per week, and a broad range of services. Health care corporations and medical practices are also responding to these changes as they extend office hours, open satellite locations, and offer more services for the convenience of patients.

Demographic Factors

A number of demographic factors will influence the demand for and use of medical services. Likely changes in the age composition through the end of the century include a decline in the under-18 group, an increase in the 30- to 44-years-old group, and a considerable increase in the 65 and older population. Some estimate that the senior citizen group will grow as much as 20% by the year 2000. The social composition in the United States will continue to change as the nonwhite-to-white ratio grows from 17 : 100 to 20 : 100 by the end of the century. The level of educational attainment in the United States has been increasing, and the trend will continue. Another demographic factor to observe is the migration rate—in the past migrants tended to be young adults, but recent patterns of US mi-

gration indicate that elderly are migrating in equal numbers to the younger groups. These changing demographic factors will influence all aspects of health services, but a few areas are likely to be more affected than others. As the population ages, office visits, hospitalizations, tests, and drugs will be used at higher rates. Whites are more likely to have office or telephone visits, whereas nonwhites see physicians in hospital emergency rooms or clinics. Nonwhites tend to use hospital resources more intensively than whites. Visits to a physician's office tend to increase with educational level. Young migrants have a high demand for obstetric care.

COST CONTAINMENT

A national survey of the US public and selected professionals in the health care field reported a general consensus that fundamental changes are needed to make the health care system more cost-effective and accessible (*Equitable Health Care Survey I, II;* 1983, 1984) The chief conclusions of this two-part report were:

The primary barrier to obtaining medical care is cost of care.

Widespread dissatisfaction exists with cost of hospitalization.

Health-care system discourages price competition.

American public is ready to accept cost-containment proposals.

Corporations support the cost-containment programs.

Physicians believe that cost-sharing would be effective and acceptable.

The third-party payment system is a major contributor to high costs.

The payers of the health care bill, industry and government, will no longer stand by as medical care costs escalate. These costs are threatening the competitive ability of business firms, and they are limiting the federal and state governments' capacity to balance their budgets. The issue is not whether the health care system will be changed but how. Cost-containment initiatives are one of the major efforts underway to limit the high cost that industry and government have to pay for health care. The following is a summary of cost-containment methods described in a *Health Cost Management Handbook* (Kolimaga, 1984).

High-Low Benefit Options

The employee is given a choice between a comprehensive package of health benefits and a less expensive package. Usually the high and low plans are offered by the same carrier, and employees are permitted to switch plans during an annual enrollment period. Generally, the employer pays part of or all the low-option plan, and those employees who select the high-option one will pay the difference through payroll deduction. The low-option plans will include many of the following features: reduction in hospital coverage, higher coverage for outpatient surgery, higher deductibles for drugs and medical appliances, copayments for emergency room visits, bonuses for early release from hospitals and shorter stays for maternity. Employees can tailor their health benefit package to their unique circumstances.

High-low plans have their limitations. Adverse selection is the tendency as high-cost users may tend to concentrate in the high-cost option. Employees and physicians may become confused about all the different options, causing uncertainty about what is excluded or included.

Choice of Health Plans

Competition among health plans is expected to lead to cost reductions. One way for employers to control their portion of the health care bill is to allow employees to choose among competing health plans. One employer could offer several health care plans, including at least one staff or group model health maintenance organization (HMO) and one individual practice association (IPA HMO). In addition to offering employees the opportunity to participate in alternative delivery systems, preferred-provider organizations (PPOs) and a high-low benefit option could be included within the standard health benefits package. Each option would contain a core set of benefits and would differ from the others in the kind of additional benefits and the premium charged. The employer contribution would be fixed, and the employees who chose a more expensive plan would pay the difference

through payroll deduction. An annual open enrollment period would require employees to choose a new plan or indicate if they wish to remain in their former plan. Normally no action is needed if they prefer to stay in their current plan.

Hospital Cost Control

With the indemnity option, hospital costs usually account for about one half of an average employer's health expenses. The surgery-related costs account for about 40% of all hospital costs. The following procedures are being recommended to reduce hospital and surgical utilization.

Preadmission Certification. These programs require patients seeking nonemergency inpatient treatment to receive prior review from an insurance carrier or review organization before payment is authorized. Preadmission certification generally is designed to reduce hospital admissions, shorten length of hospital stay, and encourage prospective review of ancillary services. The limitations of the preadmission review are obvious—it may be seen as an inappropriate intervention into the doctor-patient relationship, and reviews can be relatively complex and time-consuming.

Ambulatory Surgery. Recent developments in surgical techniques and improvements in anesthesia have led to same-day surgical admission and discharge. Inclusion of ambulatory surgery benefits is strongly endorsed as an effective cost-containment device of employers. From the payer's perspective, the most cost-effective settings for ambulatory surgery are the following, in order of priority: (1) Physician's office; (2) Independent, free-standing ambulatory surgery center; (3) Hospital outpatient surgery and testing procedure. According to standards established by insurance companies, the following procedures can usually be performed on an outpatient basis: abortion, biopsy (breast, skin, etc.), cataract extraction, circumcision, cryosurgery, cystoscopy, dilation and curettage, excision of skin tumors (both benign and malignant), tonsillectomy and adenoidectomy, and vasectomy.

PreAdmission Testing (PAT). Procedures such as routine diagnostic examinations, laboratory tests, and x-rays are more costly when performed in the hospital. Previously, hospitalizing patients for tests was encouraged by the health insurance plans because their reimbursement rates were always higher for inpatient services. The PAT may contain some qualifications, such as coverage of testing for only a limited time prior to admission or advance certification of a forthcoming admission. Health maintenance organizations use PAT as a way of holding down costs, and PATs are becoming fairly common in group health insurance contracts. Most empirical studies have found that PAT will reduce average length of stay and may save roughly 1% to 2% of total claims costs. Preadmission procedures are also intended to shift inpatient testing into a more appropriate outpatient setting and perhaps to avoid some hospitalizations completely.

Second-Opinion Surgery. Inpatient surgical procedures increased nearly 70% from 1971 to 1982. Much of this increase has been attributed to our third-party insurance system, which provides few incentives for less expensive nonsurgical approaches. Second-opinion surgery programs have been successful in deterring unneeded elective surgery, especially high-cost, frequently performed procedures such as hysterectomies and cholecystectomies. There are three types of second-opinion programs: voluntary, incentive, and mandatory. Under a *voluntary* program, 100% of the cost of second-opinion consultations is covered, but surgical costs are paid whether or not a second opinion is obtained. Under the *incentive* approach, the cost of the second opinion is fully covered, but if surgery is performed, the patient has lower coinsurance. The *mandatory* program will also pay for surgical consultation, however, payment for elective surgery is reduced, sometimes by 50% if a second opinion is not obtained. Frequently performed procedures included in second-opinion surgery programs are: foot surgery, breast surgery, cataract surgery, hemorrhoidectomy hernia repair, laminectomy, prostate surgery, coronary artery bypass, and laminectomy. Recent declines in surgical admissions may be attributed not only to nonconfirming second opinions but also to the "sentinel effect" of mandatory programs. When physicians know their recommendations will be reviewed by another physician, they are more conservative in their practice style. Despite the obvious record of success, second-opinion programs require the willingness of providers to accept the concept. Providers and consumers may think that a mandatory opinion infringes on the private domain of doctor-patient decision making.

Deductibles and Coinsurance. Another cost-containment approach shifts part of the cost to patients with higher deductibles and coinsurance. If the first dollar expenses must be paid out of pocket, similar to home and auto insurance coverage, the patient may be more prudent in purchasing health care services. A *deductible* is a fixed amount paid by the patient for services before the insurance plan pays any bills. Some companies are being encouraged to have deductibles as high as $500 to $1000 for hospitalization and surgical procedures. Under *coinsurance,* the patient pays a fixed percentage of the bill, perhaps to 25%, with an upper limit on the patient's out-of-pocket costs for a year. A *comprehensive* medical plan can combine both deductibles and coinsurance. Another approach is to use *indemnity* schedules for hospital and physician services. The plan pays a fixed amount per service or diagnosis, and the patient is liable for costs above the allowable amount. This encourages employees to locate lower-cost providers. In 1981, nearly 50% of commercial insurers were offering comprehensive plans with both deductibles and coinsurance, typically 20 percent copayment and $100 deductible. These cost-sharing plans reduce utilization and make consumers more price sensitive. However, they may delay consumers from seeking medical care. Cost sharing may also discourage patients from obtaining preventive care and diagnostic tests which can prevent more costly diseases.

Short-Stay Maternity Benefits. To reduce the costs of unnecessarily long hospital stays associated with maternity care, an incentive program has been developed that financially rewards mothers of newborns who stay a brief time. Based on a limited number of programs in operation, a short-stay maternity plan usually includes physician authorization, physical assessment prior to discharge, cash incentives, and additional covered services such as nurse visits, homemakers, and lab tests. Early discharge improves morale of mothers and promotes cost consciousness among physicians, although some physicians have voiced concerns about the risks to the infant.

Other Strategies For Cost Control

Although cost containment is directed toward reducing health benefits, some features may hold costs by expanding health benefit packages. This additional coverage includes convalescent care, hospice, birthing centers, alcoholism treatment, and mental health services. Under the appropriate circumstances and within specified limits, these options can reduce health costs.

In their book *The Physician and Cost Control* (1980), Carels, Neuhauser, and Stason outline several cost-control strategies for ambulatory and hospital care. Several of their suggestions coincide with the methods outlined in the preceding paragraphs, but they are well worth repeating.

In ambulatory care, some cost-control recommendations include:

1. **System Monitoring of Health Care Services** This monitoring would take the form of utilization review and external and internal audits. If quality of care is the objective, emphasis should be put on outcome audits. National guidelines for appropriate utilization should be established and then used as points of references.
2. **Coordination of Services** The concept of primary physician as the coordinator of referrals, diagnostic tests, and elective hospitalizations has considerable merit. Primary physicians can provide a significant deterrent effect on excessive use of health resources, especially if there is a financial incentive such as prepaid medical services or other cost-sharing arrangements.
3. **Efficient Management Techniques** These techniques can achieve considerable savings. Patient scheduling, medical records, financial accounting, and personnel supervision require management systems.

4. **Cost Awareness** It is of the utmost importance that physicians be aware of the costs of medical service. Education in costs and cost-effective decision making should be an ongoing organizational process.
5. **Substitution of Ambulatory Care for Hospital Care** When appropriate this substitution should always be an objective. Availability of ambulatory facilities for diagnostic studies prior to surgery is one component. Restructuring health insurance coverage to include fuller coverage of ambulatory services is another.
6. **Financial Incentives** Incentives for cost-effective use of medical services may need to take several forms so that physicians on fee-for-service and prepaid plans receive a financial reward for decreasing use of hospitalization and ancillary services while maintaining high-quality care.
7. **Coinsurance Provisions** These should be included in health insurance programs.
8. **Limits on Self-Referral** Self-referrals for laboratory and radiologic procedures must be limited to keep costs down and maintain quality control over small, privately run diagnostic centers.
9. **Global Fees.** These fees have considerable potential for controlling costs; they have been in existence for obstetrical services and could be expanded to other medical and surgical services.

The following recommendations pertain to cost control in hospitals:

1. The *patient* should receive a copy of itemized charges for all services. This would increase awareness of cost and allow a review to determine if all services were actually rendered. Patients should have periodic reminders to instruct them how to use their insurance benefits. They should also be advised to shop for medical service and to ask about the type and cost of care prior to treatment.
2. The *physician* should be provided with a printout of hospital utilization by physician and peer group. Data in service, costs per service, tests, procedures, and bed cases should be itemized and correlated with regional and national norms.
3. The *hospital* should assume a major role for

cost-containment programs. Hospitals must organize and manage utilization reviews, cost-control procedures, continuing education programs, and other strategies to enhance cost-effective corporate and physician behaviors.

4. The *third-party* insurance companies, government, industry, and unions should be encouraged to write contracts and benefit plans simply, emphasize exclusions and copayments so that enrollees know what is *not* covered, and build in cost-effective language for claims review as well as promoting responsibility for appropriateness of care.

PROSPECTIVE PAYMENT

In an attempt to limit the high level of government spending on health care, especially Medicare hospitalization, a prospective payment system (PPS) went into effect in 1983. This fixed-fee type of reimbursement was a radical departure from the traditional cost-based payments. The PPS sets fees based on diagnosis-related groups (DRGs). The DRG system was initially established for Medicare payments for hospital changes, but similar types of reimbursement are expected to be utilized for private insurance plans, physicians services, and outpatient costs. The PPS pays hospitals a fixed amount per discharge based on the diagnosis of the patient. All hospitals with an agreement to participate in Medicare are covered except psychiatric hospitals, rehabilitation hospitals, long-term care hospitals, and hospitals in US territories. The PPS covers all nonphysician services in the hospital, including services which may be provided by outside suppliers such as laboratory and x-rays. The AMA has published an excellent pamphlet for physicians entitled *Diagnosis-Related Groups and the Prospective Payment System* (1985). The following is a summary of the features of the PPS/DRG system discussed in the AMA's guidebook.

DRGs

The basis of payment for the PPS is the diagnosis-related grouping, which is merely a method for classifying patients by diagnosis. Diagnosis-related groupings (DRGs) are assigned to a case based on principal diagnosis, treatment performed, age, sex, and discharge status. A fiscal intermediary has the ultimate responsibility of assigning 1 of 467 distinct DRGs to the case. Reimbursement is based on the DRG, as opposed to the traditional method of payment. A three-year transition phase was established to allow hospitals to adjust to the new pricing system. Payments for each DRG are based on two factors: (1) DRG weight, an index assigned to reflect relative costs for treating a specific DRG—the weight is an indication of the relative resource consumption regardless of which hospital or region the service is provided; (2) dollar rate, determined by a combination of federally established rates and a rate reflective of the individual hospital's cost structure. The hospital rate applies only during the transition phase.

The major factor involved in assigning the DRG is the physician's assessment of the principal diagnosis. It is important that the principal diagnosis correspond to various tests, procedures, and notes contained in the medical record. Regulations require that the attending physicians attest in writing at the time of discharge or shortly thereafter to the principal diagnosis, secondary diagnosis, and procedures performed. Once the discharge sheet has been completed by the physician, the chart is forwarded to the hospital's medical records department for reviewing and coding. From the medical records department, the information is forwarded to the financial office for completion of the bill to be submitted to the fiscal intermediary. The fiscal intermediary, through use of a computer program, determines the appropriate DRG and then calculates payment to the hospital.

Special-Facility Adjustments

The PPS legislation provides for an adjustment for special facilities. These adjustments generally increase DRG reimbursement for such health facilities as sole community hospitals; special designations by HHS because of location, weather, travel, or absence of other hospitals; cancer hospitals; referral centers; and teaching hospitals. Legislation also provides that adjustments can be made to hospitals for such financial considerations as outliers (atypical) cases, transfer patients, kidney acquisitions, capital costs, and bad debts.

Peer Review Organizations

Responsibility for maintaining quality of care is assigned to a peer review organization (PRO) by the Health Care Financing Administration. A PRO is defined as an entity which is composed of a substantial number of licensed doctors of medicine or osteopathy engaged in the practice of medicine or surgery. Each state will probably be designated as a PRO geographic area. The PROs are required to review validity of diagnostic information provided by the hospital for purposes of payment; completeness, adequacy, and quality of care; appropriateness of admissions and discharges; appropriateness of care provided to outlier cases. Every hospital must have a contract with a PRO as a condition for medical reimbursement.

Implications

The most obvious impact of the PPS is that hospitals are now economically at risk. The economic incentive for a hospital is to find a way to provide services at a cost below the DRG rate. Hospitals will begin to provide the services that are the most cost-effective. Acquisition of the high-cost technology may be delayed until a positive economic impact can be documented. Hospital administrators and PRO organizations will be monitoring physicians' behavior. Physicians will be informed of their costs for treating a case and how their costs and practice patterns compare with those of other physicians treating similar patients. Potential implications of the PPS/DRG system are as follows:

Decisions about the hospital procedures, ancillary services, and lengths of stay will be made collectively by physicians and administrators. Since fiscal intermediaries determine DRG rates from the medical record, emphasis will be placed upon accuracy and timeliness of physicians' record keeping. Medical-records administrators will have in-

creasing influence on patient management and cost reimbursement.

Hospitals will encourage physicians to perform preadmission laboratory and x-ray procedures, since these procedures could still be reimbursed separately under Medicare Part B (the physician's services).

Physicians and hospitals may operate ambulatory care centers to avoid the PPS/DRG system, since at this time it is limited to hospital care. Transfer of patients to nursing homes and rehabilitation centers or early discharge may be encouraged by the hospital.

Despite an overwhelming negative reaction by hospitals and physicians when PPS/DRGs were initiated, the first full year under the prospective payment system has achieved the desired results. Government spending for Medicare has declined, whereas over 80% of the hospitals in the system have reported excess revenues as a result of their DRG reimbursement. Some hospitals have increased revenues by 15% to 20%. Hospitals that are unable to operate profitably under the PPS/DRG system are most likely to be the small, rural hospitals.

COMPETITION

Thanks to a receptive government, favorable economy, lucrative market potential, and tolerant consumers, the health care market has now become a highly competitive environment. Both the nonprofit and for-profit health care organizations are rapidly increasing in size and influence in hospital and ambulatory health care. The competitiveness of the situation is also being fueled by the increasing supply of physician and nonphysician health practitioners. Competition in the health care field will be discussed from the perspectives of corporate organizations, ambulatory care centers, and physician supply and income.

Corporate Organizations

For-profit, investor-owned organizations such as Hospital Corporation of America (HCA), Humana, Prudential, CIGNA, American Medical International (AMI), and other national and regional organizations are moving rapidly into hospital management and ownership, ambulatory health centers, and prepaid health plans. As larger, profit-oriented companies begin to dominate health care, concerns have been raised about accessibility of health services for the low-income population, sacrificing quality of care for efficiency, and the graduate medical education system.

The for-profit hospital industry generated over $12 billion in revenue in 1981, and at least three companies surpassed $1 billion in revenues. Investor-owned US hospital chains own or manage nearly 700 for-profit hospitals and 300 nonprofit hospitals. The entire for-profit industry now owns or manages almost 20% of US hospitals.

Even though the for-profit organizations are getting the most attention, other corporate structures are proliferating. The voluntary or nonprofit hospitals are expanding into large, centralized systems, usually on a regional basis. But some have also gone national, such as Kaiser Permanente medical groups. Physicians are also well-represented in the ownership and management of these larger health care organizations. The trend toward large-scale health systems will produce many different organizational affiliations.

Health care plans, including Medicare, Medicaid, and industrial health, will be contracted, with competitive bidding. Large numbers of physicians will be employees of for-profit and nonprofit organizations, with lucrative opportunities for positions in ownership and management as well as direct patient care. Traditional hospital-oriented medical centers will diversify into ambulatory care, nursing homes, home health, and ancillary service centers. Solo physicians, small medical practices, and the rural, independent hospital may be unable to survive in prospective payment and prepaid systems unless they affiliate with larger health care systems. Franchised medical practices will be as commonplace as other retail establishments.

Ambulatory Care Centers

The changing profile of the health consumer brought with it a growing demand for convenient, affordable health services. Physicians in traditional medical practices, located in the proverbial "doctors' park," were slow to recognize this new consumer orientation. Health care entrepreneurs were not! In addition, as the medical reimbursement system began to recognize that ambulatory medicine is cost-effective, a new health care field was reborn. Ambulatory care centers have grown in popularity because they emphasize what consumers and payers are demanding: accessible, quality health services at a reasonable cost.

Ambulatory centers can be operated independently by a local group, franchised by a national company, or affiliated with a hospital. Physician ownership is very common. The growth of ambulatory health centers, especially those promoting themselves as urgent care facilities, has been phenomenal. In 1983, urgent care centers recorded nearly 12 million office visits, representing nearly 10% of the primary care encounters in the United States. By 1990, more than 5,000 ambulatory health centers will be in operation, twice the current number. Despite the negative reactions by the medical establishment, ambulatory centers have been generally accepted by the public. These centers are also appealing to younger physicians who want neither the financial and managerial risks nor the excessive time demands that are synonymous with private practice.

Desirable features of the ambulatory centers from the patient's perspective are walk-in care, extended office hours at no additional cost, immediate treatment when necessary, lab and x-ray facilities available on-site, and accessible locations, usually in high-traffic areas. The positive aspects for physicians are the regular working hours, attractive salary and benefits, no capital investment unless they are owners, excellent working conditions and staffing, and limited involvement in the day-to-day administrative functions. These centers have also moved aggressively into industrial medicine, offering local industries such services as executive physicals, preemployment history and physicals, screening evaluations, worker's compensation, health promotion, and other occupational health programs.

Ambulatory centers have received a variety of criticisms. Patients may be delayed from seeking care from other more appropriate sources such as consultants or hospitals. Physicians who work in these centers are usually employed on a limited basis, and thus they may be less committed to practicing high-quality, cost-effective care. Regulations for these centers are minimal to nonexistent. Consumers may be misinformed about the limitations of these centers to perform critical care and trauma services. Reductions in patient volume may place financial viability ahead of quality patient care.

Even though the ambulatory care centers have become a very functional health care delivery system, the long-term success of these centers will depend on several factors: qualifications and expertise of medical and ancillary staff, stringent quality of care standards, sound financial base to meet current and future needs, fully equipped and maintained facility, and effective working relationships with the medical community.

Physician Supply and Income

The supply and income level of physicians have an important impact on the competitive nature of the health care industry. The number of physicians is increasing per capita, and, according to various sources, a physician surplus is on the horizon. The income of physicians, especially in the medical and surgical specialties, has risen steadily in the past decade. As Tables 1.2 and 1.3 illustrate, the increase in supply and income has not been equal across specialties. The problem may be more a function of geographic and specialty distribution than total supply. The dis-

Table 1.2 Physician Population 1963 vs. 1983

Specialty	1963	1983	Annual % Change
	(000)	(000)	
All Physicians	299.8	478.4	+3%
GP/FP	73.5	62.0	−1%
Internists	34.7	66.3	+5%
Pediatricians	14.0	30.3	+6%
OB/GYN	15.7	26.9	+4%
Medical Sub-Specialties	57.7	160.0	+9%
Surgical Sub-Specialties	23.4	49.8	+6%
U.S. Population (Millions)	189.2	238.2	+.15%

Source: Reynolds, Roger A., and Robert L. Ohsfeldt (Editors), *Socioeconomic Characteristics of Medical Practice 1984*, American Medical Assoc., 1984

Table 1.3 Physicians' Income from Medical Practice

	1973	1983	Annual % Change
All Physicians	$49,000	$106,000	10%
Specialties:			
GP/FP	$42,000	$69,000	6%
Internal Medicine	$48,000	$93,000	9%
Pediatrics	$41,000	$71,000	7%
OB/GYN	$55,000	$120,000	11%
Surgery	$57,000	$146,000	14%
Radiology	$60,000	$148,000	13%
Anesthesiology	$48,000	$145,000	18%

Source: Reynolds, Roger A., and Robert L. Ohsfeldt (Editors), *Socioeconomic Characteristics of Medical Practice 1984*, American Medical Assoc., 1984

parity between the earning potential of primary care and secondary care specialties can also be seen in Table 1.4, the statistics for which were compiled from the 1985 cost and production report of the Medical Group Management Association in Denver, Colorado. With the emphasis upon primary care and ambulatory procedures, one can conclude from these figures that the medical and surgical specialties may have the most to lose if their patient volume declines.

Table 1.4 Ratio of Charges to Office Visits

Speciality	Average Charge Per Visit
Pediatrics	$37
Family medicine	43
Internal medicine	83
Obstetrics/Gynecology	98
General surgery	135

ALTERNATIVE HEALTH SYSTEMS

During the last economic recession, business and government began to explore alternative medical plans as mechanisms to bring down expenses for the health insurance of their employees and beneficiaries. The obvious alternative to fee-for-service payment was prepayment. The two prepayment models considered most appropriate for widespread application were health maintenance organizations (HMOs) and preferred-provider organizations (PPOs). HMOs and PPOs are a dramatic departure from traditional health care delivery and financing, because they create financial incentives for health care providers and institutions to reduce the amount and type of services offered.

Health Maintenance Organizations

Since 1973, federal law has required employers to offer at least one HMO of each type to employees if the HMOs meet certain federal standards. Initially many employers were reluctant to implement this option since it was a relatively new approach, and the medical establishment and health insurance industry were not advocating this payment system. However as the employers' health care insurance premiums continued to rise and as empirical studies began to report that HMOs were less costly than indemnity plans, industry saw the light. Currently less than 5 percent of the population is enrolled in some form of prepaid health plan, but projections for the end of the century estimate this figure to be as high as 50 percent.

HMOs have five general features:

1. Contractual relationship to provide specified health services
2. Defined population enrolled for a set period of time, usually one year
3. Voluntary participation
4. Fixed payments regardless of program use
5. Assumption of a portion of financial risk by the providers.

HMOs have four basic models. The *staff* model delivers services through a group practice established to provide services exclusively to its members. Physicians are salaried employees. An example is the Winston-Salem Health Plan operated by R. J. Reynolds Company. *Group* model consists of physicians working together in shared facilities providing comprehensive health care.* *Individual practice plans* are an-

---

* Two different forms of group models are in effect. One is when patients are exclusively HMO enrollees, such as The Kaiser Permanente plan. The other group model is when the practice combines both HMO and fee-for-service patients, such as the Pru-Care, Prudential model. These models are explained in more detail later in this chapter.

other HMO model. Private physicians continue to see their fee-for-service patients but also agree to accept the risk for providing comprehensive care to enrolled members of an HMO. HMO enrollees can select personal physicians and in some cases consultants, from a designated list of physicians that the HMO has under contract. Since IPAs are less costly to establish and operate, they are growing more rapidly than the staff or group models. An important feature of the IPA plan is the *gatekeeper* concept. This means that the primary care physicians, typically family physicians, internists, and pediatricians, agree to provide all primary care services and act as the principal coordinator when referring to consultants and when hospitalizing patients. In some IPA plans, such as HealthAmerica, the gatekeeper is required to formally approve the use of consultants, hospitalizations, and high-cost procedures before payment will be made. The distinguishing features of four nationally recognized plans are summarized in Table 1.5.

Kaiser Permanente

Kaiser Permanente began as a nonprofit HMO in California in 1929. As early as 1950, Kaiser was promoting competition with other health plans. Kaiser's philosophy is that competition contains costs and is preferable to government-mandated regulations. About 90% of Kaiser's members are working people and their dependents who joined through job-related groups. The remaining 10% joined as individuals. Kaiser manages their own fully equipped health centers. Depending on the enrollment and population in a specific regional area, they may also operate a hospital. If Kaiser members require specialty referrals or hospitalization not available from Kaiser directly, then Kaiser physicians make the arrangements. All bills for hospital care, physician services, drugs, and tests, are paid by Kaiser. Paperwork and claims forms are kept to a minimum for enrollees and employers. Reimbursement claims are typically required only when a member receives emergency care from another medical source. Members can receive care from Kaiser facilities in other states.

Kaiser is heavily concentrated on the West Coast, but they are moving into other large metropolitan areas such as Dallas, Texas; Wash-

Table 1.5 A Comparison of Four Health Maintenance Organizations

Organization	Kaiser Foundation Health Plan of N.C.	PruCare	Blue Cross/Blue Shield Personal Care Plan	HealthAmerica
Type of Plan Profit/Non-Profit Reimbursement to Primary Care M.D.s	Prepaid Group Practice Non-Profit Monthly capitation per enrollee paid to Carolina Permanente Medical Group.	Group model Profit Monthly capitation per member paid to Nalle Clinic.	IPA Non-Profit Age-adjusted capitation per month per enrollee.	IPA Profit Monthly capitation per enrollee, biannual payment from consultation fund and annual payment from hospitalization fund.
Reimbursement to Specialty M.D.s	Fee-for-service paid by Carolina Permanente Medical Group.	Clinic staffed by all major specialties.	Fee-for-service paid at prenegotiated amount by Personal Care Plan.	Fee-for-service paid by HealthAmerica when authorized by primary care physician.
Holdback	No holdback, prepaid group practice at risk for expenses that exceed capitation.	No holdback, but clinic has financial incentive to keep hospital utilization below aggregate targeted amount.	20% holdback for specialty care doctors.	None, but primary care physician at risk for expenses that exceed up to 10% of capitation surplus of consultation fund returned to primary care physician two times a year.
Coverage	Prepaid plan inclusive of out-patient and inpatient services/supplemental drugs and vision, and durable medical equipment.	Comprehensive: $15 copayment emergency room, $3 prescription drugs, mental health inpatient up to 30 days 20% per payment, outpatient up to 20 visits 50% per payment.	Comprehensive coverage, $10 copayment for home visit.	Comprehensive coverage, small copayment for office visits and prescription drugs, hospitalization 100%.
Monthly Premium*	$55 individual, $150 family	$50–55 individual $150–160 family	$50 individual $140–160 family	$55–60 individual $160 family
Hold Harmless Provision	Yes	Yes	Yes, M.D. can not bill subscriber.	No
Mechanism for Review/Appeals	Internal peer controls, enrollee grievance procedure approved by Federal Office of HMOs.	Formal grievance procedure for members, medical advisory committee, and membership advisory committee.	Peer review/Professional Alliance and Medical Director.	Quality assurance by medical director and peers; Utilization review by nurses, peers and medical director.

* As of 1985.

ington, D.C.; Denver, Colorado; Hartford, Connecticut; Cleveland, Ohio; Baltimore, Maryland; Kansas City, Missouri; New York City; Atlanta, Georgia; Charlotte and Raleigh/Durham, North Carolina; and Hawaii. Kaiser enrollees receive an identification card along with detailed information about their benefits. Physicians who work in Kaiser health facilities are employees of the Permanente Medical Group Practice.

Prudential Pru-Care

Following the lead of Kaiser in the HMO market, large insurers such as Prudential, John Hancock, CIGNA, and CNA entered the prepaid health insurance field. Prudential's HMO division, called Pru-Care, began in 1974. Prudential's initial development with HMOs used the group model. In 1984, however, they opened their first individual practice HMO in San Antonio, and plans call for further expansion of IPA models. As with most prepaid plans, Pru-Care offers benefits and services with no limitations on number of days of hospital care, number of office visits, or dollar amount spent for the member's care. By 1986, Pru-Care expects to be the provider of health care benefits to 500,000 Americans, with forecasts of 1 million members by 1990. Pru-Care has health plans in 17 major metropolitan areas nationally, primarily functioning through large, well-established multispecialty group practices that have offices in several locations in the community. Two Pru-Care group models are in Richmond and Charlotte.

In Richmond, Pru-Care was selected as the HMO provider by a cost-containment task force of area businesses. Pru-Care chose an existing multispeciality group of more than 40 physicians which had served Richmond for nearly 60 years. HMO patients were integrated into the practice along with the fee-for-service patients. The clinic allows each HMO patient to choose a personal doctor from its staff. The marketing campaign to local employers and government workers emphasized comprehensive prepaid care, preventive health services, no copayments or deductibles, and a well-respected group practice. The clinic's contract with Pru-Care requires the medical group to supply all physician services to enrollees for a fixed monthly payment, negotiated annually. Pru-Care provides additional renumeration if the clinic succeeds in meeting hospital utilization targets, including length of stay, cost per day, and number of admissions per thousand patients. Pru-Care also contracted with two well-regarded Richmond hospitals to provide inpatient services but is required to pay these hospitals on a charge/cost basis. To monitor hospital utilization, Pru-Care hired a registered nurse as a full-time hospital coordinator to review admissions and discharges. One result of Pru-Care's success in Richmond was the formation of an IPA by 100 local physicians.

In Charlotte, Pru-Care is affiliated with a large multispeciality group similar to the one in Richmond. This was the first group model formed in Charlotte. Pru-Care members receive most of their primary care in a single, convenient location. Specialty care is also available within the clinic. Hospitalization or additional specialties are arranged by clinic physicians. The clinic has weekday and weekend hours and operates a walk-in clinic 12 hours a day for minor emergencies. If hospitalization or emergency services are needed outside the service area, then the local Pru-Care coordinator must be notified within 48 hours. A hospitalization coordinator is employed by Pru-Care, similar to the Richmond situation. The clinic has a primary location where all medical and surgical specialists practice and two other sites in Charlotte where internists and pediatricians provide primary care. Besides the full range of inpatient and outpatient services, Pru-Care covers preventive health services such as weight reduction classes, immunization, periodic health assessments, and other health checkups. Home health services, skilled nursery facilities, and physical therapy will be covered upon the recommendation of clinic physicians.

Blue Cross and Blue Shield of North Carolina

As a major health insurer in the state, Blue Cross and Blue Shield became involved at the earliest stage of discussion regarding HMO activity. The result was the personal care plan, an IPA model which contracts with individual physicians who provide medical services in their own offices for their regular fee-for-service patients and for the enrollees of the personal care plan (PCP) who select them as personal physicians. The PCP was the first individual practice HMO plan in North Carolina. The plan includes primary-care physicians and medical and surgical specialists and requires that referral be made by the assigned personal physician to a physician and hospital also under contract with PCP.

The initial marketing of the PCP occurred in North Carolina's three largest metropolitan areas, Charlotte, Greensboro, and Raleigh/Durham. Companies with at least 200 employees were eligible to offer the plan to their employees. Blue Cross and Blue Shield contracts with local physicians, both primary care and consultants, and then offers the list of participating primary care physicians to enrollees who select their plan. Selection of personal physician is made on a yearly basis by all enrollees. Personal physicians are typically family physicians, internists, and pediatricians. The PCP, through its participating physicians, offers 24-hour care, seven days a week, prepaid comprehensive benefits, fixed monthly fees, and a personal physician to either provide all needed services or to coordinate referrals and hospitalizations. The monthly capitation per enrollee includes office visits, hospital medical visits, immunizations, examinations, office lab tests, EKGs, and injections. Capitation rates vary depending on the age of enrollee, and monthly payments are sent to the personal physicians based on the number of enrollees. The PCP also has referral and institutional funds which are used to reimburse for consultant services and hospitalizations. If a balance remains in these funds, a portion is redistributed to participating physicians. Blue Cross and Blue Shield administers the PCP, which includes marketing, financial management, claims processing, medical information systems, and utilization and peer reviews.

HealthAmerica

HealthAmerica is a national HMO based in Nashville, Tennessee, that operates plans in over 20 states with 750,000 members. It was established initially by a group of family physicians in northeast Ohio in 1975. The Ohio plan is now functioning within the corporate struc-

ture of HealthAmerica. Currently two thirds of the plans are group HMOs and the remaining one third are the individual practice HMOs using the primary care physician network. Their primary care physician network emphasizes that the primary physician is the health care manager. The basic premise of the primary care network is that coordination of medical services for patients by personal physicians will avoid duplication and inappropriate use of services. The gatekeeper functions place the responsibility for cost management directly on the primary physician. As with most IPAs, this model allows physicians to practice independently, offering both prepaid and fee-for-service plans.

HealthAmerica promotes their primary care network throughout the country. The largest plans are in Pennsylvania, Ohio, North Carolina, Chicago, Illinois, and Seattle. Advantages to employers and employees are essentially the same as those in previously discussed HMOs. HealthAmerica requires the primary physicians to accept the overall responsibility of delivering primary care and coordinating the other health care needs. In return the primary physician receives capitation based on the age and sex of enrollees. The capitation fee covers primary health services and most ambulatory laboratory studies. Additional funds are set aside for referral services as a shared-risk pool for consultant services, with a stop loss in the range of $1,200 to $1,500 per case which limits the physicians risk to this amount. In addition, funds are also set aside for hospital care, emergency services, and ambulatory surgical procedures. The primary physician is responsible for authorizing referrals and hospitalizations and has an incentive to be judicious with both. Any surplus in the referral services fund accrues 100% to primary physicians. Any surplus in the hospital services fund is shared equally between the primary physician and HealthAmerica. Primary physicians are at some risk for overuse of the referral services fund as well as the hospital services fund. Up to 10% of the capitation fees may be forfeited for deficits in these separate funds. This penalty would apply only for inadequate patient and cost management, not for of adverse selection. A monitoring system is set up locally with the HealthAmerica medical director and the medical directors from each practice to review the financial status of the various funds and to determine if adverse selection is a factor for a particular practice's negative results.

HMO Pitfalls

Despite the growing acceptance of HMOs by industry and government, these alternative delivery systems have their limitations. Several concerns have been raised:

Plans are vulnerable to unemployment, inflation, and capital scarcity.

Many plans have not met all the requirements for federal qualification.

Health maintenance and prevention are not substantially higher when HMO care is compared with fee-for-service practices.

Cost savings may be achieved by reducing needed services and procedures

Sometimes extraordinary attempts may be made to minimize hospitalization and expensive treatments.

Primary care physicians incur significant economic risks in some plans.

Continuity in doctor-patient relationship is a lower priority in some HMO models.

Financial viability may compromise clinical decision making.

In the IPA plans, primary physicians are responsible for a considerable amount of the administrative work, including attendance at quality assurance and financial review meetings.

Multiple HMOs in one private practice may be confusing and lead to inefficiency and patient and staff dissatisfaction.

Important questions to consider when considering an HMO affiliation are:

How many different prepayment plans can one practice reasonably subscribe?

Will patients be managed differently depending on their method of payment?

Are physicians prepared to modify their treatment and consultation patterns to meet the prudent standards necessary to keep costs down?

How will the practice handle irate patients who demand excessive treatment or inappropriate referrals?

Chapter 3 discusses HMO affiliation further.

Preferred-Provider Organizations

Another alternative health care system is the PPO model which resembles both the fee-for-service and HMO methods. PPOs generally operate as an administrative mechanism to arrange for predetermined below-market fees from a panel of health care providers. Independent third-party organizations, such as insurance companies, other health agencies, or employers, may function as PPOs. Discounts for physician services and hospital care can range from 5% to 20%. The organizations review and screen claims to ensure that services are needed and that quality of care is acceptable. Like HMOs, most PPOs use primary care physicians to authorize consultants, lab, x-rays, and inpatient admissions.

There are at least three types of PPO: (1) provider-based, organized by physicians and/or hospitals; (2) carrier-based, organized by insurance companies; (3) employer-based, developed by employers for their self-insured plans. These PPOs have several common elements. They organize a panel of providers so that consumers may have a choice; the panel includes physicians, hospitals, dentists, and allied health personnel. A negotiated fee schedules is offered usually at approximately 20% below regular fees, and review committees monitor excess use of services, especially referrals and hospitalizations. Nonrestrictive clauses ensure that consumers are not limited to the panel of providers, although in some plans they must pay a premium for choosing providers outside the PPO.

The success of PPOs, as with HMOs, will depend on their ability to control health costs by reducing use while maintaining high-quality care. Discounted rates may produce cost savings in the short run, but without a use-control mechanism, providers may merely increase services or perform additional procedures to compensate for the discounted fees. To foster cost-conscious behavior, PPOs normally institute at least three measures. First they redesign benefits with added incentives for patients to use outpatient surgery, home health care, and rehabilitation and outpatient mental health services. Second, they establish use controls such as prior authorization for elective hospitalization, elimination of weekend admissions, mandatory second opinions for surgery, concurrent review of hospital care. Third, they monitor physician and hospital use and cost patterns by region and nationally.

Despite the PPO's relative newness, the organizations are growing rapidly because their start-up costs are low, they simplify administrative work, and they are compatible with fee-for-service practice patterns. Some PPOs have achieved satisfactory results in their initial stages. For example, Blue Cross's Key Care in Virginia pays physicians 85% of their usual rate and provides a bonus if the physician meets hospital-use targets. Key Care signed 500 doctors and five hospitals in less than a year. The Hanes Group in North Carolina offers a PPO in which employees who use the services of physicians on a preferred-provider list pay a maximum of $10 per visit for services covered, including outpatient surgery, x-rays, and lab work done in the physician's office. The medical plan pays the remaining portion of charges directly to the physician. Aetna's Choice plan allows enrollees to use the personal physician of their choice for routine, ambulatory care, but specialty referrals and hospital care must be provided by physicians and facilities under contract to Aetna.

Preferred-provider plans are still in their introductory phase, and their ultimate impact on reducing health costs are still uncertain. Several concerns have surfaced regarding PPO plans:

Some PPOs charge providers a start-up and monthly fee without any guarantee of patients.

Physicians may violate antitrust laws if they communicate PPO rates, prices, and costs among fellow subscribers.

Malpractice policies may not apply under a PPO contract.

Administrative and organizational responsibilities required of the physicians and their offices may not be economical unless a high volume of PPO patients are enrolled.

PPOs' discounted fees may jeopardize the price structure for fee-for-service patients; the discounted fee schedule could also be lowered by the PPO if competition became intense.

Coverage of patient claims outside the service area of the PPO may incur additional financial problems.

Health Care Coalitions

The new economic environment of health care has spawned another cost-containment innovation, health care coalitions. Coalitions are joint public and private sector initiatives for addressing rising health care costs. Because business, government, and medicine are all adversely affected by the high costs of health care, the logic behind the development of health care coalitions is that these three groups need to solve the problem jointly. Health care coalitions facilitate the communications and negotiations between consumers, payers, and providers in the allocation of health resources for a local area. As of November 1985, according to the Office of Health Care Coalitions of the American Medical Association, 151 coalitions were in operation nationally. The principals in the majority of these coalitions are businesses, hospitals, physicians, medical societies, commercial insurers, Blue Cross and Blue Shield, and labor organizations. Coalitions are functioning in 40 states, but the heaviest concentrations of coalitions are in the East and Southeast.

The activities of health care coalitions vary from data collection on health care costs and service use to supporting the development of alternative delivery and financing systems. Some of the information coalitions provide to their members includes description of benefit plans, status of health promotion and wellness programs, cost and use data for diagnoses and treatments, and results of cost-management programs. Coalitions may also provide staff and resources to assist in designing benefit plans, conducting utilization reviews, establishing HMOs, and organizing support services such as home health and hospice care. A six-member national organization known as the "Dunlop Group of Six," comprised of the American Hospital Association, American Medical Association, Business Roundtable, Health Insurance Association of America, AFL-CIO, and Blue Cross and Blue Shield is available to support the start-up of coalitions. The following section discusses some examples of coalitions that have

made significant impact upon the econo-
mies of health care in their respective communities.

Mecklenburg County,
North Carolina

The Mecklenburg County Medical Society,
through the initiation of a few physicians, invited local businesses and hospitals, the county
government, the Chamber of Commerce, Blue
Cross and Blue Shield, and United Way in the
Charlotte area to join in forming a coalition entitled the Cost-Management Council. A planning
grant from the Robert Wood Johnson Foundation and assistance from the North Carolina
Foundation for Alternative Health Systems
were instrumental in getting the coalition off the
ground.

One of the first products of this coalition
was preadmission review (PAR). Physicians in
the Charlotte-Mecklenburg area wrote a set of
criteria for various illnesses. These criteria outline when hospitalization is indicated and how
long a patient should be in the hospital. The
PAR program uses these criteria to help reduce
unnecessary hospitalization and to lower average length of stay. Within its first two years,
over a dozen employers, with nearly 30,000
workers and dependents, incorporated PAR
into their benefit plans.

Mecklenburg's Cost-Management Council's
efforts have produced many immediate positive
results. Average length of stay for uncomplicated admissions have been reduced. A majority of cataract removals are now performed
without overnight admission. Home health
agencies were organized to provide posthospi-
tal follow-up care for new mothers and infants
who left the hospital with short stays. Another
innovative program soon to be implemented is
an affordable care for the elderly program
(PACE). Hospitals and large group practices
will be offered the opportunity to hire case managers to coordinate the care of chronically ill
older people. Case managers will design an individualized service plan involving relatives,
home health, and specialized therapists. Another goal of PACE is to address the problem
of Medicare patients overstaying their DRG
limits.

St. Louis Business Health Coalition

The St. Louis coalition was established primarily by the business sector. In fewer than three
years of operation, it has enrolled 38 companies
who employ more than 100,000 workers. A major result of this coalition's effort was the reduction in hospital costs to its members and the
leveling off of health care premiums. The chief
reason reported was the analysis of utilization
and hospital charges and the publishing of these
data for review by employers and providers.
The utilization review program cost $450,000
and produced a savings in health expenditures
of nearly $5 million. The St. Louis coalition
plans to establish a prospective payment system similar to the Medicare DRG program.
Such a system is already in operation for 13
common outpatient surgical procedures. The
pricing standards were agreed on by 21 hospitals and two free-standing surgicenters.

Birmingham Steering Committee

The Birmingham Steering Committee in Birmingham, Alabama, a group of five physicians
and five business representatives, became organized to review physician practice patterns, especially the high users, and to develop strategies to resolve high hospital admission rates.
The Steering Committee developed a prototype
health benefits plan with provisions to encourage consumer and provider cost consciousness.
Approximately 20 employers in the Birmingham area either have made or are in the process
of making changes to their health benefits plans
based on the prototype plan. The efforts of the
Steering Committee have paid off. A review by
Blue Cross Blue Shield of Alabama data for
nine major employers indicates that the number
of medical and surgical admissions decreased
nearly 20% in two years. In addition the medical and surgical inpatient days used by these
employees decreased by about 20% for the
same period.

Toledo Area Consortium

The Toledo Area Consortium for Affordable
Health Care is a broad-based organization co-

sponsored by physicians, business, the Blue Cross plan, hospitals, labor, and the public sector. Since its formation in 1982, its goal was to reduce hospitalizations in northwest Ohio, where they were nearly 20% higher than the national average. To accomplish this goal, the Consortium supports the Physicians' Medical Care Foundation, a private peer review organization which developed a program called the "peer data method." Through this program, area physicians receive information comparing their hospital use patterns with those of their peers in the area and nationwide. During the program's first two years, a large number of physicians were identified as higher-than-average users, and they were then urged to adopt a more cost-effective style of practice. The Consortium is planning to expand its focus to include ancillary services and hospital admissions.

Brown County, Wisconsin

A committee comprised of leaders from business, medicine, and government was initiated in the Green Bay, Wisconsin, area through the efforts of the Brown County Medical Society. The committee was formed to pinpoint health-related problems that business and medicine could work on jointly. One of the first concerns identified was the delay in workers returning to their jobs after accidents or injuries. The committee addressed this issue through development of a standardized return-to-work form, publication of an industrial information booklet for physicians, and sponsorship of two conferences on health care cost containment. Although data for measuring the impacts of these programs are unavailable, the business representatives believe that through the joint efforts of committee members, excessive employee absences have been curtailed. In addition to this activity, the committee will continue to monitor return-to-work issues and is investigating other health care concerns that can be resolved through the cooperative efforts of business and medicine.

CONCLUSION

The economic environment of health care is changing, and all indications are that these changes will favor the consumer and payer. The majority of medical services will be offered within some aspect of large-scale organizations and in a price-competitive market. These changes have not gone unnoticed by physicians. Findings from a national poll conducted by Harris and Associates (1981) of physicians in private practice, HMOs, IPAs, and residency programs indicate that the medical community is well aware of the changing health care environment. The physicians surveyed reported that the doctor surplus was a distinct possibility. More concern was expressed by subspecialists than by family practitioners. Most physicians believed that increased competition will lead to extended hours and expanded services at lower fees. They were uncertain how competition would affect personal income. Most believed that physicians would choose less patient volume and reduced income in return for more leisure time. Fifty percent of the survey expressed doubts about the future of medical practice to such an extent that they would not recommend their profession as highly today as they would have ten years ago. Salaried physicians were much less negative than were self-employed ones. Reimbursement ceilings, influx of for-profit companies, and increased presence of regulatory controls were major reasons for dissatisfaction with medicine as a career. The survey found that while self-employed, office-based practice remains the norm, there has been a steady shift toward salaried employment. Almost all physicians in practice 30 years or more are in traditional office practice situations, whereas 40% of physicians in practice fewer than five years are in salaried positions. Preferences for group practice and salaried positions were common among women physicians and physicians in two-income families. Professional and personal priorities of women physicians are significantly different from those of their male peers. Female practitioners and residents tend to specialize in primary care and are more likely to be hospital-based and salaried. Most physicians believe an increase in the proportion of family practitioners is both likely and desirable. Physicians appear quite responsive to the introduction of physicians' assistants and nurse practitioners to provide diagnostic and therapeutic services to underserved populations. Younger physicians reported the greatest support for physician extenders.

The Harris survey also published findings specifically upon the impact of HMOs, IPAs, and other forms of prepaid practice on the practice of medicine. One half of the physicians surveyed think that their practices will be affected by prepaid plans. Physicians acknowledge that the presence of prepaid plans in their vicinity caused reduction in income, and most physicians not working in HMOs had generally negative attitudes about HMOs. Physicians working in prepaid groups endorsed HMOs as a desirable practice opportunity. Physicians gave more positive ratings to HMOs, staff and group models, than did IPA physicians. Residents had more favorable opinions of HMOs than did practicing physicians. Residents were also much more likely to give HMOs credit for containing health care costs. Most widely perceived advantages to HMO patients, reported by the physician respondents, were lower expenditures and greater accessibility to medical services. Perceived disadvantages to patients of HMOs were inferior doctor-patient relationships, patient dissatisfaction with lack of choice of providers and services, and inconvenient office locations. Closed-panel HMOs were perceived to be more cost-effective and financially viable than IPAs. However, in quality of care and quality of physicians, IPAs were preferred. Benefits of working in HMOs were ease of establishing a practice directly out of residency, reduced working hours, more vacation time, and income security. Disadvantages of working in HMOs were lack of incentives for individual initiative and lower ceiling on earning potential and less autonomy then fee-for-service practice. Most HMO physicians plan to spend their entire career in prepaid practice.

References

Arthur Anderson Co.: *Health Care in 1990's: Trends and Strategies*. Chicago, American Hospital Association, 1984.

American Medical Association Department of Health Care Coalitions, Division of Health Service: *Beginning and Building a Health Care Coalition*. Chicago, American Medical Association, 1984.

American Medical Association Division of Health Policy and Program Evaluation, Department of Health Care Resources: *Diagnosis-Related Groupings (DRGs) and the Prospective Payment System*. Chicago, American Medical Association, 1985.

American Medical Association Council on Long-Range Planning and Development: *The Environment of Medicine*. Chicago, American Medical Association, 1984.

Department of Health Care Coalitions, Division of Health Service: *Health Care Coalitions: Impact in Three Communities*. Chicago, American Medical Association, 1985.

Carels E, Neuhauser D, Stason W: *The Physician and Cost Control*. Cambridge, Mass, Oelgeschlager, Gunn and Hain, 1980.

Freeland M, Schendler C: Health spending in the 1980s: Integration of clinical practice patterns with management. *Health Care Financing Review*, Spring 1984, 1–68.

Herzlinger R: How companies tackle health care costs: Part II. *Harvard Business Review*, September–October 1985, pp 108–120.

Kolimaga J (ed): *Health Cost Management Handbook, Strategies for Employers*. Raleigh, NC, North Carolina Foundation for Alternative Health Programs, 1984.

Louis Harris and Associates: *The Equitable Health Care Survey I, II: Options for Controlling Costs and Physicians' Attitudes Toward Cost Containment*. New York, The Equitable Life Assurance Society of the United States, 1983, 1984.

Louis Harris and Associates: *Medical Practice in the 1980s, Physicians Look at Their Changing Profession*. Menlo Park, Calif, Kaiser Foundation, 1981.

Starr P: *The Social Transformation of American Medicine*. New York, Basic Books, 1982.

2
Marketing Health Services

- **What ethical principles should guide marketing in health care?**
- **How can a practice conduct a marketing audit?**
- **How can a health care organization become consumer-oriented?**
- **What are the features of a comprehensive marketing plan?**
- **What challenges must be overcome to market health services effectively?**

Since the health care industry has now joined the other industries and professions that face intensely competitive environments, excess capacity, new types of competitors, and pressure to cut costs, marketing has become more visible and acceptable than at any time in the history of medicine. Marketing is a new business function in health care organizations in comparison with other management features such as personnel, finance, communications, and public relations. Marketing in health care has taken a low profile because of the medical profession's unwillingness to promote (advertise) medical services and the physicians' attitude that their competence and reputation were enough to attract and retain patients. However, as health care moves from the small-scale, cottage-industry practice to the large-scale, corporate organization, marketing programs will become common among health care providers and their organizations.

Marketing is broadly defined as the exchange process through which patients and health care providers receive mutual benefits. As consumers, patients will benefit if their needs are identified and satisfied at a reasonable cost. Providers will benefit if they receive fair compensation for the services they render and if the work they perform is gratifying. To effect a satisfactory exchange process between health consumers and health care providers, the following must take place: (1) a systematic assessment of consumers' needs and preferences that provides information about both the current and future perspectives of patients, and about potential changes in health-related trends in the population; (2) an evaluation of the current operating system to determine how effectively the organization meets the needs of consumers and achieves a profitable result; and (3) a set of strategies that will keep the organization competitive in the future. A marketing program is the vehicle with which to achieve these objectives. This chapter discusses health care marketing from several perspectives, including the ethics of marketing, the marketing audit, consumer orientation, marketing strategies, and the challenges of marketing professional services.

ETHICS OF MARKETING

The code of behavior for physicians over the past several decades was that advertising or any other overt marketing approach was unethical. The medical professional believed that direct solicitation of patients was neither in the best interests neither of the people served nor of the individual physician's professional image. A commonly heard phrase was "Our good medicine will be our marketing program." Promoting oneself or one's practice was frowned upon because many thought this would lead to deception. Another bias often associated with marketing was that any effort or money put into marketing would detract from a physician's primary responsibility of providing quality health care. Marketing was disdained because it insin-

uated a form of manipulation and created an unnecessary step in the delivery of patient care.

In 1979 the Federal Trade Commission ordered the U.S. medical profession to "cease and desist" from restricting, regulating, impeding, declaring unethical, interfering with, or advising against advertising services. This action was followed by the adoption of a new set of principles of medical ethics by the American Medical Association House of Delegates in 1980.

As shown in Figure 2.1, the principles of medical ethics place primacy upon the benefit and protection of the patient. These standards emphasize the physician's responsibility to provide relevant information to patients and the public. The principles also establish physicians' rights to choose whom they serve and the environment in which they offer their services. An-

AMERICAN MEDICAL ASSOCIATION

Principles of

MEDICAL ETHICS

Preamble:
 The medical profession has long subscribed to a body of ethical statements developed primarily for the benefit of the patient. As a member of this profession, a physician must recognize responsibility not only to patients, but also to society, to other health professionals, and to self. The following Principles adopted by the American Medical Association are not laws, but standards of conduct which define the essentials of honorable behavior for the physician.

I. A physician shall be dedicated to providing competent medical service with compassion and respect for human dignity.

II. A physician shall deal honestly with patients and colleagues, and strive to expose those physicians deficient in character or competence, or who engage in fraud or deception.

III. A physician shall respect the law and also recognize a responsibility to seek changes in those requirements which are contrary to the best interests of the patient.

IV. A physician shall respect the rights of patients, of colleagues, and of other health professionals, and shall safeguard patient confidences within the constraints of the law.

V. A physician shall continue to study, apply and advance scientific knowledge, make relevant information available to patients, colleagues, and the public, obtain consultation, and use the talents of other health professionals when indicated.

VI. A physician shall, in the provision of appropriate patient care, except in emergencies, be free to choose whom to serve, with whom to associate, and the environment in which to provide medical services.

VII. A physician shall recognize a responsibility to participate in activities contributing to an improved community.

Figure 2.1 Principles of Medical Ethics. Reprinted by permission from the American Medical Association. Adopted by the AMA House of Delegates July 1980.

other distinction is the responsibility to participate in and improve the community.

Edward J. Shahady, MD, an experienced family physician and medical educator in family medicine, offers two ethical principles for marketing health services (1984). The first is the principle of *marketing to achieve two natural effects*. The initial and most important effect is to market for the good of society. The second effect is to market for the gain of the physician. To successfully implement this principle one must (1) conduct a monitoring system to ensure the highest level of patient satisfaction and quality control and (2) establish economic measurements to maintain fair physician compensation. *Nil marketing* is the second principle; it means that if consumers are not appropriately informed of the qualities of good health, they might wrongly obtain or avoid services and endanger their health care. Thus, physicians have the responsibility to promote their concept of good health and then provide it in an accessible and affordable manner. This principle implies that physicians and other health care professionals are obligated to market their services to improve physical and psychological well-being of their current and prospective patients.

Physicians faced with the dilemma of how to market their services ethically should consider the following questions:

Are patients' wants and needs clearly understood by health care providers?

Has every attempt been made to inform patients about ways to maintain a healthy lifestyle?

Are patients receiving adequate care from other providers?

Are physicians' fees, costs, and personal incomes appropriate?

Would patients or consumers be negatively affected by remaining uninformed about some aspect of their health?

MARKETING AUDIT

A marketing effort should begin with an audit of factors that are essential for developing a comprehensive plan to identify and satisfy consumer needs. If the practice has existed for a long time, first conduct an internal audit to determine the effectiveness of the existing organizational system. If the organization is new, then the audit should focus more on outside factors such as consumer trends, competition, economic conditions and new opportunities available for health care services. Regardless of the practice's age, a marketing audit will provide valuable information about one or more of the following (See Figure 2.2):

1. Consumer demographics and preferences
2. Number and type of competition
3. Product/service features
4. Finance and reimbursement policies
5. Location and facilities
6. Promotions and communications

The marketing audit could be conducted by an outside group. Using independent, objective consultants may ensure that the findings will be considered valid by physicians and practice staff. Consultants may also be useful in implementing the recommendations from the marketing audit. Committing the necessary resources and involving all members of the practice in the process will ensure a successful investigation. The audit report will enumerate a variety of conclusions and recommendations that can be converted into strategies that meet consumer needs cost-effectively.

CONSUMER ORIENTATION

Marketing begins with the consumer. If health care providers are to market ethically, they must be responsive to the changing characteristics and attitudes of their consumers. As these changes occur, physicians have several options. They can ignore the changes and continue to practice as they have in the past. They can drastically change their practice patterns and perhaps jeopardize their ability to practice effectively. They can integrate the knowledge of consumers' preferences with their established practice methods and modify only those areas which need to be changed. The following presents data from consumer studies and suggestions on how practices can obtain consumer information.

Prior to implementing a marketing plan a health care organization should conduct a marketing audit. The following topics and questions could be included in such an audit.

ENVIRONMENT

What are short and long-run trends in the local economy? How will these trends affect the size, age, distribution, and other demographic patterns of the population? What are the principle occupations? Are they stable? What are the public's attitudes and preferences about prepaid care, HMOs, advertising, cost containment, and other health innovations. Who are the major health care competitors? What are their strategies? How well are they accepted by consumers and payers? Are health care coalitions developing? How compatible is the practice with the criteria for joining or merging with other health systems?

CONSUMERS

What are the major market segments, and expected growth rates? How are consumer lifestyles and values changing? How satisfied are consumers and payers with health services? Who are the major payers of health services? What types of delivery and payment plans are they advocating?

ORGANIZATION

Who is responsible for the practice's management decisions? Who will direct the marketing plan? What role will consultants play in the planning, implementation, and evaluation phases? How well is the practice being managed? What problems must be solved before the marketing plan can be undertaken? What marketing actions have been tried in the past? What were the results? What organizational results will indicate the success of the marketing program? i.e. New patients, $, Industrial contracts, etc.

PRODUCT

What is the range of services now offered? Which ones are cost-effective? Which ones are not cost-effective, but will still be retained? What services need to be phased out? How much time and resources can be invested in new services? Who will "champion" the changes and innovations?

PRICE

What are the current methods of payment? Do they reflect the community trends? How many services are offered on a contract basis? What percentage of the practice revenue is prepayment? Is this acceptable? How effectively are costs managed? Are cost centers set up to monitor efficiency in various parts of the organization? How are fees set? Do they relate directly to costs? Do patients perceive appropriate value for services received? Are the fees and costs of competitors being monitored?

PLACE

Is the facility adequate for current business and clinical work? Is there space and resources for expansion? Are special facilities available for the elderly, disabled, and children? Is the practice fully equipped? Is the practice location convenient to patients' workplaces and homes? Is parking adequate and immediately adjacent to the practice? Are satellite offices in operation? Do providers work in other settings, such as industrial plants, nursing homes, etc.

PROMOTION

How does the practice promote its services and the providers? Does the practice distribute a patient brochure, a letter to new patients or a newsletter? Are patient education materials published by the practice? Does the practice sponsor, or participate in, health education programs? In what community activities do providers and staff participate? Are there any "free" services offered?

Figure 2.2 Health Care Marketing Audit

Consumer Opinions

Researchers from the Department of Family Medicine at the University of North Carolina conducted a study to determine consumers' perspectives of their health care (Cogswell et al, 1985). Diverse segments of the population such as office workers, professional men and women, retirees, young singles, minorities, and people living in rural areas discussed a variety of health care topics. Questions were open-ended so that participants would offer ideas and suggestions spontaneously. Consumers indicated what they liked and did not like about current health care services and what they wanted in the future. To dramatize the value of consumer orientation in marketing, the priorities of four illustrative groups are presented below.

Office Workers. This group was composed of single and married women, most of whom had a school-age child. Convenient access to health services is their major concern. They do not like leaving work for routine health care. They prefer a medical practice that is reasonably close—no more than 30 minutes from their home or workplace. They also desire ample parking and minimal waiting time to see the physician.

Because of their moderate income, they are cost-conscious and willing to be seen by less skilled professionals such as nurses or nurse practitioners for some of their routine care. This group is in favor of evening office hours and appointments on weekends. They feel, however, that they should not be penalized by being charged a higher fee for evening and weekend visits. This view is shared by interviewees in other groups.

This group of office workers is very conscious of exercise, nutrition, and maintaining a healthy life-style. They would welcome more information and guidelines from physicians so that they can manage more of their personal and family health care. Many commented that dentists have done a better job of prevention and health maintenance than physicians.

Mothers With Small Children. "New" mothers voice many concerns about health maintenance and prevention. This group criticized what they perceive as physicians' disinterest or lack of knowledge about nutrition for mothers and young children, exercise following childbirth, the value of breast feeding, and the emotional stresses of child rearing.

These mothers also value patient education and having a regular doctor for the majority of their family's care. When the topic of advertising was discussed, interviewees were opposed to slick media advertising by physicians. They do want physicians to inform them about the services they offer and the costs of those services. This particular group is interested in knowing the physician's professional credentials, special interests, and philosophy of practice.

Senior Citizens. The elderly consumer places a high value on doctor-patient communications and continuity with a regular physician. These consumers want a physician who spends time with them and knows their specific health care situation. Since senior citizens use medical services frequently, they also are interested in a convenient practice site. Older consumers also want more discussion about the cost of procedures and medications, especially before an examination or series of tests. Many voiced concerns about physicians' unwillingness to address the financial implications of the elderly person's health care. Those on fixed incomes are often on a limited budget and would welcome payment options and suggestions for keeping expenditures under control. Since they do not want to jeopardize their doctor-patient relationship, many of their concerns go unmentioned.

Professionals. Professional men and women voiced many strong views about their health care services. A common theme was their interest in becoming more involved in decision making, particularly with routine exams, lab tests, x-rays, elective procedures, and the use of ambulatory instead of hospital services.

Because many support aging parents, these consumers are also extremely aware of medical care for the elderly. They place a high importance on establishing a continuing doctor-patient relationship for themselves and family members. Time is important to these consumers, so they prefer convenient locations and minimal waiting time for appointments. Some even suggest that they should charge the physician for keeping them waiting.

The women voiced a strong interest in prevention and patient education. They were more oriented to self-care than men. The women also said they are willing to receive routine and follow-up exams from nurse practitioners and other nonphysician health professionals, especially if the cost were less and if the waiting time shorter.

Patient Surveys

Physicians whose patient population includes one or more of the groups mentioned above may benefit from these findings. The preceding discussion indicates how important it is to listen to what consumers have to say. Although medical practices are unlikely to organize such a consumer interview study, other methods of obtaining consumer and patient information are available. A questionnaire is effective for monitoring patient satisfaction and detecting changes in attitudes and preferences. Examples of questions to include on a patient survey are:

New Patients

How did you hear about our practice?

How far do you live (and work) from our practice?

What type of health services are most important to you?

How many members of your family will be coming to our practice?

Did you receive adequate information about the practice and your physician?

Do you have any suggestions about appointments, fees, physicians, staff, or other features of our practice?

Regular Patients

Please indicate how satisfied you are with the following:

□ Physicians   □ Waiting time
□ Office staff   □ Telephone use
□ Fees   □ Emergency care
□ Appointments   □ Hospital care

What problems have you encountered with the practice?

How can the practice provide better health care to you and your family?

Some of the most consistent findings from patient satisfaction studies indicate that patients would have the strongest attachment to a practice if the following services were provided:

Twenty-four-hour a day, 7-days-a-week availability

Advice on how to stay healthy

Treatment from a physician knowledgeable about all aspects of patient's health

Assistance in decisions about most cost-effective treatments

Treatment of health care needs over an extended time

Maintenance of all medical information, including hospital care and referrals, in one practice location

Management of health care needs of entire family

These issues were also mentioned frequently in the consumer group interviews. Obviously the public has strong opinions about the delivery and financing of health care, and it behooves physicians and other health care professionals to consider these views as they market their services.

MARKETING STRATEGIES

The changing economic environment of health care and the increased influence of consumerism will necessitate that health care providers design and offer a comprehensive set of marketing strategies. The traditional approach for implementing a marketing program involves four distinct components: (1) *Product* is the range of services offered to patients. (2) *Pricing* is determined by the cost of and payment for services. (3) *Place* is the location where the services are offered. (4) *Promotions* are the communications between providers and consumers. Because of the highly competitive nature of the health care field, each of these dimensions needs to be included in the marketing effort of a health care organization (see Figure 2.3).

Product

The product of health care organizations represents the entire range of patient care services, procedures, and tests that a medical practice offers. Product questions are what services to offer and who to serve. Since health care services are offered through people, the marketing effort involves the members of the health care team. In a sense, "the people are the product." Thus, product marketing in health care begins with the development and maintenance of an efficient and responsive organization. If patients or consumers do not perceive that the practice is effective and that its personnel are competent, then it will be difficult to market

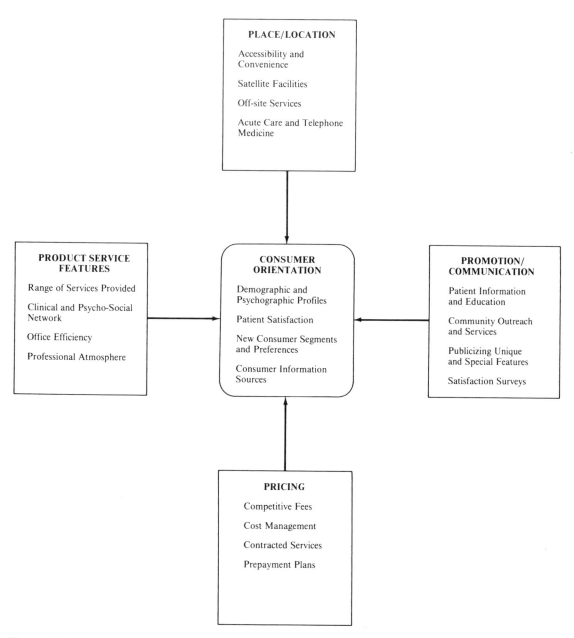

Figure 2.3 Marketing Mix Strategies

services to the mutual benefit of consumers and providers. Organizational functions such as scheduling, bookkeeping, personnel supervision, and communications must operate smoothly before any external marketing program should be implemented.

Another product-marketing consideration is the determination of unique characteristics of various segments in the patient population or the consumers at large. This is market *differen-* *tiation,* which means that services the practice offers need to be adjusted according to the preferences of major groups of patients in the practice or groups the practice wishes to attract. For instance, the qualities of at least four consumer groups are as follows.

Working Women. Working women have children in day care centers. They are often single parents and prefer convenient, low-cost services, and they are receptive to education on self-care and preventive care methods. Working women would be attracted by extended office hours, a telephone hour with physicians and psychologists, satellite offices in shopping centers, and wellness programs that promote good health and illness prevention.

Industrial Medicine. With industrial medicine, the company is the payer and sometimes the provider. Health maintenance organizations (HMOs) are attractive, especially when they can document quality services for lower fees. Industrial medicine has many avenues of entry for physicians. Companies are hiring physicians or contracting with community health centers for health maintenance programs and preventive care procedures. They are also employing nurse practitioners and other health care personnel on site and are hiring physicians as medical directors on a part-time basis to staff their medical facilities. Business firms and other larger employer groups also contract for many of their medical service needs such as preemployment physicals, executive physicals, workers' compensation cases, and diagnostic screening tests for high-risk employees.

Senior Citizens. Senior citizens live in retirement communities or in areas that are economical and convenient for them and their families. They have Medicare and usually a supplementary insurance plan. Because of their frequent use of medical services and their chronic problems, they prefer a personal physician who knows all aspects of their medical care. Costs are of particular importance to those on moderate fixed incomes. Physicians who are interested in serving the needs of senior citizens should consider affiliations with the nursing homes and skilled-nursing facilities. The chronic health needs of elderly patients also require extensive service from other health and social agencies. Physicians should be willing to take the role of organizer and coordinator for their older patients.

Professionals. Professionals are often members of dual-career couples. They have one or two children and are a relatively mobile population. They prefer the highest-quality services,

convenient locations, and minimal time for scheduling appointments. Health and fitness programs are a high priority. This group is also becoming increasingly responsible for the care of elderly parents. Professionals are seeking more of a partnership with physicians; self-care, patient education, and health maintenance are appealing to this group. The higher the education and income level of the patients, the higher their expectations for a voice in decisions that affect their care or that of family members.

Pricing

The cost of health care services and the payment process are important features that affect the marketability of a medical practice, especially since health consumers and the corporate payers for health services are becoming cost-conscious. Whether the payment system is fee-for-service or prepaid contracts, medical practices will be under pressure to operate efficiently and to establish competitive fees.

The establishment of a competitive fee schedule for physicians' services depends on at least two factors, costs of the services offered and the prices consumers pay for similar services from other providers. Managing costs efficiently requires a well-designed and -supervised practice management system within the office. Competitive fee schedules are a function of the perceived value patients associate with the service as compared with other practices.

Cost Management

The majority of health care costs, especially those in the ambulatory sector, are for salaries and benefits of the professional and ancillary staff members. The number and qualifications of personnel in a practice has a direct relationship to the cost of the services offered. The approximate ratio in an outpatient setting of physicians and staff is two staff members per one physician. Thus, big influences on costs are amount of money allocated to the salaries in relation to productivity of physicians and staff. One option that organizations are using to increase productivity is hiring qualified personnel who can perform multiple clinical procedures, such as educating patients, taking histories, giving injections, performing diagnostic tests, and operating lab and x-ray equipment. Practices are also hiring physicians' assistants and family nurse practitioners who can perform a wide range of clinical treatment services under the supervision of a physician. The benefits from this increased clinical productivity by staff members is that physicians will have time available to perform higher-level clinical care and to work in other sites such as hospitals, nursing homes, and local industry.

Another aspect of cost management is creating an efficient administrative system for scheduling, filing, billing, and other office management functions. As practices increase in size and complexity, the traditional manual techniques must be replaced with automated systems. It is not uncommon to visit practices that are overstaffed in the reception and business functions because of antiquated telephone systems, overloaded pegboard collection and billing procedures, and a "harried" insurance clerk or two who have to transcribe patient information on a multitude of forms. Computer systems are now available for patient scheduling, billing, and insurance-claim processing. Another benefit that practices derive from automated systems is the staff and patient satisfaction that result from a smoothly running organization. The biggest hurdle to office innovation is the reluctance of physicians and staff personnel to learn new methods and to adapt their behavior to the standards necessary for the new system to work effectively. Chapter 8 addresses the issue of computerization for medical practices in greater detail.

If health care organizations can increase physician and staff productivity and upgrade the office systems for finance, communications, and scheduling, significant cost savings are feasible. However, if practices do not manage their internal costs, they may find it difficult to compete with the larger health care organizations who have resources and expertise to manage their services efficiently. In the long run, consumers and third-party payers will select high-quality services for the most affordable price.

Fees

Once the organization's internal costs and productivity are at acceptable levels, the next pric-

ing issue is what fees to charge for services. Setting fees depends on two factors, the *market*—what other health-care providers are charging—and the consumers' perception of the *value* of the services they receive.

If the practice is located where health services can be obtained from several different providers and organizations, fees must reflect the community rate. Consumers often compare certain health care fees such as routine office visits, physical exams, lab and x-ray tests, and obstetrical care. If these services are essentially the same in quality, then providers have only a small variance available for them to set their fees. Insurance companies and Medicare and Medicaid payers also maintain profiles of physicians' usual and customary fees and will reimburse physicians on these rates. *Contracts* for special procedures such as employment exams, executive physicals, and health maintenance programs are important means for financing some aspects of health care. Industrial firms and other large agencies prefer to negotiate fees in advance for the services they receive. Providers are then obliged to establish a rate, usually lower than their normal fee, to provide these services to the employees of the contracted organization. The prepayment system that HMOs offer is merely an expansion of what was previously referred to as "contract medicine." By the end of the century, it is estimated that the majority of health consumers will receive their health care under some form of contract.

Since price competition is being encouraged by government and industry, health care providers must be prepared to publish their fees, negotiate contracts, and accept prepayment from third-party payers. If the quality of care is perceived as comparable, payers and consumers will choose their health plan based on price.

Place

The practice's facility and location are becoming important marketing considerations as consumer life-styles and working patterns change (see Figure 2.4). Just as product and pricing first required a look at the internal system, marketing of the physical location also requires a look

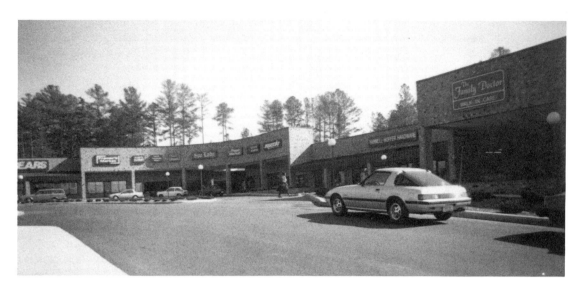

Figure 2.4 A Shopping Center Offers Patients a Convenient Location and Ample Parking. (Courtesy of THE FAMILY DOCTOR, Drs. Glenn and Jerry Withrow, Chapel Hill, North Carolina.)

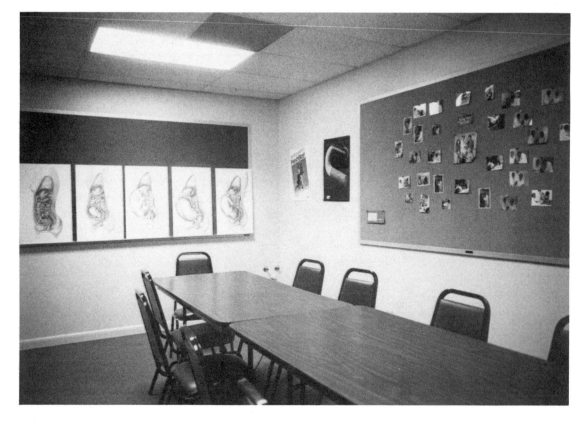

Figure 2.5 A Separate Room for Patient Education Classes and Practice Meetings Will Enhance Communications with Patients and Staff Members. (Courtesy of THE FAMILY DOCTOR, Drs. Glenn and Jerry Withrow, Chapel Hill, North Carolina.)

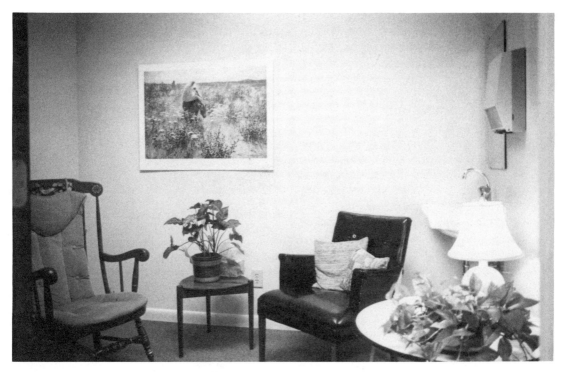

Figure 2.6 One Room in the Practice Could Be Designed for Counseling and Private Discussions. (Courtesy of THE FAMILY DOCTOR, Drs. Glenn and Jerry Withrow, Chapel Hill, North Carolina.)

at how the practice is currently functioning as a responsive, supportive medical facility.

The office can be marketed from several perspectives. First and foremost are the people who work in the practice. Physician and staff attitudes and behaviors have a tremendous impact on patients, patients' families, and others who visit the practice. Maintaining high morale and a positive working environment is a challenge. Interpersonal relations and communication skills should be a high priority in selecting and training new staff members, as should continuing education programs (see Figure 2.5).

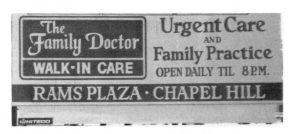

Figure 2.7 A Billboard Advertisement to Publicize the Opening of a New Practice. (Courtesy of THE FAMILY DOCTOR, Drs. Glenn and Jerry Withrow, Chapel Hill, North Carolina.)

Second to the congeniality and competence of the staff are the patient flow patterns and the interior design of the office. An attractive setting can be very therapeutic to patients and offers staff members a more comfortable environment for work. Efficiency and confidentiality are also important considerations in office layout (See Figure 2.6). Quickly channeling patients through the practice is a time saver to patients and also keeps the system operating productively. Long waiting time and unnecessary delays are just as disruptive to the staff as they are inconvenient for patients. *Keep on schedule* should be the practice motto. Physicians take heed, because you are the biggest culprits! Other locational factors should be considered only after the personnel and internal operations are working effectively.

Satellite offices, evening and weekend hours, and services provided at nursing homes, rehabilitation centers, and industrial plants are some of the strategies being recommended as part of location marketing (see Figure 2.7). Other place considerations include the adequacy of parking, opportunities for patients to be seen immediately (walk-in care is reemerg-

(walk-in care is reemerging), rapid telephone responses to patient inquiries, and networking with other health care professionals to provide additional services in the practice.

Promotions

Traditionally, physicians have promoted themselves and their practices in subtle ways: newspaper ads when opening the office, articles about the new doctor in town, patient newsletters and brochures, and participation in community activities. One-to-one communications and public relations are still the best form of promotion between health care providers and their clients and prospective clients. However, with the advent of large-scale organizations in health care, consumers and payers of health services will receive information in the mass media about the types of service available, costs of care, qualifications and expertise of professionals, and logistics of health-care facilities (see Figure 2.8).

Providers and other health care professionals will have to decide which promotional strategies are cost-effective for their specialties and locations. However, since one purpose of promotional marketing is to communicate with patients, providers have a responsibility to present relevant information to patients so that consumers can make informed decisions about their health care needs. Examples of promotional strategies which are suitable for medical practices are:

Letter to New Patients A brief information sheet about physicians, staff, policies, appointments, and special features of the practice

Practice Brochure Detailed description of clinical and financial procedures, biographical sketches of personnel, hospitals that physicians admit to, and physicians' philosophies of practice

Patient Education Handouts for reading in the reception area or in the exam rooms, health and fitness programs, special classes on chronic illnesses, or other services appropriate to the types of patients in the practice

Practice Newsletter Regular publication sent to patients in the mail and distributed in the office to publicize special events, introduce

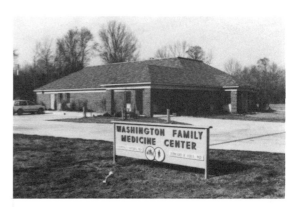

Figure 2.8 Building Design Should Include an Attractive Sign, Ample Parking, and a Covered Drive-up Area for the Handicapped and Elderly. (Courtesy of WASHINGTON FAMILY MEDICINE CENTER, Drs. Thomas Speros and Edward Hill, Washington, North Carolina.)

new personnel, and keep patients informed of changes in payment plans and other practice features

Free Health Services Health exams for athletic teams, volunteer service at health fairs, services to indigent patients, and community service

CHALLENGES

In their book entitled *Marketing Professional Services,* Bloom and Kotler (1984) state that organizations such as medical practices that provide professional services must seek a balance among the need to market aggressively, special limitations imposed by the industry, and the need to maintain client trust. Bloom and Kotler identify seven challenges in marketing professional services.

Ethical and Legal Constraints

The ethics and standards of health care professionals discourage marketing strategies which might mislead or deceive current or future patients. The temptation to make ethical compromises will increase as competition intensifies and as the surplus of physicians and other health practitioners erodes the highly personalized nature of the doctor-patient relationship.

Physicians and other health care professionals may ensure that marketing stays within ethical and legal boundaries by (1) participating in peer review or self-regulation programs, (2) educating patients about acceptable professional behavior, (3) keeping communication channels open for patients and others to inform providers about concerns and questions, (4) screening patients and perhaps discharging clients who may be excessively demanding or who desire services or benefits that are inappropriate or discriminatory.

As health care organizations and physicians become more occupied with the business of medicine, maintaining the public's trust will become important. Essential health care services are considered the right of all citizens regardless of income, age, or the nature of illness or disease. Each community will have a segment of its population that is medically underserviced, and physicians are expected to provide support to these people. Responding appropriately to these unmet health care needs is an ethical obligation for health care providers.

Buyer Uncertainty

Professional services are considered credence goods, and therefore consumers place great faith in those who offer these services. Patients are not always competent to evaluate the quality of the health care services they need, especially in urgent-care situations. Where patient uncertainty is high, professional service organizations emphasize education rather than persuasion in their marketing communications. For instance, promotional and public relations programs could be geared to teach patients when they should seek professional services, which attributes to consider in evaluating different providers, how to communicate concerns and desires, and what providers can realistically be expected to accomplish.

Buyer (patient) uncertainty is of particular concern as prepayment plans begin to take the place of the traditional fee-for-service method of payment and the indemnity health insurance programs. A completely new style of practice will evolve as physicians receive financial incentives to keep people healthy and to limit treatment for major illnesses. Physicians cannot assume that patients fully understand the implications of the prepaid health plans that require primary-physician authorization for referrals and hospitalization.

Experience and Reputation

Consumers of professional services select providers based primarily on the reputation of the provider and/or the organization. Since women use health services 1.5 times more often than men and are usually the first member of the family to seek health services, they are the key decision makers that physicians and other health care professionals should attempt to influence. Providers who are new to a community or who are offering new services should inform people personally to demonstrate their competence and to present their views about health care. A common approach by the HMOs and the PPOs is to recruit experienced physicians in the city where they will be offering their plans. Employers realize that the physicians rather than the HMO itself provide the services to their employees. Physicians should use every means available to investigate the credibility and financial viability of the prepayment plan before they consider joining.

When considering promotions, unless the advertising emphasizes the expertise of the physicians and is presented in a dignified manner, it may not benefit the practice. Offering lower fees, renovating the building, changing locations, or opening an urgent-care center should be publicized as strategies to meet consumers' changing needs and to offer cost-effective services,

Limited Differentiation

Differentiating health care services and providers may be very difficult. Patients generally acknowledge that physicians as a group are well-trained and competent, and patients tend to be loyal to their personal physicians and unaware of features that distinguish one medical practice or provider from another. Therefore, to influence patients, health care marketers have to emphasize unique and innovative attributes that appeal to health consumers. To differentiate their services, medical organizations could promote issues that may be seen as unique, such as highly qualified professional staff trained at prestigious universities, convenient services that minimize waiting time and unnecessary travel, use of state-of-the-art equipment, computers and communication systems, patient information system to assist patients and families with financial procedures and hospitalizations, and provider-initiated follow-up contacts to ensure that the referral services were acceptable.

Modified Advertising

Because the public is not accustomed to seeing or hearing advertising from professionals, especially physicians, advertising may cause negative reactions from clients and colleagues if the message and media used are too extreme for the audience or the services being offered. Radio, newspaper, and television advertising are often seen as unprofessional if they are too flashy. These media also cover a much larger geographical area than the practice serves. Since advertising results are difficult to measure in absolute numbers of new clients or new services, health care professionals should use advertising selectively and monitor the positive and negative effects of the promotional techniques being used.

Personal Approach

Because clients generally prefer promotions by the persons who actually perform the services, the personal approach plays an important role in marketing professional services. Thus the adage, "you have to sell yourself" seems appropriate. Physicians and office personnel are probably the best promoters of their practice. If patients become displeased with the attitude or behavior of anyone in the office, however, any amount of advertising or public relations is not likely to repair the damage. Therefore health care organizations should select employees who present a positive image to the public to promote their practices. Human relations programs are a must for physicians in training and for office personnel, and patient satisfaction

surveys are instrumental in determining how cooperative the personnel are perceived to be.

Time and Resources

Although there is no single formula for determining the exact amount of time and resources needed to market health services, the marketing program must have the endorsement from the senior members of the organization and the support of the management and supervisory staff. A comprehensive marketing plan requires measurable objectives, a time line for implementation, a budget for expenses, an individual assigned as coordinator, outside expertise to guide and perhaps execute the marketing plan, and a review date to evaluate results and determine what modifications are necessary.

CONCLUSIONS

Ethical marketing of health services can be achieved by recognizing consumers' needs and then offering the appropriate services to meet those needs. This chapter presented a variety of suggestions and strategies which physicians and other health professionals may employ to market themselves and their organizations in the highly competitive health care industry. First and foremost among what has been suggested is an ongoing information system to stay abreast of patient and consumer attitudes. Input from patients about current problems, concerns, and their ideas for changes will enrich the planning and decision-making processes. Gathering information from consumers at large also keeps the practice in touch with changing demographic and social trends. Another very important feature of marketing is the communications with patients and consumers about the practice. Media advertising may not be suitable, but physicians should design and publicize innovative health services such as extended office hours, cost-containment techniques, health maintenance protocols, and special efforts to serve the elderly, working mothers, industry, and other important consumer groups. The increasing complexity of health care requires affiliations with community agencies, industry, government, and other health-related organizations. These associations may provide physicians additional exposure to consumers and payers and demonstrate physicians' willingness to take their expertise and services into the community and marketplace. Whichever strategies are employed to market health services, physicians should continue to build on the traditional values of patient advocacy and contributing to the public good. Because patients want to participate in health care decisions and take more responsibility for maintaining a healthy life-style, they will be asking physicians to function as health educators and coordinators instead of the "medicine men" of the past.

The following list of the ideal characteristics of a medical practice is derived from consumer interviews and opinions and may help health professionals to assess their current marketing efforts and determine how to maintain their competitive edge.

CHARACTERISTICS OF AN IDEAL MEDICAL PRACTICE

Provides a regular health care team, which is highly recommended by friends and relatives

Makes information available about physicians' credentials and philosophy of practice

Offers education on physical fitness and nutrition to all ages of patients

Has a compassionate, communicative staff of physicians and office personnel

Takes time to discuss the consequences of medical procedures and the related costs of treatments and hospitalizations

Offers evening and weekend hours at no additional costs

Considers the patients' time and need for information as equally important as the physicians'.

References

Aluise J, Cogswell B: Closing the information gap between consumers and physicians. *Strategic Practice* 1, no. 5 (November 1985): 4-5.

Bloom P, Kotler P: *Marketing Professional Services*. Englewood Cliffs, NJ, Prentice-Hall, 1984.

Brown S, Morley A: *Marketing Strategies for Physicians*. Oradell, NJ Medical Economics Books, 1986.

Cogswell B, Aluise J, Bogdewic S, Melton J, Shahady E: A method for investigating consumers' perspectives on health care. *Journal of Health Care Marketing* 5, no. 4 (Fall 1985): 51-57.

Cooper P: *Health Care Marketing: Issues and Trends*. Germantown, Md, Aspen Systems Corporation, 1979.

Hite R: A time for re-examination: Advertising physician services. *Medical Group Management* 31, no. 2 (1984): 22-33.

MacStravic R: *Marketing Health Care*. Germantown, Md, Aspen Systems Corporation, 1977.

Manoff R: *Social Marketing, New Imperative for Public Health*. New York, Praeger, 1985.

Milone C, Blair W, Littlefield J: *Marketing for the Dental Practice*. Philadelphia, WB Saunders, 1982.

Rubright R: *Marketing Health and Human Services*. Germantown, Md, Aspen Systems Corporation, 1981.

Shahady E: Medical ethics and marketing, are they compatible? Unpublished Paper, Department of Family Medicine, University of North Carolina, Chapel Hill, NC, 1983.

Stamps P: Measuring patient satisfaction. *Medical Group Management* 31, no. 1 (1984): 36-47.

3
Practice Site

- What are the important features in selecting a community as a future practice site?
- How can a hospital be evaluated as a quality health care facility?
- What needs to be included in an employment contract?
- What are the advantages and disadvantages of solo and group practices?
- What factors will be important in evaluating membership in health mainte-

nance and preferred-provider organizations?
- How can rural practice opportunities be evaluated and planned?
- How should entrance into practice be planned for a new site? For an established practice?
- How is a practice facility planned for either new construction or renovation?

Physicians face three major decisions in their career development: whether to practice medicine as a profession, what area of speciality to pursue following medical school, and where to practice. Following the decision of what field to specialize in, the choice of a practice location may become an intermittent concern throughout one's medical education and training. Medical students realize that certain specialties are limited to large medical centers or are hospital-based. As resident physicians are recruited by communities, partners, or medical organizations, they become aware that certain factors influence practice site decisions. Deciding where to practice is an ongoing process for practicing physicians who may find that initial practice locations have become unsuitable or inadequate, thereby necessitating plans for reorganization and/or new buildings to accommodate an expanding practice.

A goal for each physician would be to choose a practice site where interests, skills, and capabilities are matched with the community's health needs and where the patient population will most closely satisfy the physician's

personal and professional needs. Subjective and objective data necessary to make the best selection include assessment of the community, medical climate, practice potential, and financial considerations. Problem areas to evaluate are demand for additional health care providers in one's specialty, restrictions upon practice autonomy, limited hospital privileges, or reluctance by the practice or community to accept the new physician's approach to health care.

This chapter addresses the many variables that affect practice site decisions, with special consideration for the needs of new practitioners. Established physicians may also find this chapter helpful if they are currently recruiting new partners or are planning changes in their existing practice.

COMMUNITY

A community may be evaluated from several vantage points. First, does it offer the personal features which will satisfy individual and family interests? Second, is it economically attractive, so that a fruitful career can be maintained over a period of 25 or 30 years? Third, is there adequate professional support to allow the physician freedom and discretion in practice? Relationships with colleagues, paramedical personnel, local officials, and patients all evolve into a community life-style, which has a distinct personality. Each of these groups should be assessed in determining the desirability of a community and future practice site.

Most physicians will probably practice in the same locale for an entire career or at least for a large number of years. Physicians should review and rank items important to their lifestyle and that of their family. For example, in considering location, seek communities that provide educational, cultural, and recreational opportunities for both present and future family needs and (if necessary) proximity to relatives and close friends. Other personal issues which may rank highly include the availability and proximity of places of worship, professional entertainment, housing, spectator sports, local politics, shopping centers, and employment opportunities for spouse and children.

Physicians will be influenced by the economic conditions of the community in which they practice. Financial security will depend on such factors as industrial growth and mix, property costs, utilities and services, mortgage interest rates, per capita income, costs of medical and office supplies, state and local taxes, population growth rates, and financial status for other professional groups.

Communities should be desirable from several vantage points. Another important dimension is the professional support. Evaluation of the professional community might consider the availability, quality, and quantity of paraprofessionals for office personnel and hospital staff; practice coverage and subspecialty consultants; allied medical support and laboratory facilities; social services agencies; hospital and extended-care institutions; emergency and acute-care resources; and legal, financial, managerial, and governmental resources.

Geographics

Before beginning on-site evaluations, determine preferences for geographical region and com-

munity size. A New England town may be considerably different from a community outside a midwestern metropolis. Professional and social status, ethnic groups, nature of nearby large cities, and the rural and urban features of the locale, will affect the geographical selection process.

Some advantages of rural communities include a generally lower cost of living, less traffic, high visibility within the community, accessible outdoor activities, stable and secure population, and access to larger parcels of real estate. Disadvantages of rural living may be isolation from personal and professional activities; limited educational facilities; longer distance from cultural, entertainment, and sports centers; lack of privacy; pressure to conform to local mores; fewer choices for shopping; and lower income potential. Whether these advantages and disadvantages are significant will depend upon physician, spouse, and family preferences.

Advantages of urban communities could include access to public transportation; moderate to high income potential; quality schools, with choices of either public or private systems; availability of advanced training and education; proximity to cultural, entertainment, and sports centers; more privacy; adequate shopping and service organizations. Disadvantages may be a longer period of acclimation; higher cost of living; less stable population; congested population; deterioration of inner city; and proximity to crime and delinquency.

Selection Process

Before your traveling begins, gather information on several communities and then select a few which appear highly desirable and therefore worth the time and expense of personal visits. The narrowing-down process could occur through correspondence from communities and potential practices, word-of-mouth references, or geographic preferences. When scheduling visits, both physician and spouse should prepare and forward agendas to pertinent individuals. They should visit together and make separate assessments, comparing notes following the visit. Figure 3.1 provides a checklist to use in selecting a community.

Figure 3.1 Selecting a Community For Practice Checklist

I. Discussion Topics

Medical Climate	Check If Accomplished	Comments

Medical Climate

1. Availability of partnerships or groups to join
2. Medical care needs of area
3. Hospital and health care resources and facilities
4. Hospital privileges and obligations
5. Medical staff organization: similar specialty and other specialties
6. Accessibility to medical school or residency programs
7. Professional relations in health care and related fields
8. Medical education programs locally and regionally

Practice Assessment

1. Demand for medical care
2. Compatibility with partner(s) — professional and personal
3. Income potential
4. Office organization: charts, billing and bookkeeping, appointments, clerical routines, third–party involvement, personnel and supervision
5. Opportunities for personal practice
6. Time utilization: office hours, night call, off–time, community agencies, and hospital committees
7. Facilities and equipment
8. Patient mix: inpatient, extended care, medicare, medicaid, welfare, age/sex
9. Professional and personal interests and obligations of partners
10. Opportunities for continuing education and/or teaching
11. Social service, welfare, and community resources

Financial

1. Compensation: salary and/or yearly income, fringe benefits, vacation and sick leave, education leave, insurance
2. Corporate structure and/or contract
3. Incentives or compensation variables
4. Pension plans and annuities
5. Seniority and privileges of rank
6. Ownership of property and assets
7. Liabilities: debts, mortgages, leases
8. Licensure requirements
9. Availability of personal financial resources: loans, mortgages, lines of credit

Personal and Family

1. Advancement of spouses' career
2. Quality of education for children
3. Religious, social, and recreational features
4. Preference for rural, suburban, or urban living conditions
5. Geographic area and proximity to family and friends

Figure 3.1 *(Continued)*

II. Information Gathering

	Check If Accomplished	Comments

Medical Climate

1. Prospective partners (individually and as a group) _____
2. Hospital administrator _____
3. Medical staff/executive committee _____
4. Attend meetings in hospital and prospective practice _____
5. County medical society _____
6. Residency programs _____
7. Read Hospital By-Laws and reports of meetings _____
8. Obtain copies of licensure documents _____

Practice

1. Attend regularly scheduled meetings — office staff and _____
   medical staff
2. Interview supervisor/manager, personally _____
3. Interview lawyer and/or accountant of the practice _____
4. Observe office during normal workday: patient flow, _____
   paper flow, and telephone routines
5. Work alongside a prospective partner for a complete day _____
6. Observe or take night call _____
7. Review *all* records, reports, and correspondence available: _____
   practice statistics, financial, medical records, patient
   communication
8. Review minutes of meetings for previous year _____

Financial

1. Meet with Bankers and Real Estate people _____
2. Review all benefits and compensation policies _____
3. Personal interview with partners and lawyers regarding _____
   contract and employment stipulations
4. Review *all* financial matters with an outside authority _____

Personal

1. Educational Institution (observe and interview) _____
2. Religious and social organizations (meet with leaders and _____
   members)
3. Visit places of interest (with and without guides) _____
4. Seek out opinions and views from "nonmedical" sources _____
5. Attend community gatherings _____
6. Obtain newspapers from previous months _____

Additional Observations and Comments

_____

_____

_____

_____

_____

Figure 3.2 Community Hospital Evaluation Form

Survey Questionnaire

TO BE COMPLETED BY
HOSPITAL ADMINISTRATOR

I. *HOSPITAL FACILITIES AND PROGRAMS*

   A. What type of governing body controls the hospital? _____

   Do physician(s) serve on this governing body?   Yes _____   No _____

   B. Personnel and services provided by hospital:

	Fulltime	*Parttime* (explain)	*Not Available*
Pharmacist	_____	_____	_____
Pathologist	_____	_____	_____
Radiologist	_____	_____	_____
Physical Therapist	_____	_____	_____
Inhalation Therapist	_____	_____	_____
Hearing Therapist	_____	_____	_____
Radiology Tech	_____	_____	_____
Dietitian	_____	_____	_____
Social Worker	_____	_____	_____
Librarian	_____	_____	_____

   C. Emergency Room Coverage:

   Staffed: Fulltime _____   Explain _____

   Parttime _____   _____

   Approximate number of ER visits a year _____

   D. Laboratory Facilities:

   1. Hours _____   3. Lung scan?   Yes ____ No ____

   2. Arterial blood gases? Yes ____ No ____   4. Pulmonary function? Yes ____ No ____

   5. Other _____

   E. Tissue Committee Reports of Normal Tissue:

   1. 0 – 5%   2. 6 – 10%   3. 11 – 15%   4. 16 – 20%

   F. Staff Physician to Bed Ratio:

   1. at least 1:4   2. 1:5 to 1:10   3. 1:11 to 1:20   4. 1:21 to 1:30   5. over 1:31

   G. Continuing Education for Physicians:

	Yes	No		Yes	No
1. Audiovisual tapes	_____	_____	4. Monthly conferences	_____	_____
2. Visiting professors	_____	_____	5. Weekly conferences	_____	_____
3. Medical students	_____	_____	6. Approved residencies	_____	_____
			Specify _____		

Figure 3.2 *(Continued)*

H. Autopsy Rate:

1. less than 10%   3. 21 – 30%   5. 51 – 75%
2. 11 – 20%   4. 31 – 50%   6. over 76%

I. Hospital Death Rate:

1. less than 5%   3. 11 – 15%   5. over 20%
2. 6 – 10%   4. 16 – 20%

J. Average Length of Stay:

1. under 5 days   2. 6 – 10 days   3. 11 – 20 days   4. over 20 days

K. Percentage Occupancy (excluding maternity):

1. under 50%   2. 51 – 60%   3. 61 – 70%   4. 71 – 80%   5. 81 – 90%   6. over 90%

L. Is there a nursing school affiliated with hospital?   Yes _____ No _____
    Do nursing students rotate through hospital?   Yes _____ No _____

M. Percentage of hospital air conditioned? _____

N. Hospital renovations in past 3–5 years _____
    _____

II. *PHYSICIAN POPULATION*

A. Specialties Represented:

	Total No.	Board Certified	Board Eligible
1. Obstetrics and Gynecology	_____	_____	_____
2. Pediatrics	_____	_____	_____
3. ENT	_____	_____	_____
4. Ophthalmology	_____	_____	_____
5. Urology	_____	_____	_____
6. Family Practice	_____	_____	_____
7. Internal Medicine	_____	_____	_____
8. General Surgery	_____	_____	_____
9. Dermatology	_____	_____	_____
10. Other _____	_____	_____	_____

B. Age Distribution:

1. 26 – 35 #____ 2. 36 – 45 #____ 3. 46 – 55 #____ 4. 56 – 65 #____ 5. over 65 #____

C. Number of new family physicians needed to meet present needs? _____

D. Number of doctors of osteopathy? _____

E. Number of physicians starting practice in past five years? _____

Figure 3.2 *(Continued)*

III. *COMMUNITY RESOURCES AND FEATURES*

A. Agencies Available:

	Yes	*No*
1. Mental health hospital	___	___
2. Speech and hearing center	___	___
3. Visiting nurse	___	___
4. Family services	___	___
5. Child guidance	___	___
6. Other_____	___	___

B. Number of pharmacists: 1. less than 5   2. 6–10   3. 11–20   4. over 20

C. Number of law enforcement officials? _____ Number of firemen? _____

D. Is there a college or university or branch in community? Yes _____ No _____

E. Is there a "medical" management consultant firm available? Yes _____ No _____

Communities that appear as likely choices should be visited at least twice, allowing ample time to meet with prospective partners or colleagues, hospital administrators and medical staff, bankers and realtors, community and school officials, and others such as religious leaders, agency directors in mental health and social service fields, and local politicians.

HOSPITAL

An important consideration in selecting a location for practice is the community hospital. Office practitioners will be involved with the hospital in a variety of ways. Practice success may not rely totally on the hospital, but this medical institution will have considerable impact on local health care and the physician's practice style. If practitioners plan to obtain admitting privileges and participate in medical staff activities, then assessing the local hospitals is imperative in deciding on a community's desirability. (See Figure 3.2.)

Meetings with administrators and medical staff could be arranged during the site visits. Topics for discussion include: the governing body, the hospital charter, policies and guidelines, size of staff and support services, teaching affiliations, medical committees, physical plant and plans for modification, occupancy, cost containment, and emergency and acute-care facilities. Information could also be obtained regarding continuing medical education programs, subspecialties represented, laboratory capabilities and costs, social service functions and staff, and recruiting programs for physician and paramedical personnel. These data can be used to compare community hospitals. Some medical standards which could be used in assessing quality inpatient care are listed in Figure 3.3.

Physicians who admit and treat patients in the hospital will apply for privileges commensurate with their training, experience, and demonstrated abilities. Incoming physicians should obtain official policies and applications from the hospital and each clinical department for which admissions will be desired. The following two subsections summarize a presentation to a National Conference of Residents and Interns by George Wolff, M.D., vice president of the American Academy of Family Physicians and chair of their Committee on Hospital Privileges.

Accreditation and Departmentalization

Hospitals may be either accredited by the Joint Commission on Accreditation of Hospitals

Gross Death Rate: The ratio of total deaths to total discharges. The average for general hospitals is 3%.

Net Death Rate: Number of deaths 48 hours or more after admission. This figure should not exceed 2.5%

Anesthesia Death Rate: Should not exceed 1 death in 5000 anesthetics.

Postoperative Death Rate: Deaths within 10 days after an operation, and due to it should be less than 1%.

Maternal Death Rate: Number of maternal deaths compared to number of obstetrical discharges. This should not exceed 0.25%.

Infant Death Rate: This should not exceed 2% of all births and the majority of the deaths should involve premature infants (under 2500 Grams).

Autopsy Rate: A minimum of 20% of deaths should be followed by autopsy. 25% of all deaths must be autopsied for the AMA to approve internship and residency programs in a hospital.

Consultation Rate: 15-20% Consultations should be held in the following cases: critically ill patient, when doubt exists about diagnosis and/or therapy, when complications arise, when major surgery is performed, cases of multiple pregnancy or other difficulties in delivery, psychoses, coronary occlusion, cerebravascular accidents, etc.

Complications: Complications should not arise in more than 2–4% of all cases treated.

Infection Rate: This should not exceed 1–2% of the patients. There should be precautions taken to control infections by controlling patients, visitors, personnel, procedures.

Average Length of Stay: The average length of patient stay in nonfederal, short-term general hospitals is 6–10 days.

Percentage Occupancy: (excluding maternity) Flexibility and adequate patient separation will be hindered if the occupancy is more than 80–85%.

Tissue Examination: Existence of a tissue committee and a policy of examination of all tissue removed in surgical procedures. The normal tissue removed, including hernia sacs and circumcision, usually should not exceed 10% of all operations.

Medical Audit: Existence of a medical audit committee which reviews records comparing diagnosis, treatment, and outcome and recording the results of its deliberations.

Staffing: Appropriate staffing is about 1 physician for every four beds, with at least the following: a qualified surgeon available at all times, qualified radiologic technician, registered pharmacist, qualified pathologist and anesthesiologist.

Figure 3.3 Hospital Medical Care Standards

(JCAH) or nonaccredited. Accredited hospitals must comply with published guidelines for screening medical staff applications. Nonaccredited hospitals must at best have a constitution and bylaws in which hospital privileges are assigned.

Hospitals may establish two types of structures to govern medical staff: nondepartmentalized and departmentalized. A *nondepartment* structure refers to a hospital in which the medical staff as a whole acts to carry out the medical affairs of the hospital, including approval or disapproval of privileges, bylaws, and constitution. This structure might be found in smaller hospitals or privately managed institutions. Even though a less bureaucratic system there may have certain advantages, a nondepartmentalized hospital may also be rigidly controlled by a few individuals. A newer physician may have minimal decision-making responsibilities in such an organization. A hospital which is *de-*

partmentalized will divide its medical staff into various departments by medical specialty and subspecialty, depending on the number of the physicians in the respective specialty. Thus, the approval or disapproval of an individual's privileges and the governance of medical affairs is decentralized and delegated to departments and their chairs.

Application and Provisional Procedure

Regardless of accreditation status, a new physician should request a copy of the hospital's constitution, bylaws, and policies regarding medical staff organization. If a department has been established in the physician's specialty, this would clearly be the place to make initial contact and application. However, all departments for which admissions and privileges are considered should be contacted personally, through meetings with departmental chairs, and then through a formal application.

The JCAH recommends that initial appointments to the medical staff be provisional for a period to be designated by the medical staff bylaws. This provisional period should be equal for all new medical staff personnel. Each newly appointed medical staff member will be assigned to a department or service where performance and clinical competence shall be observed by the chair, chief, or a designee. If at the end of the provisional time the physician has not satisfied requirements for staff eligibility, provisional status may be terminated, and written notice of entitlement to procedural rights will be specified.

Full privileges are based on a physician's demonstrated current competence, on all verified information available in the applicant's or staff member's credential file, and on the recognition that specialty board certification of eligibility, as defined by the appropriate board, is a benchmark to serve as the basis for privilege delineation. The JCAH states that privileges should relate to an individual's documented experience and to the results of treatment. Granting of privileges requires continuing experience to ensure proficiency and safety. Clinical privileges are hospital specific and are not necessarily the same among hospitals, even in a similar locale.

Physicians in residency training are strongly encouraged to document their training experience by maintaining detailed information on admissions, work-ups, diagnosis, and other clinical procedures which will indicate their competency and enable them to obtain privileges.

GROUP PRACTICES

Group practices are becoming the most attractive form of medical practice. When several physicians and paramedical staff members work as a team, they offer increased health services and can establish a system of support and cooperation. Physicians interested in group practice should know its advantages and disadvantages for both patients and the medical staff.

Group practices may be classified as single-specialty or multispecialty. Single-specialty groups tend to be small, primary-care-oriented practices, usually with three to four physicians. Physicians may start solo or in partnership and then expand their physician staff. Multispecialty groups provide a wide spectrum of medical care and tend to be much larger in size, averaging seven to ten physicians. Dermatologists, general surgeons, internists, and neurologists tend to practice with multispecialty groups.

Some groups contract with patients, either directly or indirectly, to provide medical care not on a fee-for-service basis but rather on a "prepayment" basis. Although many prepaid groups are sponsored by a third party, some of the larger groups are independent. The prepayment mechanism is based on the idea that illness is predictable for a larger population and therefore can be budgeted for. Discussions of prepayment plans are included in Chapter 1 and in a later section of this chapter.

Advantages and Disadvantages

When a physician becomes a part of an organization, he or she relinquishes a measure of autonomy. Proponents of group practice emphasize several benefits to the patient as well as the advantages for physicians; however, some flaws in the group setting affect both physician and patients.

Advantages for patients include the availability of various specialists and/or technical services in one location, better assurance of emergency services and 24-hour coverage, accumulation of patient's complete medical history in one file, and access to trained administrative and medical personnel. Disadvantages for patients using a group practice may include dilution of the patient-doctor relationship, higher probability that one or more of the other physicians may not be acceptable, and the possibility that personal or emotional needs may not be dealt with sufficiently.

Advantages which accrue to physicians in group practice include regular work schedules, both in the office and hospital; the opportunity to leave one's practice for such purposes as professional meetings, continuing education, and vacation with confidence that patients will be seen; access to extensive facilities and qualified assistants; professional stimulus from

group relationships; minimum initial cash outlays and more immediate financial security and
fringe benefits; and the opportunity to devote
time to research and administrative functions.
Disadvantages which physicians should be prepared for if they choose group practice include
slow acceptance by some of the physicians or
office personnel; adherence to established policies and procedures, with little opportunity to
make changes; sharing with all group members
the errors of associated or staff members; and
the potential for disagreements over distribution of income, expenditures, investments, personnel management, and some aspects of patient care.

Negotiations With a Medical Practice

During negotiations with a medical practice, a
physician should follow a systematic process
that includes formal correspondence, curriculum vitae (see Figure 3.4), working visits, and
contract negotiations. The correspondence
phase can include telephone and written communications to determine the general acceptability of the position being offered. If candidates wish to be seriously considered, they
should send a curriculum vitae. As the practice
opportunity is further explored, one or two
working visits should be scheduled. The working visit could include the following:

Working directly with physicians and staff
Meetings with administrative and clinical super-
    visors
Meetings with accountants, hospital officials,
    and other key outside sources
Visits to community agencies and major referral
    sources
Review of practice financial statements, medi-
    cal records, practice policies, personnel job
    descriptions, and other pertinent documents
Review of appointment and coverage schedules
Attendance at practice meetings, and hospital
    meetings
Attendance at a meeting with all physicians of
    the practice
Tour of hospital and other health care facilities

The working visit could also include meetings
with one or more of the physicians to begin the
negotiation process. At this stage the back-

Name
Address/Phone
Social Security Number
Medical Specialty and Licensure
Board Status
Education: College; Medical School; Residen-
    cy(s); Fellowship
Professional Experience and Achievements:
    Clinical Practice; Publications; Research; Pre-
    sentations; Awards; etc.
References

Figure 3.4 Curriculum Vitae

ground and qualifications of the candidate have
been reviewed, and the prospective employee
has decided upon his or her personal and professional goals.

As the negotiation process continues, the
discussion should focus more on the compatibility of the practice with the current and future
needs of the prospective employee, and from
the practice's perspective how the new physician will fit into the organization. Discussion
topics for these continuing meetings could include future plans for practice expansion; financial viability of the practice; competitive environment and how the practice plans to respond;
opportunities for the new physician to build a
practice, especially if the new physician wishes
to pursue a unique area of interest; possible
changes in the facility, equipment, personnel,
and office procedures; and long-term plans of
the other physicians, such as retirement, teaching, research, or other professional pursuits.

If the preliminary meetings are positive and
both parties agree that negotiations should continue, then a written contract should be prepared. Depending on the practice's experience
in recruiting physicians, contract revisions
should be anticipated. Figure 3.5 presents the
key stipulations that need to be included in an
employment contract.

After the compatibility issues are resolved,
the discussion will naturally turn to the question
of the prospective's salary. The "going rates"
are quite variable, depending on specialty,
board certification, location and size of practice, and the financial obligations of partners.
All prospectives should conduct surveys of recent graduates in their respective specialty to
ascertain *current market value*.

Whether joining a small group practice or a larger health care organization, the following list of features should be considered in an employment contract.

Length of term
Compensation—Salary and Fringe Benefits
Malpractice and Disability Insurance
Productivity Incentives
Financial Investment (short and long term)
Expense/Overhead Sharing
Vacation and Sick Leave
Disability Provisions
Professional Liability of Partners
Practice Management Authority and Responsibilities
Hospital Affiliations
Third Party and Industrial Contracts
Conflicts of Interest
Other Sources of Income
Buy-In Arrangements
Liquidation and Termination Clauses
Working Hours, Coverage Responsibilities, and Other Time Commitments
Insurance Policies: Health, Life and Dental
Continuing Education Leave
Pension Plan and Deferred Income

Figure 3.5 Employment Contract Stipulations

There is much more to compensation than salary. A complete compensation package should include hospital and medical society dues, major medical and disability income insurance premiums, pension and profit sharing, and life insurance and malpractice liability coverage. Vacation and off-walk time are compensation factors. Time should be allowed to prepare for boards, to attend medical conventions, to teach and precept, and to fulfill other professional obligations and interests. Malpractice insurance policies for prospectives also represent a compensation benefit. While not traditionally thought of as compensation, malpractice premiums are often paid by the practice. The most advantageous clause would be that the group will pay the prospective's malpractice coverage, regardless of premium cost.

Cautions

Be aware of *purchase obligations*. It is more advisable to have a purchase *option* for accounts receivable, facilities, and equipment. The real worth to the prospective should be carefully studied. A financial advisor should be consulted to assist in determining a fair value, discounting inflated costs, and providing a statement of collectable receivables.

Another important provision that is often omitted from the employment contract relates to the prolonged sickness or disability of the established physician(s). Physicians should be on their guard against exploitative practices that employ junior partners for a few years and then limit financial and professional growth, resulting in turnover of younger physicians. It is possible to research the turnover rates for a practice or community to determine how receptive the medical staff is to the integration of younger physicians.

The essential point in negotiating an employment contract involves the *long-term* affiliation. Serious questions should be directed toward status three years later, potential for partnership, participation in ownership of facilities, and pension plans. Long-term contracts, as an employee on a fixed-income basis, should be avoided. There is no reason for a prospective employee to accept a five-year contract. In most specialties, an equity position in the practice should commence in the second or third year.

Closely related to the discussion of a prospective's equity interest in the practice is the problem of the established physician's possible *disability*. This is a particularly acute problem in a smaller practice. The best advice for a prospective partner is to develop a contractual agreement regarding a possible case of death or disability. A long-term purchase agreement can be based on an escalating price for the practice, with such a price increasing periodically as the younger partner develops a closer relationship with the practice and its resources. Thus, if the original owner becomes disabled or dies, the practice value is determined and a new purchase agreement can be worked out within a reasonable time.

Other Potential Problems

A few other miscellaneous problems may arise during contract negotiations. These problems essentially relate to contract law, but they may take on added significance in the context of a medical employment agreement.

Managerial Control Beware of senior partners who offer, say, 50 percent of the practice profits after a few years but insist upon retaining "managerial control." Management of personnel, finances, and patient care policies should be shared among all partners.

Restrictive Covenant Quite often a clause will be written to the effect that if a partner leaves the practice after a period the departing partner agrees not to open a new practice within a reasonable radius (10 to 30 miles). Such a clause is ordinarily enforceable as a matter of law, provided that the clause is reasonable. Any restrictive covenant is potentially dangerous.

Suspension of Senior Partner To protect the newer partners, it is advisable to ask for a provision stating that if a senior partner is suspended from the practice of medicine the newer partner has the right to withdraw from the practice, notwithstanding the terms of the employment agreement.

This section has presented an introductory view of the contractual negotiation process. Actual negotiations and specific mechanics in planning and signing a formal employment contract are more complicated and vary for each situation. It is advisable to retain a lawyer, especially when such topics as tax consequences, leases and mortgages, buy-in arrangements, and other legal and financial clauses are included.

JOINING A HEALTH MAINTENANCE OR PREFERRED-PROVIDER ORGANIZATION

Professional association with HMOs and PPOs will require physicians to enter into a formal contract for their services and compensation. To assist physicians in sorting through the new legal maze of third-party affiliations, the American Academy of Family Physicians has prepared a *Compendium of Information on Considering a Contract*. Another valuable source of legal information for practicing physicians is the Department of Contract Evaluation/Negotiation Services of the California Medical Associa-

tion, 44 Gough Street, San Francisco, California, 94103, 415-863-5522. The following is a summary of some of the contractual issues presented in publications by the above associations as an aid to physicians contemplating a relationship with an HMO or PPO.

Physician Participation Agreement

Contracts with HMOs and PPOs usually take the form of participation agreements. Once signed, such an agreement becomes a legally binding contract for services and a specified compensation plan. Before finalizing the association with a third-party financial organization, physicians should thoroughly research the company and its offer, consult a medical-legal advisor, and discuss the stipulations with colleagues both inside and outside of the practice (see Figure 3.6). A toll-free hot line is available to the California Medical Association for any questions or concerns about a contract or organization. The number is 800-242-2020. The major considerations which should be evaluated by physicians before entering into a health provider contract are as follows.

Scope of Services. A clear definition of the scope of services covered by the contract is necessary to evaluate the level of risk associated with the provider's assumption of the contract.

Scope of Practice. Physicians must carefully evaluate any clauses which seek to define or limit the scope of the physician's services. Such clauses may limit services that physicians are otherwise licensed and qualified to perform and restrict use of health care facilities and referrals of patients to other physicians.

Unit of Payment. The two most common payment systems are fee-for-service and capitation. Under the fee-for-service plan, physicians are paid for the service they provide at the price they choose to charge. Variations of fee-for-service payments are discounted fees, contracted services, and limitations on increases. Capitation obligates the provider to perform services for a fixed premium while assuming the financial risk for all necessary services regard-

Relationship of Parties
Physician-Patient Relationship
   Agreement to accept members
   Transfer of members
Financial Considerations
   Allocations of funds for medical services
   Primary physician capitation—services covered and risk
   Individual referral services fund—services covered, authorization process, stop-loss, incentives and risk for referrals
   Shared risk fund for referral services—services covered and risk
   Hospital services fund—services covered, stop-loss, incentives and risk
   Special financial considerations—review of reimbursement for funds
   Financial review committee—scheduling reviews, basis of financial review, review of deficit
   Retroactive member cancellation
   Offset for liabilities incurred by physician
Physician services to members
   Services provided by primary physician
   Office location
   Sole source of payment
   Medicare enrolled members
   Charges for excluded services
   Approved and optional preferred providers
   Collection of members' copayments
Inspection of services and facilities
Records
   Physician records and procedures
   Reporting requirements to the HMO
Standards of care
   Principles of practice
   High quality cost-effective care
Insurance
   Liability insurance requirements
Solicitation of members
Term and termination
   Automatic renewal and notice required to terminate agreement
   Default on agreement
   Bankruptcy or other insolvency
   Loss of license
   Rights of parties upon termination
Assignment
Amendments
Representation and warranties of physician

Figure 3.6 HMO Physician Agreement and Contract Stipulations

less of cost. Physicians should know the costs of their services and the demand for same by the enrolled population when they agree to a prepayment rate.

Liability. Any clauses dealing with liability, either of the physician or of the third-party organization, should be examined carefully. If the contract requires the physician to indemnify the carrier against liability, known as a "hold harmless clause," most professional liability insurance policies do not provide coverage for contractually assumed liability. The physician might, therefore, be held personally liable for any damages against the insurer.

Cost of Services. When negotiating a price for services under a contract, each provider should compute the total cost of doing business as accurately as possible. Historical and health care trend data will sharpen the financial estimates and may prevent a loss of income to the provider.

Contract Review

Regardless what organization is considered, the following questions will be important in evaluating the contract:

What obligations would be imposed upon the contracting provider?

Must the provider abide by unspecified "medical policies"? Ask for all policies and requirements affecting the providers to be in writing.

How will malpractice coverage be affected?

Are limitations on hospitalizations and referrals realistic?

What other ancillary health services are prearranged?

What are the termination provisions and what are the obligations after termination?

What are the requirements for prior authorization?

How are disputes handled?

What obligations does the provider have to patients seen by other physicians?

Must all patients assigned or referred be accepted?

A more detailed list of questions to review prior to signing an HMO or PPO contract is presented in Figure 3.7.

1. Are all the parties to the contract clearly identified by name?
2. Does the contract contain any blank spaces?
3. Under what circumstances can the physician terminate the contract?
4. How much advance notice is required for the physician to terminate the contract?
5. Does the contract attempt to incorporate by reference into the contract documents which the physician has not seen or reviewed?
6. Does the contract require that the physician hold harmless and indemnify the business entity and/or any intermediary from any liability arising from the physician's rendering of professional services?
7. Is the contract an exclusive contract, prohibiting the physician from contracting with competing business entities?
8. Does the contract restrict the physician's traditional referral patterns by requiring that referrals be made only to contracting physicians and to contracting institutional providers?
9. Is the physician familiar with the referral resources available under the contract?
10. Does the contract require that the physician maintain a specified dollar amount of professional liability insurance?
11. Does the contract contain an open-ended utilization review clause requiring the physician to follow unspecified review policies?
12. Does the contract allow for the contract to be unilaterally amended by the business entity without the agreement or assent of the physician?
13. Do all provisions in the contract relating to medical records comport with state law?
14. Does the contract require that a physician participate in peer review activities for the business entity?
15. Does peer review immunity granted to physicians under state law extend to physicians who perform review for a business entity rather than a medical society or hospital staff?
16. If a contract specifies that review functions will be performed by non-physicians, does the contract describe the professional qualifications required to be a review coordinator?
17. Does the contract require that each physician member of a partnership or a professional corporation execute the agreement?
18. Has the contract been reviewed by the physician's professional liability insurance company to determine whether the contract affects the physician's existing insurance coverage?
19. Does a contractual requirement that the physician submit to arbitration any contractual dispute and/or professional liability dispute affect the physician's existing professional liability insurance coverage?
20. To what extent does a contractual agreement to arbitrate disputes preclude the physician from pursuing a course of action through the courts?
21. Does the contract automatically roll over from year to year without the physician indicating a willingness to continue the contractual relationship?
22. What impact does the termination of the contract have upon the physician/patient relationship?
23. Does the contract require that the physician keep proprietary information confidential?
24. Does the contract contain any contractual restrictions upon the physician's ability to practice medicine consistent with prevailing standards of care?
25. Does the contract make vague reference to "practice cost effective medical and surgical care" and/or "innovative cost containment techniques"?
26. Has a representative of the business entity made any oral or written representation concerning the physician's contractual relationship which is not embodied in the written contract?
27. Does the contract require that the physician notify patients of the physician's decision to terminate the contractual relationship?
28. If the contract contains a grievance procedure, does the contract fully explain all the steps and requirements of such a grievance procedure?

29. If the contract provides for a grievance committee, are members of the grievance committee appointed or elected?
30. Does the contract require the physician to pay application fees or annual dues?
31. Does the contract limit referrals to "contract" laboratory and/or x-ray facilities?
32. Does the contract limit the physician's independent and professional judgment regarding the involvement of an assistant surgeon, anesthesiologist, etc.?
33. Does the contract limit the time for the submission of claims?
34. Does the contract provide for payment of claims to the physician within a specified time limit?
35. Does the contract provide for a penalty if payment to the physician is delayed?
36. Does the contract specifically provide that the agreement will be governed by the law of another state?
37. Does the contract provide some readily available method of identifying patients under the contractual relationship?
38. Does the contract require that the physician call and verify patient identification prior to each consultation?
39. Is the business entity bound by its verification of eligibility of a contract patient?
40. Does the contract clearly define and specify non-covered services?
41. Does the contract provide that the patient is liable for payment of non-covered services?
42. Does the contract allow the physician's name to be used on brochures, other advertising, radio and/or T.V.?
43. Has the physician reviewed carefully any and all documents referenced in the contract?
44. Does the contract require written and/or other prior authorization before the commencement of specified procedures?
45. Does the contract list the specific procedures which require prior authorization?
46. Does the contract provide for the physician to receive prior authorization in a timely and reasonable manner?
47. Does the contract require the physician to modify existing office procedures and/or billing systems?
48. Does the contract require that the physician's status as a "contract" physician is conditioned upon the physician maintaining medical staff privileges at one or more contracting hospitals?
49. Does the contract obligate the physician to provide any services after the contract is terminated?
50. Does the contract allow for the fee schedule to be unilaterally changed without prior notice to the physician and/or without the prior assent of the physician?
51. Does the contract limit the number of patients the physician may (or must) serve over the course of a year?
52. Does the contract require the physician to be available on a 24-hour basis?
53. Does the contract require that a "contract" physician arrange for another "contract" physician to cover during absences and vacations?
54. Does the contract refer to unspecified medical policies?
55. Does any party to the contract have the right to unilaterally change medical policies?
56. Does the contract provide an opportunity to examine the experience and qualifications of "contract" referral physicians?
57. Does the contract require the physician to accept all patients referred under the contractual relationship?
58. Does the contract limit the right of a physician to contract with any other third party?
59. Does the contract permit termination if the contractor becomes insolvent?
60. Does the contract place cost concerns ahead quality concerns?
61. Is the contract an arrangement of potentially competing physicians who have joined to fix prices, divide markets or boycott others?
62. Does the contract specifically exclude from coverage services rendered by any recognized specialty?
63. Does the contract provide for a "gatekeeper" approach to the delivery of health care?

Figure 3.7 Questions to Ask About a Contract (From REVISED Physician's Contracting Handbook, January 1985. Reprinted by permission from the California Medical Association).

RURAL PRACTICE

Over one fourth of the nation's population reside in parts of the United States designated rural. They live in every region—Northeast, Appalachia, coastal lowlands, hill country of the south plains, and mountains to the west. Many of these rural inhabitants lack essential goods and services generally acknowledged to contribute to "quality of life." One of the most crucial of these essentials is access to health care.

Recruiting Physicians to Rural Communities

A publication by the Department of Health, Education and Welfare entitled *Finding a Doctor for Your Community* (DHEW No HSA 77-6005), reported on a number of factors which affect a physician's selection of a rural setting.

Some factors work *against* the rural community: Health care has become more specialized, and rural communities often cannot support several physicians with different specialties; support services and institutions—hospitals, laboratories, etc.,—are not readily available in many rural settings; physicians often feel the rural situation affords fewer opportunities for continuing medical education; many physicians often find it more convenient to accept a partner in an ongoing practice rather than manage their own; and an increasing percentage of physicians have grown up in urban environments and have become accustomed to them.

Factors which *favor* and appear to encourage the growth of rural practices include: the development of the family practice specialty, which is producing more physicians geared to small rural practice; numerous incentive programs and fundings for physicians and communities in areas short of health workers; use of physician extenders and other supporting personnel, which allows physicians to serve a larger population; accessibility to backup services and continuing education to remote areas; and the increasing desire of physicians and their families to live in rural settings.

Even though more physicians are becoming available for rural practices, it remains a challenge for any particular community to capitalize on this potential. Steps which a community can take to attract physicians are outlined in Figure 3.8.

Rural Practice Project

The Robert Wood Johnson Foundation funded the Rural Practice Project in 1975. The project focuses upon problems in rural areas of the country where communities are too small to support an assortment of specialists but large enough to support a group practice of at least three primary care physicians. The fundamental features which this program offered to rural communities included:

* Delivery of primary health care for the general population of a definable rural community regardless of age, sex, ethnic, or economic factors
* Program of services reflecting concern for broader preventive health needs of the community
* Initial team staffing for medical care of two or three physicians in addition to intermediate-level associates such as physician's assistants and nurse practitioners
* A qualified, nonphysician administrator to share leadership responsibilities with the physicians and meet the management and program planning needs
* Continuous critical self-examination through use of an efficient management information system and regular self-assessment of the quality of care provided
* Extensive involvement of the community in the practice program to improve awareness of community health issues
* Establishment of linkages to hospitals and other specialized medical care services for diagnostic backup, referral of patients, and continuing education of the professional staff

The Rural Practice Project's strategy is based on the importance of leadership, identifying individuals with talent, commitment, energy, and ideas. These factors will help in establishing community-oriented medical practices which can stand as innovative national models. The project fostered the principle that rural communities can provide a challenging opportunity for physicians, administrators, and other health personnel.

The project has completed its developmen-

I. Organize Community-wide
Form a community group
Determine Types of Services Needed—Physicians, Dentists, etc.
Survey Health Organizations
Identify Sources of Patients, Support Services and Income

II. Schedule And Visit
Plan for Physician, Spouse, and Family
Arrange for Visits to Hospitals, Health-related agencies, Schools, Public Service, Business Firms, and other special interests
Incorporate personal and social aspects
Provide assistance in real estate, loans and mortgages, legal and financial counseling, spouse employment

III. Questions Most Frequently Asked By Prospective Physicians
Local Medical Situation
Why is there a need for a new practice?
What is current health status of the area?
How do physicians in area work together?
Practice
What geographic area will practice serve?
Where will office be located?
What resources are available—office personnel, medical equipment or furnishings, social services, etc?
Where is nearest hospital? Mental health center? Extended care facility? Emergency transportation? Consultation and referral?

What opportunities exist for continuing medical education?
How will practice be publicized?
Community
What is socioeconomic status of the area?
What are the housing, school, churches, shopping conditions?
What social activities, recreation, entertainment and leisure opportunities are available?

IV. Post-Visit
Establish a follow-up and evaluation procedure
Appraise desirability of the physician
Plan for return visit
Develop a negotiations package—contracts, agreements, compensation, benefits, incentives, subsidies, etc.

V. When The Physician Accepts
Continue frequent contacts and acclimate physician and family
Participate in practice planning and development
Assist in recruitment of office personnel, facility design, purchase of equipment and supplies, hospital privileges, and building patient volume.
Advise physician on community health planning
Remain available for periodic support—selecting personnel, recruiting a partner, patient advisory groups, etc.

BE PREPARED FOR "POST-HONEYMOON" PERIOD

Figure 3.8 Community Recruitment Effort

tal stage, and there are 13 rural practice sites serving the following communities: Paoli, Indiana; Hindman, Kentucky; Leeland, Michigan; Isle, Minnesota; St. Ignatius, Montana; Bakersville, North Carolina: Jackson, North Carolina; Reedsport, Oregon; Pacolet, South Carolina; Toole, Utah; Plainfield, Vermont; Surry, Virginia; and Scarbro, West Virginia. These communities are now enjoying high-quality health care provided by physicians and other health professionals who have made long-term commitments to these respective underserved areas.

Office of Rural Health Services

The state of North Carolina has established one of the few state agencies to meet new physi-

cians' needs and the medical care needs of rural populations. The Office of Rural Health Services (ORHS) provides support services to more than 100 North Carolina communities who desire increased health care facilities and practitioners. The technical staff and community developers also offer assistance to prospective practitioners by providing information about specific communities which match physicians' interests. The office's objective is to help with the development of new or existing practices in rural communities by assisting with recruitment as well as the establishment of the practice and necessary support systems.

The ORHS staff also coordinate their activities and consultative resources with the four medical schools and nine area health education centers throughout North Carolina. Thus, the new practices and health providers will be ensured ample referral services and continuing education during all stages of practice development.

The staff of the ORHS provide a variety of expertise in the following areas: community development, health center development, facility design and planning, management and office systems, and financial planning. Even though it has been operating only a few years, the ORHS has successfully altered many of the underserved areas of the state by providing new facilities, nurse practitioners, and physician assistant sites and by recruiting more than 100 new physicians to rural North Carolina. A close affiliation is also maintained with the National Health Service Corps and several other federal and private funding sources as a further aid to communities and physicians in their health care planning and development.

Interested physicians, community leaders, or health care planners may wish to contact the Office of Rural Health Services, PO Box 12200, Raleigh, North Carolina, 27605.

NATIONAL HEALTH SERVICE CORPS

The National Health Service Corps was established in 1972 by amendments to the Emergency Health Personnel Act of 1970 to provide care to people living in designated shortage areas. Providing health care through recruitment and placement of health teams is the immediate objective of the corps. Helping communities to build their own health resources and to develop systems that attract and keep health professionals is the longer-range objective. By 1980, over 1000 physicians will be located in rural and urban sites across the United States.

Applicants for the NHSC must meet medical, citizenship, and professional entrance requirements. Entrance may occur through scholarships and by volunteering. When a physician decides on a community, the corps pays up to $500 travel expenses and sends the prospective physician for a site visit, for one to five days. A regional recruiter follows up the site visit with phone calls to the physician and the community board. If both say yes, a match is made.

An NHSC assignee will hold an appointment either in the commissioned Corps of the US Public Health Service or the Federal Civil Service.

Persons Eligible. Physicians must be eligible for licensure in the state which is chosen for assignment. Dentists have a similar licensure policy. The NHSC recruits nurse practitioners locally and gives preference to local nurses for training in the field. Physician assistants must have completed an AMA-approved assistant-to-the-primary-care-physician program. Nutritionists, dental hygenists, social workers, and other paramedical and paraprofessionals may also be recruited.

Criticism. EVen in its earliest stages, the NHSC has been subject to criticism. Nearly $500 million in federal funds have been expended (1972–1977), and to date the retention rate for doctors remaining in shortage areas is lower than expected. In addition, communities have not become totally committed because of the transient nature of the physician, especially those who are merely serving out a two-year obligation because of the medical school scholarship. Even though the impact of the NHSC program has not been completely felt and may be difficult to evaluate, it does attempt to address the health care needs of the underserved.

Regional Offices. Requests for information should be addressed to NHSC Regional Program Consultant, DHEW Region (I–X) at the appropriate regional office listed in Table 3.1.

National Information Program on Rural Health Center Development

The Health Services Research Center of the University of North Carolina and Office of Rural Health Services of North Carolina's Department of Human Resources compiled a series of practical guidebooks designed to provide rural community leaders, government officials, health care providers, and professional technical assistance personnel with the information they need to (1) determine whether a new health-practitioner-staffed primary health center is an appropriate, feasible alternative, and, if

Table 3.1 National Health Service Corps Regional Offices

Address and Phone Number	Region	States Served
John Fitzgerald Kennedy Federal Bldg Boston, Mass 02203 (617) 223-6647	I	Maine, Vermont, New Hampshire, Connecticut, Massachusetts, Rhode Island
26 Federal Plaza New York, NY 10007 (212) 264-2547	II	New York, New Jersey, Puerto Rico, Virgin Islands
PO Box 13716 Philadelphia, Penn 19101 (215) 596-6686	III	Pennsylvania, Maryland, Delaware, Virginia, West Virginia, Washington, D.C.
50 Seventh St, NE Atlanta, Ga 30323 (404) 526-3877	IV	Kentucky, Tennessee, North Carolina, South Carolina, Mississippi, Alabama, Georgia, Florida
300 South Wacker Ave Chicago, Ill 60606 (312) 353-4613	V	Wisconsin, Michigan, Illinois, Indiana, Ohio, Minnesota
1200 Main Tower Bldg, Rm 1740 Dallas, Tex 75202 (214) 729-3031	VI	Texas, Louisiana, New Mexico, Arkansas, Oklahoma
601 East 12th St Kansas City, Mo 64106 (816) 374-2916	VII	Iowa, Nebraska, Missouri, Kansas
11037 Federal Bldg Denver, Colo 80202 (303) 837-2483	VIII	Montana, North Dakota, South Dakota, Wyoming, Utah, Colorado
50 United Nations Plaza, Rm 301 San Francisco, Calif 94102 (415) 556-8671	IX	California, Nevada, Arizona, Hawaii, Guam, Trust Territories
Arcada Plaza 1321 Second Ave Seattle, Wash 98101 (206) 442-7240	X	Washington, Idaho, Oregon, Alaska

so, (2) implement that alternative to the maximum benefit of the community. The subsections of the guidebook include such topics as overview on medical care in rural America; business and management; facility development; legal problems of rural health clinics; role relationships and clinical aspects of care in a rural clinic; and medical record and index systems for community medical practice.

The Health Services Research Center of the University of North Carolina at Chapel Hill and The Office of Rural Health Services, Department of Human Resources, State of North Carolina, Raleigh, North Carolina have spearheaded an innovative and challenging endeavor and are available to assist other educators, planners, practitioners, and developers in similar efforts. The need of the rural United States and other underserved communities is great, and the resolve will require a high level of expertise and dedication.

TIMETABLE FOR BEGINNING PRACTICE

Preparations for medical practice cannot begin too soon. The initial phase of one's career deserves advanced planning. A reasonable timetable should be developed which will allow for adequate information gathering and careful analysis of alternatives before commitments are given (see Figure 3.9).

The following paragraphs describe a sequence of events beginning approximately 18 months before entrance into practice. This sequence was adapted from actual accounts of physicians' practice preparation.

Eighteen Months Prior to Practice

During initial practice planning, keep in mind personal goals, family needs, and geographical

```
┌─────────────────────────────────────────────┐
│               12 to 18 Months                │
│  Select Practice Location                    │
│  Determine Starting Date (allow for delays)  │
│  Apply for Hospital Privileges               │
│  Determine Facility Requirements (build,     │
│     lease, renovate)                         │
│  Prepare a Capital Budget (building and      │
│     equipment)                               │
│  Consult Financial Advisors                  │
│  Contact Financial Institutions              │
│                                              │
│                9 to 12 Months                │
│  Select Practice Site                        │
│  Finalize Financial Arrangements for Capital │
│     Needs                                    │
│  Work with Architect and Builder (if         │
│     appropriate)                             │
│  Shop for Equipment and Furnishings          │
│  List Practice in the Phone book             │
│  Arrange Meetings with Hospital Officials,   │
│     Local Physicians, Third-Party            │
│     Organizations, Local Medical Society     │
│  Contact Pharmaceutical Companies and        │
│     Medical Equipment Companies (they may    │
│     provide start-up assistance for new      │
│     physicians)                              │
│                                              │
│                6 to 9 Months                 │
│  Order equipment and furnishings             │
│  Negotiate leases                            │
│  Select or Design Medical Records            │
│  Select Computer System for Financial and    │
│     Clinical System                          │
│  Prepare Annual Overhead Budget              │
│  Negotiate Line-of-Credit to Cover First     │
│     Six Months Expenses                      │
│  Obtain Licenses                             │
│  Join Local, State, and National Associations│
│  Purchase Practice Insurance Policies        │
│                                              │
│                3 to 6 Months                 │
│  Develop Personnel Policies                  │
│  Develop Office Procedures Manual            │
│  Begin Personnel Recruitment                 │
│  Select Telephone System                     │
│  Establish Financial Policies and Fee        │
│     Schedule                                 │
│  Design Practice Information Documents        │
│  Consult with Financial and Legal Advisors   │
│  Contact Local Industries and Other          │
│     Institutions for Possible Contracts      │
│                                              │
│                Last 3 Months                 │
│  Hire Office Staff                           │
│  Conduct Staff Training                      │
│  Set-up Supply Inventory System              │
│  Set-up Appointment and Coverage System      │
│  Begin Scheduling Patients                   │
│  Distribute Practice Promotion Materials     │
│  Obtain Prescription Forms, Referral Lists,  │
│     Business Cards                           │
└─────────────────────────────────────────────┘
```

Figure 3.9 Entering into Practice Timetable and Checklist

preferences. In addition, future practitioners should be formulating their own views on the philosophy of practicing medicine and what is a desirable life-style as a novice physician. Before cross-country trips are made, take ample time for conversation with spouse, family, and advisors, discussing options in these and related topics, Specific issues for consideration at this stage include practice type—sole, partnership, group, or prepaid association; location—rural, suburban, or urban; size of practice and number of partners; and personal practice preferences.

Initial visits should be preceded by information requests to potential sites such as communities which are actively seeking physicians and have formalized their recruiting effort. Also, this is an appropriate time to gather factual data from local and state organizations and seek consultation from advisors. Letters and questionnaires provide information within a relatively short period and may assist in the ranking and prioritizing of potential practice opportunities.

Whatever method selected, community contacts and visitations should commence at an informal level with both personal and professional interests on the itinerary. As a community and practice becomes more desirable, then begin formal meetings with prospective partners, colleagues, administrators, and community officials.

The suitability of a community may also be determined by availability and cost of medical office space and used or reasonably priced equipment and by the availability of families and patients who could be attracted in the initial months. In addition, hospitals may be offering subsidies or guarantees for the first year of practice, which will allay large financial commitments.

At this point in the site selection process, it may be important to narrow the decision to a specific region or state and practice type. This will allow time for more thorough evaluation of potential opportunities and for appropriately communicating positive and negative responses to communities following recruiting visits.

Twelve Months Prior to Practice

Within the last 12 months, the choices should be narrowed to the top three or four. This will enable physician, spouse, and family to spend time in each location assessing housing, schooling, community life, and other personal features. It is important to allow spouse *and* family to participate in the selection process before committing to a practice or community. This is also a key time to evaluate the medical climate of a potential practice and the community in general. Locum tenums or preceptorships could facilitate this learning process. There will be no better way to determine future practice conditions than to work in the setting for a brief period. Both office practice and hospital should be included in this experience.

If a working arrangement is not feasible, then at least one or two days should be spent investigating office setting, including records, work routines, personnel, financial productivity, practice demographics, and hospital and community relationships. This perspective will also provide an occasion to use the last months of residency as a final preparation of medical knowledge and skills that relate to the needs of the community and practice you plan to serve. There may also be time now to develop office systems and records to incorporate into the practice. If you are to start a new practice, you must begin the process of office design and layout, as well as planning space, equipment, and supplies during these 12 months. A community that is actively recruiting should provide considerable support and assistance in these developmental efforts.

Six Months Prior to Practice

Decision time is now! Planning and evaluation must now culminate in the decision—where and with whom to practice? This will be the time for licensure requests, contract negotiation, agreements, applications for admitting privileges, purchasing a home, and obtaining a mortgage. The more time allowed, the higher probability of acceptable results. If a new practice is to be established or an existing one modified, then equipment and medical supply companies will need to be contacted and orders placed. Advanced purchasing may secure price reductions and discounts.

Decisions may also have to be made about professional incorporation, billing systems, of-

fice organization, and personnel, all of which will require discussion with business and legal specialists. Therefore, relationships will need to be established with lawyers, bankers, realtors, future colleagues, partners, office personnel, and community resources. A certified public accountant and lawyer may be valuable consultants as practice decisions are being finalized.

Three Months Prior to Practice

During the last few months a checklist of "things to do" should be prepared. This could include membership in local, state, and national societies; contacts with IRS, Medicare, welfare, and third-party payers; personal and professional insurance policies; salary and fringe benefit negotiations; personal and professional budget for first year's expenses; establishment of bank accounts, with separate checking account for professional use; contacts with moving companies; and closing out of affairs in current location.

If a new practice is to be established, then the list would also include selecting office personnel, taking out appropriate employer's insurance, designing financial and patient flow systems; contacting printing companies, medical and office suppliers, and pharmaceutical firms; and making arrangements with local utilities, especially the telephone company.

Whether joining an established practice or beginning new, now is the time to initiate patient recruiting. Referral sources should be contacted personally. These include local medical societies, emergency rooms, colleagues who have closed their practices, and community agencies. A telephone number could be obtained to take names of prospective families and patients. If an established practice is in existence, then it may be possible to spend a few days seeing patients and beginning to develop a personal practice.

One Month Prior to Practice

If adequate time and effort have been allowed in the preceding months, then the final month can be set aside for incidentals and personal needs. Changing residences, employment, and geography can be traumatic, especially if strong roots have been established. Therefore, a transition phenomenon must be anticipated and allowed to occur. To cushion the shock of uprooting, all family members should attempt to stay together as much as possible to share and help each other work through the sadness of leaving one location and the anxiousness of moving to a new one.

Final preparations at the new location could include interviews by local newspapers, advertisements, patient appointments for the first four to six weeks, hiring at least one employee to start a few weeks before opening the office, and checking with vendors and suppliers. Personal visits to medical and community resources as well as financial and governmental institutions would be advised for a new practitioner. Files could be prepared of these organizations describing key individuals to contact and the policies which will affect medical office practices.

If possible, at least a few weeks should be allowed between residency and beginning full-time office practice. This will provide needed time for transition into new surroundings. There will be many demands upon time, and whenever possible all family members should be available to assist each other in the acclimation phase.

Final Preparation Checklist

The following is a list of necessities which should be obtained within several weeks of opening or joining a medical practice.

Physician
- State license
- Federal tax number
- Blue Cross and Blue Shield provider code
- Malpractice insurance
- Disability and loss-of-business insurance
- Attorney and/or tax consultant
- Business checking account
- Personal and business telephone numbers
- Announcement and business cards
- Line of credit from local bank

Office Practice
- Fire, theft, and liability insurance
- Linen and housekeeping service
- Independent laboratory service
- Telephone system and answering service
- Stationery and other business forms
- Magazines for reception area
- Schedule of fees and charges
- Rubber stamps with signature, name, and address of practice
- Appointment book and return visit cards
- Duplicating machine

PRACTICE FACILITY DEVELOPMENT*

The marketability of medical care involves several features, one of which is the facility where patients, physicians, and staff interface in the health care triad. An adequate medical facility contains office space and design so that each component of the health triad will meet its respective needs.

Facility development may involve either construction of a new building or the renovation of an existing office. Essential elements in facility development include planning, budgeting, financing, architecture, design, and construction.

Planning

A timetable for medical facility development would begin with the initial planning discussions and span all events until occupancy. A realistic start-to-finish time frame would be a minimum of six months to as long as one to two years. Timetables may be developed by consulting with colleagues who have designed similar facilities, commercial spatial designers, and medical building specialists. Planning should commence with physicians discussing their preferences, needs, anxieties, and apprehensions. Other people who may contribute to early plans are spouses, colleagues inside and outside medicine, office personnel, and medical management consultants.

---

* Information in this section was obtained from David Johnston, *Primary Care Centers, Design and Construction,* 1977.

If physicians are in group practice or are planning to join together in a new building, then delegation of various aspects of the planning should be considered. These could include selection of an architect, mortgage financing, office design layouts, and visits to similar facilities. An adequate planning phase could take several months. This will allow time to formulate ideas, gather and analyze relevant information, and present plans to other physicians. Group meetings should be scheduled at least weekly to keep everyone informed and to stimulate each person to prepare a progress report on activities.

Budgeting

During construction planning it is imperative to prepare a cost analysis. This may determine the ultimate feasibility of a new or renovated facility and will have an impact on subsequent plans and decisions. Factors which affect cost are land values; interest rates; building design; construction approach; local, state, and federal standards; and other issues such as provisions for expansion, ecological and environmental interests, and multifaceted applications.

Figure 3.10 is a sample budget for a new medical practice facility. The 5,000 sq ft facility could be suitable for a three- to five-physician group practice. A checklist for controlling costs would include the following items:

1. Hire an architectural consultant or seek advice from an experienced building designer so that the facility makes the best use of the lot or available space, preferably in medical office practices.
2. Establish a reasonable budget before starting design, and require the designer to stay within budget.
3. Review applicable building codes and state and federal construction standards. Ensure that requirements are met but that the building is not designed to a higher standard than necessary.

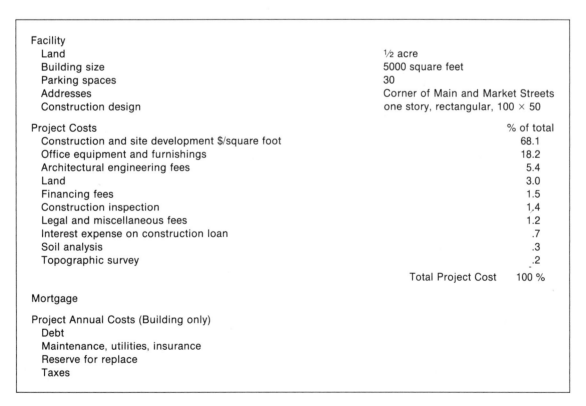

Facility	
Land	½ acre
Building size	5000 square feet
Parking spaces	30
Addresses	Corner of Main and Market Streets
Construction design	one story, rectangular, 100 × 50

Project Costs	% of total
Construction and site development $/square foot	68.1
Office equipment and furnishings	18.2
Architectural engineering fees	5.4
Land	3.0
Financing fees	1.5
Construction inspection	1.4
Legal and miscellaneous fees	1.2
Interest expense on construction loan	.7
Soil analysis	.3
Topographic survey	.2
Total Project Cost	100 %

Mortgage

Project Annual Costs (Building only)
Debt
Maintenance, utilities, insurance
Reserve for replace
Taxes

Figure 3.10 Financial Budget Components: Initial Project and Yearly Costs

4. Determine square footage for the facility without sacrificing function and efficiency.
5. Site the building on the property in such a way as to minimize drainage problems and reduce the construction required for roads and parking.
6. Choose building and office systems that have reasonable operating costs and require low or moderate maintenance. Energy conservation should be a high priority.
7. Avoid unusual and expensive materials with difficult shapes and configurations.
8. Avoid unnecessary delay in getting the project under construction, since construction costs are constantly increasing and unexpected delays quite probable.

Financing

Financial planning should be an integral part of all development discussions. Bankers and other financial advisors should be contacted throughout the planning and budget preparation stages. An attorney should be involved throughout financial negotiations. All contracts need to be reviewed with or by a lawyer, as do title abstracts, performance bonds, construction insurance, and building permits that specialize in real estate transactions.

Selecting funding sources and loan negotiations requires time and careful evaluation. Loans may be procured for construction, mortgage, and equipment. Each has distinct stipulations and requires separate contracts. The Small Business Association should be contacted as a possible source of partial or complete funding. In addition, if the practice site is to be located in rural or high-need areas, state or federal monies may be available.

Financial plans could also include a proposed budget for the practice, including physician and paramedic salaries, medical and office expenses, and other costs to sustain the operation. In addition, projections should be made for monthly and yearly revenue from patient care and any other income sources. Revenue projections can be compared to project costs and operational budgets to determine the length of time to retire debts and build equity into the practice.

Financial management will require discussions with tax accountants to plan appropriate measures to minimize the cash outflow and take advantage of all tax-related options.

Architecture

There are several architectural options for medical practices. These vary from the physician designing office layout formats to complete delegation to an architect or medical building design firm. In addition, there is modular construction which is fabricated in a factory, trailers which can be attached and mounted on a foundation, and renovation and modernization of an existing building.

The following is a brief summary of the construction approaches. Several of these should be considered in determining the appropriate alternative for a medical facility.

Design/Competitive Bid Produces a custom building, gives more owner control, and is most flexible. It may take longer to complete at higher cost than other approaches.
Design/Build Produces a custom building, controls cost, and reduces completion time. The contractor assumes more responsibility and has more control which usually means less day-to-day involvement by the owner and few in-progress changes.
Modular Is often less expensive and quicker to build. Design is standardized and almost inflexible, which may result in the acquisition of more space to compensate for inefficiencies in the layout. Cost can increase unexpectedly because of unforeseen problems with site, access, foundations, zoning, and building codes.
Trailer Facilities Quickly constructed and least costly, but they have inefficient functional layouts and have relatively short useful lives. They are most suited for temporary or satellite health facilities.
Renovation Should be considered if an adequate basic structure is available. The cost, time of construction, and functional adequacy depend on the basic structure. A detailed feasibility study is particularly important before initiating a renovation project.

Leasing May be attractive if acceptable space is available without extensive renovation. The lease approach is usually faster and requires less initial investment, but annual operating costs are likely to be higher. Functional design and space requirements frequently must be compromised to utilize the available lease space.

SELECTING AN ARCHITECT OR CONTRACTOR

Planning a facility involves evaluation of sites and funding sources, analysis of building design and construction, and various feasibility studies. Architectural and contracting firms should be selected for their expertise in all these functions, from both planning and development aspects.

Selection of an architect or contractor is an important step in the facility development process. The most qualified firms should be invited to make formal presentations to the decision-making group. Competition between firms should be based upon capabilities, qualifications, experience, cost, and responsiveness. The company which is most preferable should be notified formally by letter, subject to satisfactory negotiations of a contract. The firm should then be requested to submit a written contract proposal. Proposals and presentations will be helpful in deciding upon the construction approach and eventual firm to employ.

Office Design

Design and functional layout of an office practice should incorporate efficient, economic, private, and comfort considerations for physicians, staff, and patients. The design process should integrate practice philosophies, services, and other functional needs. Floor plan layouts are included in the appendices.

Building design is a compromise between limitations imposed by the site, functional requirements of the program, exterior appearance, and budget limitations. In designing a medical practice facility a major concern should be use of staff and resources. Fiscal success may depend on an efficient design for patient flow and office systems.

Reception Area. This area is most visible to patients and will influence many of the initial impressions. Attractive and comfortable seating will be keynote. Receptionist and nursing personnel need direct access to this area. A few standards for size and seating are: 180 square feet per physician; 10 square feet per patient; and a total number of seats for at least a one-hour patient volume. Other factors to consider include: additional seating or play area for children; special considerations for elderly or disabled patients; space for coats, umbrellas, etc.; drinking fountain and pay telephone; proximity to restroom; and music, magazines, and pictures. Figures 3.11 and 3.12 show two examples of good design for the reception area. Receptionists should be in constant eye contact with all people in reception area.

A subreception or screening room is also a consideration, especially if there will be a high incidence of patients with communicable diseases, trauma, or in different degrees of distress.

Business Office. The business activity area is one of the nerve centers for the practice (see Figures 3.13 and 3.14). This area could include

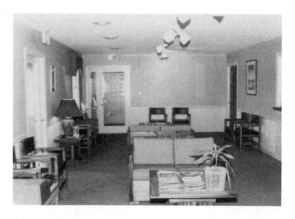

Figure 3.11 Single Seating Is Considered Most Desirable for the Reception Area. (Courtesy of WASHINGTON FAMILY MEDICINE CENTER, Drs. Thomas Speros and Edward Hill, Washington, North Carolina.)

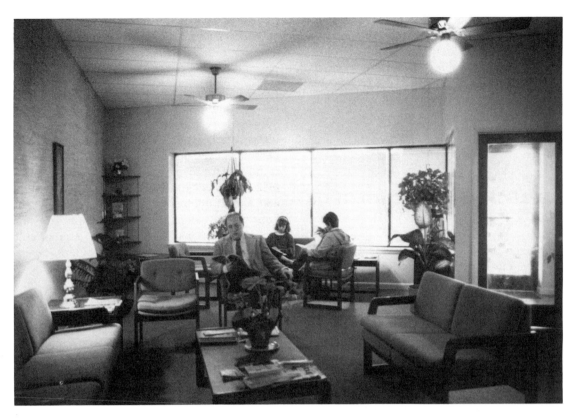

Figure 3.12   The Reception Area Should Have Comfortable Seating and a Pleasant Atmosphere for All Types of Patients. (Courtesy of WASHINGTON FAMILY MEDICINE CENTER, Drs. Thomas Speros and Edward Hill, Washington, North Carolina.)

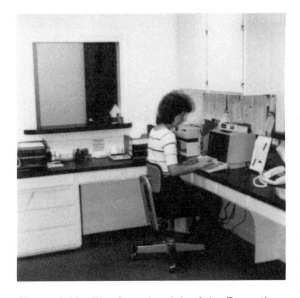

Figure 3.13   The Complex Job of the Reception-ist Deserves a Separate Work Area. (Courtesy of WASHINGTON FAMILY MEDICINE CENTER, Drs. Thomas Speros and Edward Hill, Washington, North Carolina.)

appointment system, collection window, tele-phone, files, and medical records, insurance and business forms, copying machine, and re-lated activities. There may be several people working in this area. A general space standard is 120 square feet for one employee and 80 square feet for each additional person.

Separate windows or areas should be de-signed to greet patients and dismiss them. This will provide privacy to collect payments and reschedule office visits or make appointments with referring physicians.

Medical records and financial files should be in separate rooms or areas where security and safety can be maintained. Filing or shelving which can be locked should be a consideration. Figure 3.14 presents one way to incorporate these features.

Dictating and bookkeeping may also neces-sitate separate rooms or working space. Patient volume and office work schedules may deter-mine the how, where, and when of these func-

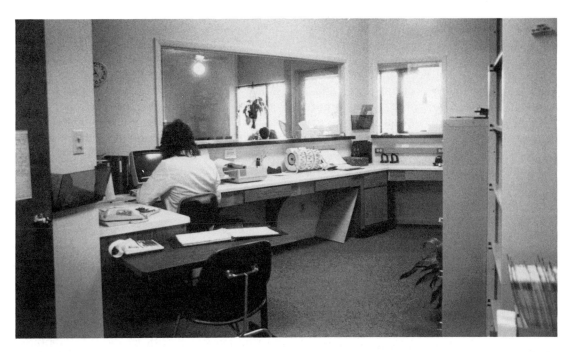

Figure 3.14 Office Personnel Need Adequate Working Space to Perform Their Many Different Tasks. (Courtesy of THE FAMILY DOCTOR, Drs. Glenn and Jerry Withrow, Chapel Hill, North Carolina.)

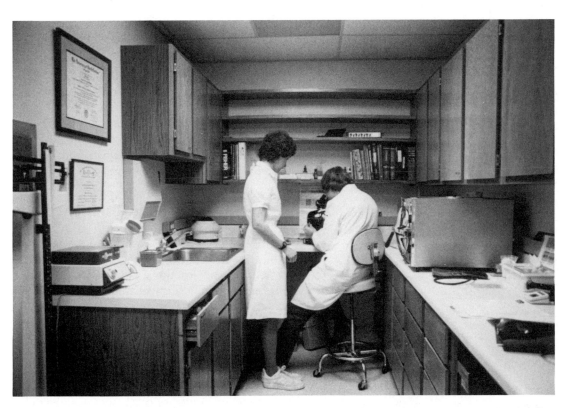

Figure 3.15 Clinical Work Stations Provide Nurses and Physicians a Convenient Location for Conducting Lab Tests and Discussing Results. (Courtesy of THE FAMILY DOCTOR, Drs. Glenn and Jerry Withrow, Chapel Hill, North Carolina.)

tions when individual space for these activities is not available.

Examination Rooms.   An examination room is the physician and nurse working space, and design will depend upon practice preferences, types of patients seen, and procedures to be performed. A typical size would be either 8 × 10 ft or 9 × 11 ft.

Examination rooms could also accommodate ambulatory and wheelchair patients, one or two additional family members, patient education materials, and wall-mounted instruments.

A minimum of two exam rooms should be available to each physician seeing patients. Three rooms may be more desirable especially in primary care or if nurses are participating in pre- and postexamination routines. In a four exam room module, one or two physicians and a nurse could be time efficient and maintain close proximity for communications.

There may also be a need for a consultation/examination room, surgical/treatment room, or a screening/patient education room. Regardless of special purposes, caution should be taken to keep space flexible, so that valuable and costly square footage is fully utilized.

Other factors to consider when designing examination rooms include: partitions for patients to undress and dress; soundproofing; doors opening away from patients; instruments within short distance from physician; space for writing charts or prescriptions; heating and ventilating systems; lighting and bright colors. Each examination room should be self-sufficient so that physician or nurse does not have to leave the patient for routine procedures.

Medical Work Station.   A convenient space should be designed to allow nurses, physicians, and other paramedical staff to complete medical records, dictate, prepare injections and medications, and answer phone messages. This space may be at the end of the corridor or within the confines of the examination rooms. This may also be combined with an in-office laboratory area.

This work station should have extensive counter space, microscope, incubator, sterilization apparatus, and drug samples (see Figure 3.15).

Additional Space.   Depending upon the size of staff and practice type, space may need to be designed for a staff lounge, an x-ray facility (see Figure 3.16), a separate laboratory, additional restrooms, and a supervisor's office (Figures 3.17 and 3.18).

In addition, a separate room for each physician should be considered. This could also be a consultation room for patients and families.

Interior Construction

Physicians need to be aware of and may wish to have some input into several facets of interior building construction. These include interior design, plumbing, mechanical, electrical, and staff-support systems.

Interior Design.   The building should present a dignified appearance and require minimum maintenance. Facilities with fewer than 20,000 square feet should be planned on one floor, unless land is limited or expensive. Ceiling height should generally be 8 ft. Bulk storage should be available, with roughly 50 sq ft per full-time physician. At least one door to each room—34

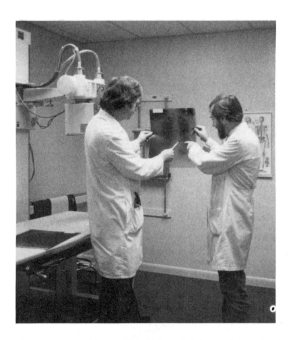

Figure 3.16 X-ray Facilities Add an Important Feature to the Ambulatory Services Offered by Community Practices. (Courtesy of THE FAMILY DOCTOR, Drs. Glenn and Jerry Withrow, Chapel Hill, North Carolina.)

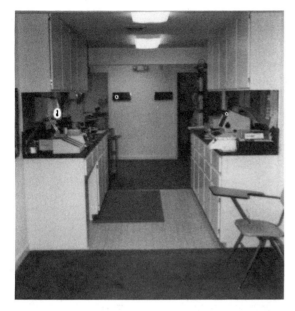

Figure 3.17 Nurse and Laboratory Work Stations Should Be Centrally Located in the Patient Flow System. (Courtesy of WASHINGTON FAMILY MEDICINE CENTER, Drs. Thomas Speros and Edward Hill, Washington, North Carolina.)

in. wide to accommodate wheelchairs. Doors 1.75 in. thick are preferable. Corridors should be at least 5 ft wide.

Vinyl wallcovering and semigloss paint should be used in exam and treatment rooms, toilets, and corridors because they are easy to maintain. Vinyl asbestos tile should be the primary floor covering considering both initial and life-cycle costs. It should be used in exam rooms, treatment rooms, work areas, and storage rooms. Carpet could be used to reduce noise in high-traffic areas such as offices, consultation rooms, lobbies, reception area, and corridors. When carpeting is used it should be a dense low pile commercial type with antistatic properties. Nylon has a longer life and is less expensive than most other fibers.

Plumbing System. Lavatories should be provided in each examining room. They should be equipped with single-lever faucets so that they can be operated without use of hands. A stainless-steel sink should be provided in laboratory and at nurses' work stations. A service sink should be provided in the building for janitorial and cleaning purposes. A plaster trap is usually desirable in one sink to accommodate casting.

The treatment room sink is typically used for this purpose.

Mechanical System. Exhaust fans should be provided in toilets, laboratories, and other areas as required by building codes. A control duct down a corridor with branch ducts to each room is most desirable for reducing sound. Heating, ventilating, and air conditioning should be carefully sized to avoid overdesign, with adjustable controls to regulate temperature in each room and work area. Heat pumps which use outside air are more economical.

Electrical System. Adequate lighting would be one 48-inch, four-tube fluorescent fixture per exam room of 1000 square feet or less. Offices, laboratory, and other work areas should have adequate lighting or be in proximity to windows. Examination rooms should have two three-way switches that control lights, one at the door and the other on the wall closest to the

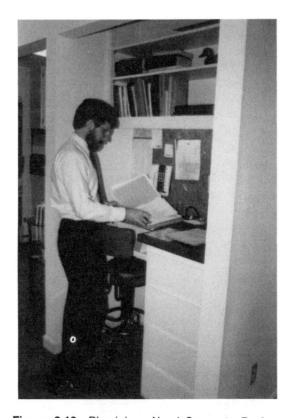

Figure 3.18 Physicians Need Space to Review and Dictate Medical Records. (Courtesy of WASHINGTON FAMILY MEDICINE CENTER, Drs. Thomas Speros and Edward Hill, Washington, North Carolina.)

exam table. Electrical outlets should be provided on each wall and for each 5 ft of counter. Battery-operated emergency lighting should be installed as required.

Staff Support Systems. Support systems in a medical office practice include intercom, dictation, nurse call and room status lights, telephone apparatus, rotating files, and computerized data. The investigation and subsequent design and implementation of these systems should be considered for present and future applications.

Equipment and Supplies

The practice facility will only be as efficient as the equipment and supplies which are used to design and maintain the operations. The exact specifications will vary depending on size, practice type, structural features, physician preferences, and procedures performed. However, regardless of equipment needs, quality and durability should not be compromised. Emphasis should be placed on reputable manufacturers and reliable distributors who will provide quality products and services over the life of the practice.

Local medical and office equipment suppliers should be contacted initially to determine availability and prices. Service after sale will be very important, and a local firm may be more responsive and flexible in negotiating contracts and accepting complaints.

The following is a listing of equipment and furnishings which are suggestions for each location in the practice. This checklist is a guideline which may have to be modified to fit the individual practice.

Examination Room

☐ Blood pressure cuff, wall mounted
☐ Bulletin boards
☐ Cabinets, writing, built-in sink
☐ Exam table
☐ Intercom
☐ Lab coats
☐ Lamp, gooseneck
☐ Mirror
☐ Ophthalmoscope-otoscope, wall-mounted
☐ Peds scales/table
☐ Scales
☐ Side chairs
☐ Soap dispenser
☐ Stool
☐ Towel dispenser
☐ Wast receptacle

Treatment Room

☐ Anoscope
☐ Audiometer
☐ Black light
☐ Cabinets, built-in
☐ Cast cutter
☐ Clothes rack/hooks
☐ Crash cart
☐ Cryo unit
☐ EKG Mark 5 Burdick
☐ Flat-top exam table
☐ Gomco compressor/suction
☐ Instruments
☐ Ishiara's color-blind test book
☐ Intercom
☐ Mayo instrument stands
☐ Modular cabinets
☐ Nail holer, electric
☐ Portable O_2 tanks, mask, carrier
☐ Power table Trend IV
☐ Scrub sink
☐ Side chairs
☐ Sigmoidoscope
☐ Snellen eye chart
☐ Stool
☐ Surgical lamp
☐ Tonometer, Shiotz
☐ Trays:
  ☐ Eye
  ☐ Ear
  ☐ Surgical
☐ Utility carts
☐ Vision tester-Titmus
☐ Waste receptacle
☐ Water Pic

Laboratory

☐ Alcohol lamp
☐ Autoclave
☐ Cabinets, built-in
☐ Centrifuge:
  ☐ Urine
  ☐ Blood
☐ Chairs
☐ Chemicals
☐ Dop tone (minidop)
☐ Eye tone
☐ Fetoscope
☐ Flashlights
☐ Hemogramometer
☐ Incubator
☐ Intercom
☐ Microscope
☐ Punch biopsy
☐ Refrigerator
☐ Sinks
☐ Soap dispensers
☐ Stools: elevated, counter
☐ Tape dispensers
☐ Towel dispensers
☐ Urinometer
☐ X-ray view box

Business Office

☐ Blackboard
☐ Bulletin boards
☐ Calculator, adding machine
☐ Chairs, secretarial
☐ Charts
☐ Clocks
☐ Copy machine
☐ Desk, built-in modular
☐ Dictaphone
☐ Filing cabinets
☐ Lamps
☐ Ledger card holders
☐ Medical dictionary
☐ Medical record file system
☐ Pegboard system
☐ Rolodexes
☐ Safe
☐ Stools with backs
☐ Supplies, office
☐ Telephones
☐ Telephone-answering device
☐ Typewriters
☐ Vertical Files
☐ Waste receptacles

Consultant Room/Physician Office
□ Chairs   □ Desk file, lateral
□ Clock   □ Dictaphone
□ Credenza   □ Lamp
□ Desk   □ Shelves, built-in
□ Desk chair   (bookcase)
                               □ Telephone

Conference Room
□ Audio/video equip-   □ Desk tops, built-in
  ment   □ Intercom
□ Cabinets   □ Shelves, built-in
□ Chairs   □ Table
□ Clock

Nursing Stations
□ Blood pressure cuff   □ Peds table/scale
□ Counter tops   □ Scales
□ Intercom   □ Telephone
□ Measuring tapes

Reception Room
□ Chairs   □ Chairs
□ Lamps   □ Toys
□ Magazines   □ Treasure box
□ Magazine rack   □ Tables
□ Peds area   □ Waste receptacle

Staff Lounge
□ Coat rack/hooks   □ Refrigerator
□ Chairs   □ Shelves, built-in
□ Closet   □ Table
□ Heating plates   □ Telephone
□ Kitchen utensils

Storage Area
□ Fire extinguishers   □ Shovels
□ Janitorial supplies   □ Sink
□ Mops, brooms   □ Soap dishes
□ Shelves   □ Vacuum cleaner

CONCLUSION

Physicians select sites for office practice based on several factors. These include family and personal needs, geographic preferences, community desirability, practice opportunities, professional colleagues, hospital facilities, medical and social service resources, financial security, and capabilities for professional growth.

A selection process should begin early and allow for evaluation of several alternatives. Topics for evaluation include hospital privi-

leges, patient population, commitments and responsibilities within and outside the practice, compensation and benefits, contracts, and continuing education opportunities. Spouses may be assessing housing, educational programs, recreational and leisure activities, and other factors affecting family life and personal career development.

If a new practice is being considered, then more intense planning will be necessary. Construction of a medical office involves land surveys, office-site design, extensive financial arrangements, development of medical and financial systems, recruitment and training of personnel, building a patient population, and initiating relationships with medical and community resources.

The challenge is to select a community and practice that (1) provides continuing motivation with opportunities for professional stimulation and (2) enables the spouse and family to develop and grow as individuals and a unit.

References

Alford T, Barnhill T: Components of faculty development—renovation and new construction. Presentation, Raleigh, NC, 1978.

Brooks EF, Madison DC: Primary care practice: Forms of organization. In *Primary Care and the Practice of Medicine,* Noble J. (ed). Boston, Little, Brown, 1976.

Cooper JK, et al: Rural or urban practice: Factors influencing the location decision of primary care physicians. *Inquiry* 12 (1975):18–25.

Eisele CW (ed): *The Medical Staff in the Modern Hospital.* New York, McGraw-Hill, 1967.

Graves G: The medical group urgent care center. *Medical Group Management* 31, no. 3 (1984):48–53.

Group Practice: Guidelines to Joining or Forming a Medical Group. Chicago, American Medical Association, 1970.

Hillmer H: Buy-in/buy-out: Is your plan in shape? *Medical Group Management* 31, no. 5 (1984):30–37.

Hollowell EE: No insurance—no privileges. *Legal Aspects of Medical Picture* 6, no. 4 (April 1978):17–19.

Johnson D: *Primary Care Centers, Design and*

Construction. Washington, DC, Appalachian Regional Commission, 1977.

Kurtz M: Selecting the right physician for your group. Medical Group Management, 1984; 31(1):24–31.

McGibory J: *Principles of Hospital Administration.* New York, G. P. Putnam and Sons, 1969.

Maugel L: Selecting a community for practice, timetable for beginning practice, financing and designing a practice. Unpublished Report, Family Practice Center of Akron, Ohio, 1977 and 1978.

Meyer L: Emergicenters—opportunity or threat? *Medical Group Management* 30, no. 3 (1983):30–49.

Organization and Management of Family Practice. Kansas City, Mo, American Academy of Family Practice, 1970.

Stewart W: Evaluating locations for medical practice. Course syllabus, Springfield, Il., Southern Illinois University School of Medicine, 1974.

What role for GP's in group practice? *Medical World News,* November 15, 1976, pp 47–48.

Wolff G: Hospital privileges and departments. Presentation to the American Academy of Family Physicians, Kansas City, Mo, October 1977.

4

Financial Management

- What function do budgets play in financial management?
- What types of insurance are necessary to minimize financial risk?
- How can investments solidify a financial portfolio?

- How are financial statements prepared and interpreted?
- What are the ramifications (costs, taxes, legal) of professional incorporation?

Financial management is of critical importance in reaching the personal and professional goals that a physician has established. Financial management involves far more than bookkeeping. It requires planning and decision making which can affect the economic and legal viability of the organization. Since the financial aspects impact directly on the physician's personal finances, the first part of this chapter addresses the personal dimension of finance, such as budgeting, investments, insurance needs, estate planning, and income tax. The second part of the chapter deals with similar topics from an organizational perspective. The last section covers the professional corporation, in terms of its economic and legal advantages, and the conversion of partnerships to professional corporations.

PERSONAL FINANCIAL PLANNING

Budget

The purpose of a budget is to plan for a future period to reconcile income with planned expenses. Personal budgets usually cover a one-year period, although shorter periods can be used during periods of transition, such as moving to a new location or purchasing a home. A budget is more than a planning device used to reconcile income and expenses. It can be used like a compass, to keep one's expenditures in line with the ability to pay them.

Actual expenditures should be recorded and compared with planned expenditures. If actual expenses are greater than planned, then corrective action becomes necessary. It may be important to revise the original budget by reallocating planned expenditures, or it may indicate a modification in purchasing. The budget should include all planned expenses, even highly discretionary ones such as vacations and gifts. Although investments are not expenses in that funds are generally available for actual consumption at a later time, they should be included in the budget as expenses or outflows so that the total income is allocated to the total expenses. Figure 4.1 presents the items which could be included in a personal budget.

Insuring Against Hazards

Individuals face a variety of hazards to themselves and their property. Among these hazards are:

Disability, which might seriously impair earning ability

Loss of life, which obviously terminates income earning

Large medical expenses, which may create substantial obligations

Liability for damages to others

Loss of property because of fire, theft, vandalism, automobile accidents, and other circumstances

Since any of these major types of risk might create a financial obligation too large for an individual to bear but their frequency and severity among a large number of people can be predicted with reasonable accuracy, these risks are insurable. A basic principle of insurance is that a large number of individuals can pool their funds with an insurance company so that the claims which occur can be paid from this pool. In this way, each individual exchanges a known small loss (premium) for protection against a possible large loss. Since various types and sizes of losses have different impacts on various individuals, the purchase of insurance is an individual matter. The following paragraphs discuss several types of *personal* insurance; each should be carefully considered in financial planning.

Life Insurance   Life insurance is one of the more complex issues in developing a personal

Income:
1. Salary
2. Dividends
3. Interest
4. Borrowings
5. Spouse's Salary
6. Moonlighting Income
7. Proceeds from sale of capital assets and/or securities
8. Gifts
   Total

Expenses:
1. Home Mortgage or Rent
2. Car Payments
3. Car Upkeep and Gas
4. Food
5. Clothing
6. Federal, State and local tax
7. Personal property tax
8. House upkeep
9. Furniture and Home Improvements
10. Loan Payments and interest
11. Utilities-gas, electric, water
12. Telephone
13. Banking services-safe deposit box, etc.
14. Personal attorney
15. Personal accountant
16. Medical and Dental out-of-pocket costs*
17. Insurance
    a. Life*
    b. Disability*
    c. Hospitalization*
    d. Major Medical*
    e. Auto
    f. Homeowners
    g. Personal Liability
18. Nonreimbursed Professional Expenses
    a. Books
    b. Dues
    c. Licenses
    d. Entertainment
    e. Travel
19. Recreation, Entertainment, and Vacation
20. Contributions and Gifts
21. Personal Investments
    Total

*Often paid for by the organization

Figure 4.1   A Personal Budget

financial plan. A decision to purchase life insurance should be made only after evaluation of personal and family financial needs and with assistance of a qualified insurance agent. Some of the life insurance needs which should be considered are financial obligations to creditors following the insured's death; financial obligations created by death, such as funeral costs, estate settlement fees, capital gains, and taxes; possible needs related to business associations; and prospective cash and income needs of the insured's family.

Life insurance for other family members might be considered to replace the economic value of a spouse working at home or to guarantee the future insurability of children. All forms of life insurance are variations of the types of policies discussed below.

Term Insurance. A form of life insurance similar in concept to renting a place to live is term insurance. It is often called "pure" insurance or protection, because it provides only one benefit: payment of a certain sum at death during the policy term. The premium for term insurance is a combination of mortality cost (probability of death) and the insurance company's operating costs. Since the probability of death becomes greater as one gets older, term insurance premium rates increase at older ages. Since the cost is increasing substantially, more healthy people begin to discontinue the payment of premiums, leaving the insurance company with a group of less healthy insureds. When this occurs, the mortality statistics used for the original premium calculations become inaccurate, and more deaths occur per thousand than would have been forecast. Because of this problem, most insureds allow their insurance plans to be renewed only to age 65 or 70.

Whole-Life Insurance. Whole-life insurance can be likened to purchasing a home, with the cash value of the policy being compared to the equity in the home. Since this cash value grows free from income taxation, it is an excellent means of savings for a liquid emergency fund. Premiums on the various forms of whole life may be paid on a modified basis, i.e., lower during a initial period and increasing to a level payment thereafter or on a shortened basis where all premiums might be paid within a specified period of time such as 20 years, or to age 65. The insurer sets aside a reserve for each policy so that all claims can be paid in the future. To establish these reserves, the company calculates a level premium (approximately

equal to the average of the term premiums from issue age to age 70) for the policy. Thus in the earlier years, the insured is making a larger payment than is required to cover mortality and operating expenses. This excess creates a reserve, or cash value, in the policy, which has the effect of reducing the company's risk at later times. This cash value accumulates during the term of the policy and is available to the owner of the policy.

Endowment Insurance. This type of insurance is designed to build a cash value equal to the death benefit by a specified age. Thus, an endowment at age 65 with a $10,000 face amount will have a cash value at age 65 equal to $10,000. At this point there is no "insurance" left and the cash value will be paid to the insured. Endowment premiums are higher than those for whole-life or term insurance.

Disability Insurance. In the absence of substantial assets either having been accumulated or inherited, all financial plans depend on one's ability to earn an income. The incidence of disability is substantially greater than the incidence of death at most ages, and disability creates an even greater economic problem, since the disabled person must still be provided for. Disability insurance sufficient to cover business and personal (family) income requirements should be purchased. Individual, noncancellable policies are available. These policies, once insured, cannot be modified by the insurance company. The definition of disability is very important, and the timing of the start of disability payments is flexible. Benefits are almost always limited to a specified percentage of earned income.

Group and Association Insurance. Insurance coverage available through an employer group or a professional society affiliation is group or association insurance. Premiums for such plans are almost always subject to change by the insurance company, and many plans allow cancellation by the insurer. The waiting period before benefits begin and the length of payments following this are frequently determined by the plan or the insurance company rather than the insured. Most association plans have lower premiums at a given starting age than comparable noncancellable policies, with provision for increases as specified ages are reached. Usually, association insurance plans do not restrict benefits based on income. Frequently, a combination of individual noncancellable coverage and association coverage is the best way to provide for disability needs.

Medical Care Insurance. Medical care insurance includes coverage for hospitalization, surgical, medical procedures, physician care, and major medical problems. It is difficult to compare policies due to many combinations of deductibles, coinsurance percentages, exclusions, and limitations. Each health insurance policy must be examined carefully. Physicians may receive professional courtesy from colleagues and thus may not require physician care coverage, but most hospitals do not waive their charges, and hospitalization coverage becomes necessary. Professional courtesy does not always extend to spouse or children, and coverage for family members might only be obtained if the family head also purchases a policy. Often health insurance is provided through a group health plan established for employees of a practice.

In order to keep premium costs realistic in terms of needs, a careful evaluation of medical care insurance needs should be made. Some physicians' professional associations have plans which provide for hospital and nursing expenses without reimbursement for physician's fees (where professional courtesy is frequent). Using deductible provisions and/or coinsurance provisions (where the insured pays part of each claim) helps to keep premiums lower. If an individual can afford to pay a certain level of medical expenses out of pocket, it is wise to establish this level of self-insurance in the medical care plan. See the section on professional incorporation for additional discussion of this topic.

Personal Liability Insurance. Liability for damages to others may arise from use of an automobile, infringements on the rights or property of others by you, your family members, or your pets. Automobile liability insurance is required in nearly all states, but the minimum levels required are usually far below the awards which might be made in an accident involving a physician or his family member. Additional coverage should be sought. Some homeowners insurance policies include coverage for personal liability (see next section).

Homeowners Insurance. An important personal protection policy is homeowners insurance. A house is more than a dwelling. It represents a sizable investment, both for owner and mortgage lender. Insurance against fire and other forms of damage does more than guarantee that repairs can be made to the dwelling. It also protects the investment against major loss, hence many lenders require that the property be adequately insured. Homeowners insurance policies can also provide protection to personal property, both in the home and while you travel, and can provide liability insurance for suits which originate from an injury occurring on one's premises.

Homeowners insurance does not always pay the full cost of any damage. Full coverage of property requires a policy of at least 80% of its value. Due to rapid rise in real estate prices which increases the value of a home, some policies now automatically increase coverage by a percentage that represents inflation in housing prices. However, local factors may cause this to be less than the necessary increment. Homeowners policies need to be examined periodically to determine if coverage is adequate.

Investments

In addition to protection against unpredictable or unforeseen risks, the physician also needs to accumulate assets for other reasons. Some of the considerations for establishing an investment program are the need for savings to be available for emergencies, future financial opportunities, and major purchases; the need to meet major cash requirements, such as college education; the need to provide income for retirement or to transfer capital to other family members.

An investment program will be an important feature in a financial plan. Income should exceed expenses, even at the early stage of a medical career. An investment program should be developed which contains a balance of short-term and long-term holdings with a steady monetary growth. The earlier investments begin, the greater the potential for increased asset value and dividend income. Just as with insurance, there are many pros and cons of investments. A decision to purchase one form of investment over another should be made after careful evaluation and consultation with trusted advisors. An accountant can provide advice on the tax consequences of different forms of investments and assist in determining what types of investments have the best benefits from a tax perspective. An attorney is a valuable resource when investments involve real estate and other forms of long-term holdings. Contracts, financial commitments, and risks should be discussed with an advisor who has nothing to gain by the decision.

Savings Account. An obvious form of investment is the savings account at a commercial bank or savings and loan association. These accounts pay a fixed interest rate, and funds are insured up to $100,000 by an agency of the federal government. There is virtually no minimum balance, and funds can be withdrawn very quickly. In recent years, commercial banks and other investment firms have offered certificate accounts. These pay higher interest than regular savings accounts but require that funds be left in the account for a fixed period (ranging from several months to years) with a minimum balance of $1,000 or more.

Money Market Funds. Money market funds pay a higher yield than do savings accounts and are very liquid. Brokerage firms, banks, and savings and loan associations offer these investments, with insurance up to $100,00. These funds usually require a minimum balance, several hundred dollars, and have some limits to the amounts that can be withdrawn.

Securities. Investing in the stock or securities market is often considered after sufficient liquid reserves have been accumulated. Only a broker can buy and sell financial securities. Brokers are registered and regulated; in addition to providing the services to buy and sell securities, they provide advice and guidance. All transactions involving financial markets involve charges which are usually based on a percentage of the transaction. A commission is paid to the brokerage firm on each transaction, regardless of whether the security is bought or sold.

Common Stock. This is the investment which many people associate with the securities market. Each share of common stock represents ownership of some fraction of the company and so entitles the owner to vote for the board of directors and receive dividends. The owner of stock is not personally liable for any action of the company.

Preferred Stock. Preferred stock is similar to common stock in that it represents a share of ownership, but preferred stockholders have prior claims on assets and dividends of the company over common stockholders. Preferred stock is usually issued at a fixed dividend rate and dividends for the current period must be paid before any payment to common stockholders.

Bonds. Bonds represent indebtedness of a company or government. Each bond carries a fixed interest rate. Prices of bonds fluctuate with changes in interest rates and investors' perceptions of the company's ability to pay the principal at due date. Bonds are secured by physical assets of the company. Debentures are also corporate obligations paying a fixed interest rate and promising to pay a fixed sum at a future date.

Commercial Paper. Commercial paper is another form of corporate obligation. It is similar to debentures in that it is not secured by physical assets, but the denominations of commercial paper are much higher than bonds of debentures, ranging upward from $100,000. The maturity period of commercial paper is much shorter than bonds or debentures.

Mutual Funds. Mutual funds are also known as open-ended investment companies, and they sell and buy shares which represent their own portfolio of securities. When they receive cash for shares they have sold they use it to purchase additional securities. Mutual funds differ in terms of the method by which they pay the manager and advisor of the fund. The difference represents the sales fee. In a no-load fund the price for buying and selling shares are the same. The management costs are charged to the fund and are paid from dividends received by the portfolio's securities. Mutual funds specialize in types of securities, such as tax-free bonds, growth stocks, preferred stocks, and other securities.

Nonsecurities. Several types of nonsecurity investments can be made. The most common of these is real estate. Real estate prices have increased at higher rates than the interest on many investments. Tax provisions on mortgages make real estate an attractive investment. Real estate must be maintained and insured to protect against loss. For substantial real estate investments, syndications or limited partnerships are made up of a number of investors. In the limited partnerships, losses generated through interest deductions and depreciation may be passed through to the individual partners for personal income tax purposes. Another form of investment is the small business. Many small businesses look for financial support, often by incorporating as a closed corporation in which stock is available not to the general public but only to selected investors on a private basis. Investing in small businesses may contain a higher risk because financial return will depend on a decision by a small management group or the success of the company in selling its products or services at a profit. A third form of investment which does not involve financial securities is the franchise. Franchises can be purchased that do not require the owners to be operating managers. Investing in franchises involves the same risk as investing in a small business.

Risk, Return, Liquidity

Investments should be analyzed from three perspectives: risk, return, and liquidity.

Risk. This refers to the possibility that the original investment will not be recoverable in full. Deposits in savings accounts and certificates of deposit are without risk if the balance is kept to less than $100,000. Cash values of life insurance are guaranteed by the companies issuing the policies, which are closely regulated. Bonds issued by the federal government are also considered to be riskless. But almost every other form of investment has some risk. Com-

mon stock is subject to the risk that every business faces. Bonds can vary in their risk, even those that are backed by governments. Real estate is also subject to risk. The housing and land market in an area may collapse, or a fire may cause total damage.

Return. This refers to profit on the investment, which could be expressed in terms of annual percentage increase. Savings accounts have low rates of return, averaging from 5% to 7%. Some stocks offer little or no dividends but increase in market value because of demand by other investors. Many stocks offer yields of 7% or higher. Rate of return is related to risk. The greater the risk, the higher the potential rate of return. An uncertainty which stocks encounter is that each investor has their own estimate of future risk and return. Thus, stock value is susceptible to fluctuations in demand by both small and large investment groups. The tax treatment of the return must also be considered.

Liquidity. Liquidity refers to conversion of investments to cash within a relatively brief period. Liquid investments can be bought or sold in a matter of hours or days, whereas nonliquid investments may take weeks or months to sell. Stocks and securities are relatively liquid, whereas real estate properties and small business are nonliquid. Evaluation of future risk, return, and liquidity are often based upon subjective assessments. Experienced advisors such as accountants, stock brokers, and bankers may offer useful advice about investment decisions.

Estate Planning

Regardless of the composition of a financial portfolio, the existence of personal assets produces an estate that requires planning. Initially, estate planning involves a will. The cost of a will is usually very low, often less than $100 for a basic will. When a person has died without leaving a will, the courts will decide on the allocation and distribution of the estate. Without a will the courts may require the administrator to post expensive bonds. Allocations made by the court may be contrary to expectations that existed before death. A will should be considered a necessity for secure financial planning. A will also allows parents to nominate guardians for their children if both parents die. Trusts, or trust funds, are legal agreements in which assets are retained and managed by a reputable institution, normally a bank, for the benefit of the creator of the trust or a third party. Trusts are frequently set up at death through the will. A will normally distributes assets to the heirs after all claims, fees, and taxes have been paid. A trust can delay and control the distribution of the property for many years after death. In this way funds can be provided at specific times for specific needs of the heirs. Trusts avoid probate, and settlement costs are reduced. Trusts can be constructed so that the tax burden is reduced. In preparing wills and trusts, expert advice should be sought from an attorney and bank trust officer.

PROFESSIONAL FINANCIAL PLANNING

Professional financial management is similar to personal financial management, since both involve budgets, insurance, investments, and taxes. As with personal management, expert advice from an accountant, attorney, and banker are essential for maximizing financial return from professional activities.

Budget

Professional budgets should be developed as a planning instrument which will guide management decisions and assist in evaluating fiscal performance. Budgets should be revised during yearly planning meetings. They will serve as continuing reminders of current plans and programs, and facilitate periodic examination of results. The process of drawing up a budget requires an accounting of expenses and delineation into major and minor categories.

Both income and expenses should be outlined in the budget. In addition, a monthly and year-to-date reporting method should be followed. Figure 4.2 presents a budget for a medical office practice. The categories listed are the essential ones and may vary depending upon size and type of practice.

Income
Professional Services
a. Dr. A
b. Dr. B
c. Dr. C
d. Dr. D
Diagnostic Services
laboratory, radiology, and EKG)
TOTAL

Expenses
Professional Salaries
a. Dr. A
b. Dr. B
c. Dr. C
d. Dr. D
Staff Salaries
Wage Taxation and Insurance
a. Social Security Contribution
b. Unemployment Insurance
c. Workmen's Compensation Insurance
Benefits
a. Hospitalization
b. Major Medical Insurance
c. Disability Insurance
d. Life Insurance
e. Medical and Dental Reimbursement
f. Pension Plan
Facility
a. Mortgage/Rent/Lease
b. Repairs/Maintenance
c. Utilities-gas, electric, water, garage
d. Telephone/Intercom
Supplies
a. Drugs and Medical
b. Clerical
c. Postage
d. Laundry/Uniforms
e. Laboratory Expense
Administrative
a. Billing Expense
b. Attorney
c. Accountant
d. Banking Services
e. Dues/Subscriptions/Library/Licenses
f. Meetings/Conventions/Entertainment
g. Automobile Expense
Insurance
a. Premise Liability
b. Building
c. Equipment, Furniture, and Fixtures
d. Business Interruption
e. Malpractice
f. Umprella
Interest Expense
Business Taxes
Capital Asset Purchase
Dividends

Figure 4.2 A Professional Budget

Insurance

A major practice expense is insurance. There are at least ten professional insurance needs. Whether any or all are purchased will depend upon scope of the practice and physicians' assumption of risk as office practitioners. The greater the risk one is willing to assume, the less insurance that is required.

Workers' Compensation Insurance. Required by most states, this insurance covers medical payments for employees injured or sustaining an illness while working.

Building Insurance. This protects the physical facility against damage due to fire or other natural causes. When a facility is financed by a mortgage, such insurance is required by the lender.

Equipment, Furniture, and Fixtures Insurance. This protects the contents of the facility against damage, theft, and burglary. When equipment or furniture are leased the lender will again require that such insurance be obtained.

Premises Liability Insurance. This insurance protects the physician against property damage and personal injury, including death, which results from ownership, maintenance, or use of the premises. This insurance does not cover liability due to professional activities but involves liability for accidents happening on the professional premises that are not part of the professional services (such as someone falling on the steps or slipping on the sidewalk).

Business Interruption Insurance. This protects the professional practice against temporary loss of income because of damages to the building or its contents.

Partnership Insurance. Partnership insurance is life insurance taken out on each practice member by the other practice members. The insurance is used to pay a lump sum amount to the beneficiaries to purchase that partner's share of the practice, in terms of their interest in the facility and its contents. The insurance may also be set up to pay an income continuation for a period of one to five years. This income con-

tinuation payment represents the partners' investment in goodwill in the practice and uncollected fees. By having the partnership pay the premiums and being the beneficiary of the insurance, it is assured that the funds will be available to purchase each share.

Since the Tax Reform Act of 1976, the purchase and sale of a partnership interest will be subject to capital gains treatment to the estate of the decedent, if the purchase price is greater than the decedent's tax basis (original purchase price minus depreciation) in the property being transferred. Because of this, many professional partnerships are reevaluating their buy and sell provisions to allow for the purchase and sale only of the physical assets in the partnership. The decedent's share of accounts receivable at the time of death may be paid in installments monthly or annually, as those receivables are collected. This will have a tendency to spread the taxable income over a number of years to the estate and/or heirs, rather than lumping a large payment into one taxable year.

In many cases, it is felt that there is not a substantial amount of goodwill which will benefit surviving partners, so that the buy/sell agreement makes no provision for large amounts of goodwill.

Disability Insurance. Disability insurance has been discussed in the section on personal financial planning. In a multidoctor practice, however, it is imperative that provision be made in the partnership agreement describing what income would be paid by the partnership to a disabled partner. Frequently, a full pro-rata share might be paid for a period of, say, 90 days, followed by a reduced draw or share for up to one or two years following the onset of disability. In the absence of such a provision, a partner who is totally disabled might still be able to legally demand a proportionate distributive share of partnership income. For these reasons, it is necessary that individual disability insurance be coordinated among the partners.

Professional Overhead Expenses. Since a physician has only one income but two sets of expenses, i.e., personal and professional, it is necessary to also have disability coverage for professional overhead expenses. Depending on the makeup of the group practice, a physician might become disabled but still have to meet lease payments on office and equipment, payroll costs, utilities, and so forth. Generally, business overhead expense insurance provides payments for up to one to two years as a reimbursement for overhead expenses actually incurred during a period of disability. Since this need is usually shorter than personal disability insurance, its purchase will not usually reduce the amount of personal disability coverage which may be available.

Professional Liability (Malpractice) Insurance. Malpractice insurance rates have become a major issue in recent years. Within a few years, rates have doubled or tripled. Several insurers stopped operating in many states, and public attention was focused on this difficult aspect of medical insurance as a result. While the medical malpractice crisis appears to be resolved, the problem still remains. Malpractice insurance is very expensive due to the high jury awards (high out-of-court settlements are often agreed to) and the varied interpretation by juries of what constitutes malpractice.

Malpractice insurance is an agreement in which the insurer will pay on behalf of the physician all sums which the physician becomes legally obligated to pay. Damages may be awarded in a suit because of injury arising out of the rendering of, or the failure to render, professional services by the physician or any person for whose acts or omissions the physician is legally responsible. When a physician is practicing in a group setting or in a hospital, the institution is also subject to malpractice suit, and the group practice or hospital must also have malpractice insurance. This extends to partnerships. In a two-physician group each must have their own policy and the partnership must also have coverage.

Malpractice insurance rates vary with geographic region and scope of the physician's work. Physicians who do not perform obstetrical procedures, surgery, or ordinarily assist in surgical procedures pay lower rates, while certain surgical specialists, such as neurosurgeons and plastic surgeons, pay the highest rates. Malpractice coverage usually extends to only the first $600,000 or $1,000,000 in claims. For extra coverage, umbrella insurance is necessary.

Umbrella Insurance. Umbrella insurance protects the physician against catastrophic and potentially ruinous claims. Umbrella coverage can be obtained in amounts ranging from $1,000,000 to $5,000,000. The insurance covers any liability that exceeds the other insurance in force. To obtain umbrella insurance, the physician must carry, at certain levels, basic professional liability, premises liability, and personal automobile and homeowner liability coverages. The umbrella insurance covers all losses after the underlying insurance is exhausted. As with any form of insurance, individual umbrella policies differ in their deductibles and exclusions.

As can be seen, the number of different insurance policies necessary for sound financial management is great. Five types of coverage should be considered for personal needs—life, disability, medical care, liability, and property, with additional life and health policies for spouse and children. Ten coverages may be needed for professional practice, with additional professional liability policies needed if the practice setting involves a group arrangement. Structuring an insurance portfolio requires professional consultation from insurance brokers, attorneys, and accountants. There are specialized consulting firms that combine all of these professions and develop for the physician or partnership a comprehensive plan that covers both individual personal and professional needs, as well as covering the insurance needs of the group.

Since the cost of these programs will be extensive, physicians should evaluate different insurance agents and brokers and obtain bids to compare costs. Since several insurance policies will be purchased, physicians should take advantage of the competitive nature of the insurance industry.

Investments

Professional investments have similarities to personal investments, but there are considerations which limit the extent to which monies can be invested in risky or speculative assets. Unlike one's personal investments, professional investments are assets generated from work and retained in the practice to finance further growth. These investments may include equipment, services, renovations, new building, or additional personnel. For this reason, excess revenues should be invested in secure and liquid securities or in tangible assets which have a high potential for financial return. This tends to eliminate real estate from consideration, unless the real estate is going to be used as a site for a professional facility. It also tends to eliminate long-term (four to six years' maturity) savings certificates. The result is that professional investments that are not facilities or equipment tend to be relatively short-term low-risk securities, such as savings accounts; large denomination, short-term certificates; very secure bonds with a large market; or possibly preferred stocks.

When an investment is being considered in a practice facility or in equipment, the practice has alternatives. Practice funds may be invested into the projects, or outside assistance from a lending or leasing institution may be sought. When a facility is being constructed, it is often advisable to obtain a mortgage from a bank for part of the facility cost. Such borrowing does not deplete practice funds and allows for a larger facility to be built than may have been constructed otherwise. While a mortgage may carry large interest payments, these become a cost of operating the practice.

When equipment is being considered, it is possible to have a lease/purchase arrangement with the manufacturer and a financial institution. It is also possible to purchase the equipment and then collateralize the equipment, borrowing funds from a local institution. An accountant and lawyer will be valuable resources for these transactions.

Pensions, Annuities, and Keogh Plans

One of the most difficult items of financial planning for physicians is the selection, design, and funding of an appropriate retirement plan. Perhaps part of this is the psychological attitude of physicians who think they might never be forced to actually retire. In addition, there is the problem of having denied oneself many luxuries during a long period of training, and the immediate desire is to make up for lost time with heavy spending. Once the young physician begins to enjoy all income in luxury expenditures, it is difficult then to make the sacrifice to set aside money for a later time.

Since 1962, when the original Keogh Act was passed by Congress, many advances and improvements in pension legislation have been made. Most of these improve the benefits available to the professional who wants to establish a retirement plan for the physician and employees. The plans are not without restrictions, however, as benefits available to the doctor must also be available to employees, who also depend on the physician for their livelihood.

Individual retirement annuity or an individual retirement account (IRA) is available to anyone. Individuals can also set up other qualified retirement plans with annual contributions up to $2,000 ($2,250 for a spouse-IRA).

A *Keogh Plan* is available to unincorporated self-employed people. A money-purchase Keogh Plan allows the self-employed individual to deposit the lesser of 15% of earned income or $30,000 each year. The annual deposit is deductible from earned income, and contribution reduces taxable income. These funds may be invested with an insurance company, bank, trust company, stock broker. Some latitude in investment decisions may be given to the account holder.

Interest earnings and capital gains in the account are not taxable until money is withdrawn from the plan. Since the basic purpose of the plan is for retirement funding, there are penalties for withdrawal of funds prior to age 59.5. Plan assets distributed in a lump sum at retirement receive benefit of a special ten-year forward-averaging rule, while installment payments are taxed as ordinary income in the year received. Death benefits paid in a lump sum receive the ten-year forward averaging for income tax purposes and are also subject to estate tax. Amounts payable after death which do not qualify as lump-sum distribution are free from estate taxation but subject to regular income tax as received.

Under a Keogh Plan, a contribution must be made for all full-time employees with three years or more of service. This contribution must bear the same proportion to employees' earnings as the physician's contribution does to personal income. An employee's benefits are fully vested when contributed, so a terminating employee may withdraw the total sum which has been deposited for him or her. If at least one common law employee is covered by a Keogh Plan, additional voluntary contributions may be made by the self-employed. These voluntary contributions are subject to a limit of 10% of earned income or $2500, whichever is greater. These voluntary contributions are not deductible when made, but accrue interest tax-free until withdrawal. The contributions themselves (but not interest attributed to them) may be withdrawn prior to age 59.5 without penalty.

In addition to the money-purchase plans described above, it is now possible to establish a defined benefit Keogh Plan. Such a plan may allow larger Keogh contributions than the above mentioned limits for a high-income physician age 45 or older. Because of the actuarial calculations involved in such a plan, these would be most readily available from insurance companies and agents.

Other forms of retirement plans available to corporate entities will be discussed under Professional Corporation.

Payroll Taxes

There are several different payroll taxes which any employer must pay to federal, state, and local governments. On the local level, many large municipal areas have payroll taxes. These taxes are sometimes a flat yearly amount, such as $10 per employee. More often they are like state and federal unemployment compensation taxes, which are 3% and 5%, respectively, of the first $4,200 of each employee's wages. Workers' Compensation insurance is calculated on the basis of total wages, such as 51¢ per $100 of wages. The employer must also pay a share of the social security tax, 5.85% of the gross wage. In addition to paying these taxes, employers also withhold from employees' wages federal, state, and local income taxes and social security tax. Each of these tax withholdings must be reported to the employee with each paycheck.

Financial Statements

There are three basic financial statements: the balance sheet, the income statement, and the revenue and expense report. These statements can be prepared from daily, weekly, and monthly financial information generated in the practice. Advisors may design these statements and audit them periodically. If the practice is incorporated, it is advisable to have an accountant prepare the financial statements.

Financial statements may be used in several ways. The balance sheet may be examined to determine if the practice is relying too heavily on creditors to finance operations by comparing assets to liabilities. The asset usage can be studied by comparing the amount of resources allocated to inventory and cash. The practice may be stocking a high inventory, paying for it promptly with cash, and not receiving any interest on the money tied up in the inventory. The practice could then increase its cash position by buying and stocking less inventory or by not paying its inventory bills as promptly. The income statement describes the components of the costs of the practice. Too low an income may indicate excessive costs, an unrealistic fee schedule, or low collections. The expense and revenue report displays information concerning costs and revenues and pinpoints items which are deviating from planned budget.

Balance Sheet. A balance sheet is a description of the financial position of the practice at one point in time. All resources are expressed in monetary units. Each resource is considered an asset owned by the practice. In addition, the balance sheet reports all liabilities, which are debts of the practice owed to others. Equity of the practice is also presented in the balance sheet. Assets have been purchased with funds supplied by the owner or creditors. Thus, total assets must equal the sum of liabilities and owner's equity. A balance sheet lists assets in one column and liabilities and owner's equity in another column. The sum of the columns must balance. Figure 4.3 presents the types of assets and liabilities that are typically included on a balance sheet.

Income Statement. An income statement presents the overall financial process and outcome that has occurred in the practice over the past accounting period (usually a year). In the income statement all revenues that have been generated are presented and summed, all costs practice against national averages. The information is presented for an individual physician, so groups can just multiply the figures by the number of physicians in the group.

PROFESSIONAL CORPORATION

The professional corporation has become a financial innovation for practicing physicians. The corporation provides advantages of both sole proprietorship and partnership, because a physician is both an owner of shares of the corporation and an employee of the corporation. The corporation can also structure itself to be nonprofit, if this meets the humanitarian or tax considerations of the physician. This section will begin with the definition of a professional corporation, followed by legal requirements of the corporation, especially those which pertain

---

ASSETS

Current Assets
　Cash
　Supplies
　Accounts Receivable
　　Allowance for Bad Debts
　Total

Fixed Assets
　Building and Land
　Furniture, Equipment, Fixtures
　　Accumulated Depreciation
　Total

Total Assets

LIABILITIES AND OWNERS EQUITY

Current Liabilities
　Income Taxes
　Payroll
　Payroll Taxes
　Accounts Payable
　Total

Long-Term Debt

Total Liabilities

Owner's Equity (current value of practice investments)

Total Liabilities and Owner's Equity

Figure 4.3　Balance Sheet

---

that have occurred are presented and summed, and then the difference between revenues and cost is taken. This reveals the profit (or loss) of the practice. Figure 4.4 presents the various items that would be included in a practice income statement. The income portion should distinguish between cash collected and charges that are still uncollected. The practice overhead rate should be calculated by comparing actual expenses with cash collections. This gives a more accurate picture of the financial condition for the period.

Income and Expense Budget.　An income and expense budget combines an income statement and budget for an accounting period. An income and expense summary based on data from the Medical Group Management Association is shown in Figure 4.5. This information may be useful for comparing the financial activity of a

---

Income
　Professional Services—Cash Collections
　Diagnostic Services—Cash Collections
　Total

Expense
　Professional Salaries
　Staff Salaries
　Wage Taxation and Insurance
　Benefits
　Facility
　Supplies
　Administration
　Insurance

　Subtotal

　　Allowance for Bad Debt
　　Depreciation
　Total

Income before Interest and Taxation

Interest Expense

Income before Taxation

Taxation

Net Income

Dividends

Income Retained for Investment in Corporation

Figure 4.4　An Income Statement

	Family Practice	Internal Medicine	OB/GYN
Gross Patient Charges	$226,000	$300,000	$363,000
Revenue (Cash Received)	$218,000	$293,000	$340,000
Overhead (as A % of Revenue)			
Employee Payroll	25.9%	22.8%	20.3%
Data Processing	2.0	1.5	n.a
Lab Expenses	3.4	3.5	3.2
Radiology Exp.	2.1	3.2	n.a.
Med. & Surgical Exp.	3.3	3.2	1.9
Building & Occupancy	7.0	5.5	5.2
Furniture & Equipment	1.7	2.0	2.0
Office Supplies	2.1	1.8	1.6
Telephone Expenses	1.3	1.2	1.2
Insurance Premiums	2.7	1.7	6.2
Other Expenses	6.6	4.8	5.7
Total Overhead Expenses	58.1%	49.6%	47.3%
Physician Benefit Expenses	7.3%	8.9%	9.3%
Income Available	$75,000	$122,000	$148,000

Source: The Cost and Production Survey Report—1985, Medical Group Management Association, Denver, Colorado

Figure 4.5 Income and Expense Summary, 1984, average per MD family practice, internal medicine, and OB/GYN

to ownership and liability. Another discussion topic will be the conversion of a partnership to a professional corporation. The last section will present advantages and disadvantages of the corporation form of practice, from both tax and nontax perspectives.

Definition

Professional corporations are the result of legal statutes in each state. There is no uniform statutory framework in the United States, and so this discussion of professional corporations must be compared with the appropriate laws which apply in the state where the practice will be developed.

A corporation is a legal entity or person. A group of individual practitioners known as incorporators, with the assistance of an attorney, develop a document known as the articles of incorporation or charter. This charter contains provisions of the organization, including name, term of existence, powers and purposes, capital stock and management structure, and registered office agent. Since the corporation is a

legal person, it can be sued, and can sue, and so in the charter, the corporation must designate a person and place where judicial and other legal papers can be served or presented to the corporation. The charter is signed by the incorporators, filed with the state government, and after various fees are paid, the corporation begins its existence. In some states, charters that involve the practice of medicine are sent to the state board of medical examiners for review and approval.

In addition to the charter, the corporation must have a set of bylaws which state the operating principles and provide additional details about internal structure. If it has been incorporated as a nonprofit corporation, then no stock is issued and physicians involved with the corporation are considered members of the corporation, not stockholders.

Legal Aspects

Legal aspects of a professional corporation and the process of developing a charter require the services of an attorney. Initially, only a few states allowed professional corporations, but by 1973 all states had passed enabling legislation. The Internal Revenue Service (IRS) oversees the legal aspects of a professional corporation, regarding personal income tax and other financial matters which affect taxable income of physicians and the corporation. Two specific legal issues which physicians must assume are ownership and liabilities.

Ownership. An important issue in professional corporations is ownership. Because it is the corporation that is practicing medicine, and only physicians can practice medicine, state laws require that only physicians can own shares of a professional corporation. Any ownership by a nonphysician results in termination or dissolution of the corporation. The corporation can provide medical services only through authorized physicians, and so each physician owning shares in the corporation and/or practicing in the corporation must be licensed in the state. If a physician retires from the practice of medicine or becomes disqualified from practicing medicine, in most cases, it will be necessary to terminate connection with the corporation, regarding both practice and ownership.

Management of the corporation must be assumed by the stockholders. A board of directors will be elected by the stockholders, and may include the stockholders themselves. The directors will then appoint the officers of the corporation: president, vice president, etc. These officers may be the stockholders and/or directors. Thus, each physician in the corporation may be wearing four hats at any given time: as a physician employee of the corporation providing medical care, as president of the corporation responsible for the day-to-day management of the corporation, as a director of the board responsible for major policy decisions, and as a stockholder expecting financial gain from his ownership of shares. The officers of the corporation may decide, however, to hire a business manager and delegate certain authority and responsibility for business decisions.

Liabilities. Two types of liabilities face any practice. First, there are liabilities which occur from the operation of any business—the premises liabilities. Second, there are liabilities that occur from the provision of medical services—

professional or malpractice liabilities. In most situations, corporations are liable for the actions of their employees. Corporations also have limited liability, and so the combination of these two legal aspects would seem to mean that a physician is not liable for professional malpractice and that the corporation has only limited liability in these cases. However, the professional standard of the physician's accountability for a patient, based on the close personal relationship between physician and patient, requires that the physician remain directly liable to the receiver of medical services.

State laws which permit professional corporations have resolved this conflict by requiring that only physicians may provide services through the corporation, that the physicians and the corporation are subject to the standards of the medical profession and thereby subject to regular disciplinary action if the standards are violated, and that the physician remains liable for any professional malpractice. The limited liability of the corporation is eliminated and liability involves the employee-physician. Unlike a partnership, however, a stockholder-physician is not personally liable for professional liability of employees not under direct supervision, such as other physicians.

At the same time, those aspects of the professional corporation that do not involve the practice of medicine and malpractice remain under the conventional laws concerning limited corporate liability. In other words, premises liability involves the corporation only, and any suits charging liability but not malpractice involve just the corporation. For these reasons, the professional corporation must have premises liability insurance, whereas physicians must each carry personal malpractice insurance.

Costs

Four costs are usually included in the price of incorporation. Orientation sessions in which legal aspects are discussed with physicians costs approximately $250–350 for a two-physician practice and $350–500 for a three- or four-person practice. The actual incorporation papers and bylaws range from $350 to $500. When very low quotes are received, it is often only for these first two services. The drawing up of the pension or profit-sharing plan is the single largest cost, between $660 and $1,000. Some attorneys may not draw this until the corporation has been in existence for six months or a year, but it is a cost that will occur eventually.

The cost of the pension or profit-sharing plan may be alleviated by use of a prototype or master plan. A prototype or master plan is one which has been designed, generally by a bank, mutual fund, or insurance company, for the use of its clients. In nearly every case the use of a prototype or master plan assumes that at least a substantial portion of the retirement plan assets will be invested through the plan sponsor. The employment contract and the buy/sell agreement will cost between $300 and $600. There are other expenses that do not go to the attorney, but rather are the fees, stock certificates, and so forth, which will cost between $100 and $250, and the accountant's fee will be between $250 and $600. Total cost for incorporating may range between $1,800 and $3,450.

Some additional costs that should be considered. Throughout the first year an attorney may become necessary for other matters. The retainer for one year may range from $250 to $750. An insurance consultant or actuary may be needed to develop the pension programs at a possible cost of $500. The services of an actuary and a consultant may be provided free of charge by an insurance company interested in obtaining the business of the corporation. When a professional corporation purchases its own facility and major amounts of equipment, it is sometimes advisable to establish a separate partnership, corporation, or trust to own those assets. This second partnership or corporation may have owners who are not in the professional corporation. These may be spouses or children of the physicians. The cost of establishing the second corporation may be between $600 and $1000. Lastly, the attorney may feel that it is necessary for a major legal review at the end of the first year. This service costs between $200 and $600. This service may be included in the retainer, if the attorney agrees to it. These additional optional costs can total from $1,050 to $2,850, bringing the total cost from $2,800 to $6,300. This cost may seem extreme but it is due to the many different services involved in incorporating. The exact fees will depend on exactly what services are desired.

Incorporation

The process of forming the corporation after a lawyer has been selected begins with choosing the incorporators. The incorporators in many states do not have to be physicians. Lawyers can serve as incorporators but only to perform legal procedures. The incorporators sign the charter or articles of incorporation, which is filed with the office of the secretary of state where the practice is to be located. The charter includes a corporate name, which is often highly regulated by state law. Corporate stock is distributed to physicians who are owners of the corporation. Incorporators who are not physicians do not receive any stock. The corporation then enters into an employment agreement with the physician-owners. This agreement is a written document that defines the relationship between the physician and corporation in terms of salary, medical, and managerial considerations. The agreement does as much or more than the charter and bylaws in creating the impression that the corporation and the physician-employees are distinct and separate. Further, the employment agreement defines the scope of employment in terms of duties, hours, and responsibilities, and defines fringe benefits and compensation.

The compensation plan is of critical importance to the functioning of the corporation. The IRS carefully examines these plans to determine whether compensation is reasonable or unreasonable, and to review the criteria of the plan. If, upon investigation the IRS rules that the compensation plan is actually a disguised dividend plan, then the corporation and employees as stockholders are liable for extra taxation. This problem may be avoided by designing a salary system that is totally independent of ownership. IRS bases reasonable compensation upon physicians' talents and qualifications, difficulty of work, prevailing economic conditions, compensation paid by other professional corporations to similar physicians, and previous income of the physician. If the compensation is unreasonable, the IRS can declare compensation to be a disguised dividend and double taxation will result. There are many different possible salary and bonus systems. *The Medical Group Management Association Digest of*

Medical Group Employment Contracts and Income Distribution Plans contains samples of various agreements used in partnerships and corporations. Most of these plans involve a base salary, with adjustments for seniority, administrative work, and continuing education, and bonus payments determined by bookings, collections, or other productivity-related measures.

Conversion of a Partnership

There are three considerations which may occur when converting a partnership into a professional corporation: (1) transfer of accounts receivable, accounts payable, goodwill, and other liabilities; (2) income bunching in the first year; and (3) the transfer of Keogh retirement plans.

Transfer of Assets. Transferring accounts receivable, goodwill, and liabilities such as accounts payable from the partnership to the corporation can involve complex tax issues. Because tax laws are ever changing, consultation with an attorney and accountant on this subject is crucial in making any plans to incorporate. Accounts receivable can be transferred, but transfer of accounts may result in some taxation. If owners of the accounts receivable (members of the partnership) remain in control of the new corporation by owning at least 8% of the stock, then the transfer can be tax-free.

Accounts payable can also be transferred, but a problem develops if the accounts payable are greater than the accounts receivable. A solution to this is for the partnership to pay all the accounts payable prior to transfer. It is also possible to obtain a closing agreement from the IRS in advance of the transfer which serves as a ruling in advance as to whether there will be any tax liability due to the transfer of accounts.

Income Bunching. Individuals operate on a calendar-year basis for taxation, but partnerships and corporations operate on a fiscal year of their own choosing. The result can involve taxation on as much as 23 months' income, even though the physicians may only receive a salary for 12 months. For example, if a partnership with a fiscal year from February 1 to January 31 decided to incorporate on February 1,

1978, the allocation of the partnership's income from February 1, 1977 to January 31, 1978 will be included in the partner's tax return for 1978, along with their corporate salary for 1978. There is no best solution to this problem, but two alternatives can limit the burden. Each has its own drawbacks.

First, reduced salaries can be paid during the first year of the corporation. This can involve quarterly payment of salaries on the first day of the next quarter, yearly payment of the first year salary on the first day of the next year, or paying the first year salary over several years. All these involve a decreased cash flow to the physician—cash which is necessary to pay taxes. A second approach is to continue the partnership that existed prior to the formation of the corporation. The continuing of the partnership to receive the funds due from accounts receivable, pay accounts payable, and distribute profits, along with a low salary from the corporation, may reduce the income bunching. However, the increase in salary from the corporation after the first year may cause the IRS to question the reasonableness of the salary, and this method also leaves the corporation with very little cash flow or income during the first year. Both these alternatives involve low salaries in the first year. This can require young physicians to borrow during their first year against their future first-year payments. The first year can be very disadvantageous from a tax perspective, but the following years will tend to have many more tax advantages which will compensate for first-year loans.

Transfer of Keogh Plan. A third issue involves the transfer of the existing Keogh plan from the partnership to the corporation. If the plan is terminated, the distribution is considered premature and is subject to taxation. Assets can be transferred to the new corporate plan, but this requires that the Keogh accounts be distinct and their assets remain subject to Keogh rules. This can be costly, as special plans are required in this situation. The best alternative is to freeze the plan. Although this produces two distinct retirement accounts for each former partner, tax benefits are worth additional bookkeeping in retirement. Due to changes in tax laws, any decision to freeze a plan or transfer it should be discussed with appropriate consultants.

Joining a Professional Corporation

When joining a professional corporation and becoming a part owner of that corporation, the following areas must be scrutinized: alternative methods of acquiring stock, the financial condition of the corporation, the employment agreement, the shareholders agreement, and the negotiating process.

Methods of Stock Acquisition. Depending on the different ways that stock is acquired, there may be different tax consequences. The best approach for the physician joining the professional corporation is to purchase authorized but unissued stock from the corporation. When the corporation sells this type of stock, there is no taxable gain to the corporation and no taxable liability to the shareholder. The purchase price of the shares is generally based on the book value. Book value is determined from the balance sheet. In determining book value, no value should be attached to accounts receivable or goodwill. Life insurance owned by the corporation insuring the life of the stockholders should be valued at their cash-surrender value plus the unearned portion of any premiums.

Corporation's Financial Condition. Prior to joining a professional corporation, review all pertinent information concerning the organization and its financial condition. These documents include the certificate of incorporation, bylaws, balance sheet and income statements, and minutes of board of director meetings. A check should also be made into any financial obligations such as taxes, debts, and other liabilities. The pension plan and profit-sharing requirements should also be evaluated to determine if the new partner could be at a disadvantage. The lease for the office premises should be read to ascertain whether it is in the name of the corporation or shareholder(s).

Employment Contract. The employment contracts of the shareholders should be examined, particularly provisions regarding termination, financial investment, benefits, and other issues which could affect the new shareholder. The important consideration is how will the new shareholder relate to the board of directors and

to what extent is the new member involved in decision making. Other factors which could be included are severance pay, base salary and supplements, expenses paid by the corporation, disposition of accounts receivable, disability payments, restrictive covenants, vacation, and leaves of absence. A termination provision is a must. Special consideration should be given to a provision in the event of death or divorce of a shareholder and its effect on the ownership of the corporation's assets and funds.

Stockholder's Agreement. Items to be carefully reviewed in a stockholder's agreement are: rules relating to shareholder action and election to the board of directors; loan provisions; malpractice insurance provisions; provisions relating to the disposition of the corporation assets; and limitations on the issuance of new stock.

Negotiating Process. Younger professionals are not in a position to obtain a status in the corporation equal to that of the shareholders who built the practice. Based upon the seniority of the physicians, shareholders may differ in the amount of stock holdings, salary, benefits, pension, and/or profit-sharing benefits. Potential trouble spots will be the contributions to pension plans and insurance programs. Depending on age, life-style, and financial worth, there may be a wide difference in need between the new shareholder and the senior physicians.

Advantages and Disadvantages of Practice Corporation

As has already been demonstrated, the creation of a professional corporation involves considerable taxation and legal questions. Cost may be a factor, and numerous problems may arise in the conversion. The advantages and disadvantages to operating a practice in the corporate form involve tax and nontax considerations. Some of the tax disadvantages, such as transfer of accounts and income bunching, have already been mentioned. The following paragraphs present some general advantages and disadvantages of professional corporations.

Tax Advantages

Fringe benefit deduction and reinvestment are two major tax advantages of professional corporations (see Figure 4.6).

Fringe Benefits Deduction

All normal business expenses of operating the corporation, including fringe benefits for employees, are deductible from corporate revenues for income tax purposes. Such fringe benefits can include automobiles or allowances, continuing education, justifiable dues and memberships, and any of the following.

Group Term Life Insurance. A plan of group term life insurance covering the employees of the corporation, including the physicians, is deductible from corporate income. The first $50,000 of such coverage is free, in that no income is reportable by the employee for the economic benefit of such coverage. Amounts over $50,000 generally result in some taxable income to the employee, usually less than the actual premium charged. There are special require-

Corpora-tion	Entity	Partner-ship
460,000	Total Billings	460,000
	less	
(180,000)	General Overhead	(180,000)
(32,000)	Qualified Plan	0
(8,000)	Insurance	0
(219,488)	Salaries	0
20,512	Profit	0
(4,512)	Federal Tax	0
16,000	Retained Capital or Distributable Revenues	280,000
	Individual	
54,872	Salary Distribution	70,000
19,582	Federal Income Tax	(27,720)
0	Retirement Savings	(8,000)
0	Insurance	(2,000)
0	Capital Contribution	(4,000)
35,290	Net Income	28,280

Figure 4.6 Tax Benefits of Professional Corporation

ments for a group plan covering fewer than ten employees to qualify.

Medical Reimbursement Plans. Group health care covering employees is fully deductible by the corporation, and the premiums are not taxed as income to the employees. In addition, the corporation may pay certain medical expenses for its employees such as the cost of routine annual physicals, dental and orthodontic work for family members, and expenses not covered by the group health insurance plan. For such a plan to qualify, it should be written with defined limits as to the amount of reimbursement which might be available.

Some medical reimbursement plans include provision for reimbursement of personal disability insurance premiums paid by certain employees of the group. A well-written medical reimbursement plan provides substantial advantages to the employees, as all medical expenses can now be paid with before-tax dollars rather than with only those in excess of 3% of adjusted gross income, as is the case with partners and sole proprietors.

Disability Insurance and Sick Pay Plans. A corporation can pay and deduct the premiums for disability insurance covering some of or all its employees. The premiums themselves are not included in taxable income for the employees, but the benefits when received are subject to income taxation. A sick pay exclusion is available so that a portion of these benefits may be excluded from taxation. The maximum sick pay exclusion is $100 per week if adjusted gross income during a period of disability is not in excess of $15,000 per year. There is a dollar-for-dollar reduction in the exclusion if adjusted gross income exceeds $15,000, so that benefits in excess of $20,200 per year of disability will be fully taxable as ordinary income.

Retirement Plans. There are three basic types of retirement plans available to the corporate entity. For each of these, the corporation may purchase and deduct the cost of the qualified plan, and the contribution therefore will not be included in the taxable income of the employee until the benefits are received. The basic types of plans are described below.

In a *profit-sharing plan,* the board of directors of the corporation may determine that they would like to contribute a percentage of profits at the end of each year for the purposes of accumulating retirement funds for employees. These funds will be accumulated tax-free until each employee's retirement. The plan must have a definite allocation formula among the covered employees, usually based on that employee's percentage of salary to total payroll. Contributions may be made on a purely discretionary basis and can be omitted in years of low profits at the discretion of the board of directors.

Since Social Security provides a substantial retirement benefit relative to income for lower-paid employees, the profit-sharing plan may allow a contribution based on earnings in excess of the Social Security limit before allocation to all employees across the board. This will allow a larger percentage of the total contributions to be allocated to the higher-paid employees, including the physicians. Vesting of employees' benefits may be spread out, so that an employee terminating after a short period of employment cannot take all contributions upon termination. The forfeitures arising from these nonvested accounts are typically reallocated among those who remain in the plan. The funds may be invested in life insurance, annuities, stocks and bonds, or any of a number of other investments at the discretion of the trustees (who may or may not be involved directly with the corporation).

A *money purchase pension plan* is similar to profit sharing in that contributions are generally determined as a percentage of payroll, and the ultimate benefit at retirement is equivalent to whatever the sum of contributions and interest will provide. Although the Internal Revenue Code does not impose a specific limit on how much the corporation can contribute and deduct each year, the practical limit in most cases will be 25% of payroll up to $30,000. A money purchase plan is subject to the minimum funding requirements, which means that contributions must be made each year according to the plan's contribution formula, regardless of the existence of profits. A waiver may be allowed because of substantial business hardship, but the waived amount must be deposited over not more than 15 future years.

The third type of retirement plan available to corporations is a *defined-benefit plan*. Such a plan determines contributions actuarially after determining what final benefit is desired, that is, retirement benefit equal to 50% of average monthly salary in the five years immediately prior to retirement. Using certain assumptions as to interest rates, a contribution limit will be established and funding will be required each year to keep the plan on target in order to provide the promised benefits. Defined-benefit plans usually allow larger contributions for individuals over age 45 at the inception of the plan, whereas money purchase formulas generally benefit younger employees.

This is only a brief description of the types of plans available. There are many variations available in retirement plans as far as types of funding, sources of plans themselves, vesting of benefits, eligibility rules, and government regulations. Only a qualified pension expert should be enlisted to help design the plan.

Reinvestment

The second major tax advantage of corporations involves capital accumulation and reinvestment. The corporation can retain profits and reinvest them in the practice. The tax rate on these retained profits is less than the rate paid by the physician-owners on their salary. Under a partnership arrangement profits would have to be paid out and taxed at a higher rate before being reinvested. Within the corporation less taxes are paid on the same reinvestment. Depending upon equipment purchased, some special tax credits may also be available.

Tax Disadvantages

Several tax disadvantages should be discussed with the attorney and accountant before making a decision to incorporate. Some are small or avoidable, but they must be taken into account in developing financial plans.

Social Security. When a physician becomes a corporate employee, the tax treatment of FICA withholding, social security taxes, changes. On the maximum income of $17,700 subject to the tax in 1978, the rate is 12.10% or a total tax due of $2,141.70. One-half of this is paid by the corporation and is deductible from corporate revenues, but the effect is still greater than the comparable tax on self-employed physicians, which in 1978, was $1,433.70, based on a rate of 8.10% on the first $17,700 of income. This discrepancy will increase over the next ten years. By 1987 the yearly difference between corporate employee and self-employed social security will be $1,831.80.

Taxes. State and federal unemployment taxes will be greater for a corporate employee than for a self-employed physician. The workers' compensation insurance rates will also be higher. In addition, the corporation will be subject to state franchise taxes, although these are not great. Many states and localities have corporate income taxes. Because the corporation will be paying most of its revenues as salaries and benefits and will therefore have little profit, these taxes will be of little consequence. However, the corporation will have to file these tax returns regardless of amounts owed. Thus, professional corporations are faced with filing additional returns and a more complex tax burden.

Taxable Dividends. Corporate profits are taxed, and out of these profits dividends are declared, which, when received by the owners, are taxed as income. This double taxation may seem a major drawback but, as pointed out concerning state and local taxes, the professional corporation, after paying all salaries, operating costs, fringe benefits, and then needing to retain profits for reinvestment, will not have sufficient remaining profits to declare dividends. This will minimize the double taxation burden.

Excess Accumulation. There is an IRS regulation that corporations cannot accumulate more than $150,000 in profits, unless the corporation can demonstrate that it is for reasonable business needs. While most professional corporations may not encounter this problem, it can be resolved by increasing fringe benefits or prefunding a stock redemption agreement. These may not be deductible from revenues, but they can be used to reduce unreasonable accumulations. There is also the personal holding company tax problem. This tax would result if more than 60% of the contracts entered into by the corporation allowed the client to stipulate which employee of the corporation would perform the purchased services. This only occurs when half of the stock is held by five or fewer individuals. This can be avoided by not allowing any written contracts that allow patients to designate which physician they prefer to treat them. The expectation of patients as to which physician will treat them is not considered to be a designation.

Reasonable Compensation. Another major tax disadvantage involves the issue of reasonable compensation. Even though compensation from a corporation may be the same as or less than that received from a previous partnership, the corporation should expect that the IRS will make a thorough examination of the compensation agreement and records of the corporation and preexisting partnership. Although these tax disadvantages are potential problems, careful planning and professional consultation prior to incorporation should reduce them to manageable levels.

Other Advantages

There are five major nontax advantages to professional corporations. Two of these advantages affect the management structure of the practice, and the other three affect legal consequences.

Management Structure. A corporation, compared to a partnership, has more centralized and defined management structure. The charter and bylaws of the corporation place ultimate responsibility with shareholders. This is manifested through the board of directors, the officers of the corporation, and the executive committee of the board. Those members of the corporation not interested in management can delegate responsibility for management to those with an interest in this aspect of practice management. In a partnership, all members are supposed to be equally active in the management of the practice.

Fiscal Planning. The second effect of a corporate structure is that fiscal planning can be successfully pursued. A formal budget should be developed for each fiscal year to correctly allocate revenues to salaries, overhead, pension programs, fringe benefits, and retained profits for future development. Cash flow will be of major concern, since it will be the basis for salaries and bonus payments. Budgeting will focus physicians' attention on expenses of operating the practice. Separate accounts will clarify operational costs. While a physician in solo practice or several in a partnership could have maintained independent financial records, formation of a corporate structure requires a composite of financial records.

Liability. A corporation possesses limited liability that is not present in a partnership. This limited liability does not cover professional liability, but it does cover other obligations. In a partnership, the entry of any one member into a contract binds the other partnership members as well as the partnership itself. In a corporation, only an officer of the corporation, acting within the bounds of authority given to him or her by the board of directors, can enter into a contract, and only the corporation becomes liable. This liability only affects assets in the corporation not assets of shareholders.

Practice Continuity. A partnership ends when a member dies or leaves. A corporation survives termination of members. When the corporation has a prefunded buy-sell arrangement, death of each member causes shares of that member to be sold to the corporation for a prearranged price. The estate receives cash, not shares, which prevents ownership by nonphysicians, (which could cause the dissolution of the corporation), and the corporation continues with remaining members. A new physician can join by purchasing shares owned by the corporation. Because the corporation possesses financial and medical records, practice continuity is ensured.

Transfer of Ownership. Although only a physician can own shares in a professional corporation, it is still much easier to transfer such shares between physicians than it is to transfer the interest of one physician in a partnership to another. It is much easier for a physician, on retirement, to sell shares to a younger physician than it is for the older physician to bring in a new, younger partner prior to retirement. It is also possible for two professional corporations to merge into one corporation. Two partner-

ships would have to dissolve and a new partnership would have to be formed.

Other Disadvantages

There are eight disadvantages which may arise from the corporate forms of practice which are not tax related. These may not appear to be disadvantages to some physicians, but to others they may be serious enough to abandon any interest in incorporation.

Costs. As has been described, costs of incorporation can range from two to six thousand dollars. A major cost may be relocation of offices. Physicians in a corporation must have offices that are in close proximity to each other, if not sharing a single large suite of offices. The IRS can rule that a corporation is not in fact a corporation if this is not done. Costs of finding and remodeling a large office space and moving two or more practices in together can be very costly. A minor cost is that the corporate name must be on all stationery and forms used by the practice. The corporation will have to file more tax reports than a partnership and will have higher accounting and legal fees. The bookkeeping system of the practice may have to be upgraded, requiring trained clerical staff.

Regulation. It has already been mentioned that corporations have to file more tax returns than a partnership and that the practice will be under IRS scrutiny during its first years. The corporation may have to disclose more of its internal operations to the public than would be required of a partnership, due to governmental regulation. A corporation may have to comply more with Occupational Health and Safety Administration and Office of Economic Opportunity regulations than would be the case with a private practice.

Advisors. Tax and legal complexities of the corporate form of practice require a greater reliance on accountants, attorneys, stock and insurance brokers, and bankers than in a partnership. The prevalence of these issues will require the establishment of ongoing, working relationships with attorneys and accountants. These relationships require time and a commitment to fully understand the organizational and financial functions pertinent to operating a corporation.

Control of Investments. A physician's personal savings for retirement are replaced by corporate contributions to a pension plan. Although this produces substantial tax savings, it does have a drawback for physicians who enjoy financial speculation. Even though physicians are free to make investments out of their personal salary, they are limited as to how much can be invested, since their salary is reduced by the funds contributed to the corporate pension program. Because of the fiduciary responsibility of an investment committee, an insurer, or bank trust department, corporate investments may not be as speculative as those considered by individual physicians. So, for those physicians who prefer financial speculation, this aspect of corporate practice may be a disadvantage.

Wage-Price Restrictions. The possibility exists that a future wage-price freeze may affect only professional corporations and not solo practitioners or partnerships. In that case, incorporated physicians may be more disadvantaged. A properly-drafted employment contract may alleviate this problem.

Ethics. Even though the practice is a corporation, the patient-physician relationship remains confidential and inviolate. The corporate structure may appear to break down the closeness of the professional and personal relationship.

Younger Physicians. The professional corporation provides substantial benefits to the physician by purchasing extensive benefits and making pension contributions which are deducted from revenues before a salary is paid. Younger physicians may have considerable debts and be reluctant to begin extensive long-term savings and retirement programs. Their financial needs will be short term and may be inhibited by charters of the corporation.

Business Discipline. A difficult feature of corporate practice is development of business and organizational discipline. A different style exists in corporate practice compared to solo or small partnership practices. Physicians sacrifice some of their independence when they form a corporation and become employees of it. Arrangements must be scheduled with other physicians and management of the corporation for vacations and study periods. The contract specifies various obligations and responsibilities which employees must fulfill. If the contract is violated, the physicians may have to pay damages to the corporation or face possible termination. In a corporation, the physician receives a specified salary, so it is not possible to borrow funds from the practice account to pay for a vacation, as in a partnership or a solo practice. To some extent, the discipline extends into personal finances. Membership in a professional corporation attracts IRS audits. To avoid personal tax problems, physicians in a corporation should hire accountants to prepare their personal returns.

Audits of Professional Corporations

The following table summarizes the IRS audits of 350 professional corporations. The major categories of problems were: (1) automobile, travel, and entertainment; (2) qualified retirement plans; (3) unreasonable compensation, and (4) miscellaneous. The types of audits listed below may be helpful to understanding the implications of professional incorporation.

Audit Category	Audits	
	Number	%
Automobile, travel, and entertainment	76	22
Qualified retirement plans	49	14
Unreasonable compensation	7	2
Miscellaneous	218	62
Totals	350	100

Automobile, Travel, and Entertainment
- Reduced business percentage of corporate-owned auto
- Disallowance of auto expenses, country club dues, and boat expenses
- Christmas gifts exceeding $25
- Auto expense where 100% of auto is written

off with reimbursement on a mileage basis by professionals for personal use
- Entertainment facilities
- Depreciation taken on automobiles

Qualified Retirement Plan:
- Discriminatory qualified retirement plan
- Pension deductions disallowed on the theory that retirement age of 55 was too early
- Examination of profit-sharing trust loan
- Practice of borrowing from employee's profit-sharing trust
- Unreasonable compensation
- Compensation–fringe benefit plan
- Compensation paid to stockholder's children
- Corporate expenditures determined to be personal expenditures
- Compensation to a nonprofessional employee

Miscellaneous
- Disallowance of wife's travel overseas and meeting expenses
- Disallowance of capitalization of repairs
- No corporate bank account
- Unreasonable rent of land and building from stockholder
- Disallowance of excessive ordinary insurance
- Disability insurance proposed for disallowance because of discrimination in favor of officer-employees and lack of plan
- Disallowance of depreciation in furniture and fixtures

Lawyers and physicians should be mindful of the IRS when establishing a professional corporation as well as during the preparation of fringe benefit programs and retirement plans. Local IRS agents may be valuable advisors at the planning stages, as a prevention for future audits which are both costly and time consuming.

CONCLUSION

The financial aspect of practice is a fact of life. If physicians recognize this early in their careers and are committed to understanding fiscal matters, then the primary goals of quality health care and personal and professional growth will not be compromised.

Financial expertise will require the understanding of budgets, insurance, investments, income and other forms of taxes, and pertinent fiscal issues relevant to the private practice of medicine. Along with a base knowledge of these financial matters must evolve: (1) an ability to design and interpret documents and reports and (2) willingness to select and incorporate advisors into decision making and problem solving. Physicians should always maintain their presence in financial affairs and fully participate in both analysis of information and formulation of decisions.

The professional corporation is a legitimate option for practicing physicians. The features of an incorporated practice should be investigated, regardless of years in practice, number of partners, and financial income. Converting a solo practice or partnership to a corporation has many ramifications and will require expert advisors and consultants.

Since physicians may have minimum time for financial or legal orientation and education, the choice of well-qualified advisors is imperative. There should be ample time spent with the advisors during planning sessions so that advisors can effectively represent the physician and recommend decisions which will meet both personal and professional financial requirements.

References

An unprecedented look inside America's best managed private medical practices. *Physician's Management* 17 (March 1977):17–30.

Anderson B, McCoy J: Caution: leases can hide dangerous curves and clauses. *Health Care Management,* October 1985, pp 24–37.

Baird GW, Jr: Income distribution in group practice: An overview and four factors to consider. *Medical Group Management* 22 (March-April 1975):14–22.

Beck LC: *The Physician's Office.* Princeton, NJ: Excerpta Medica, 1977.

Berman HJ: How reports can help you manage working capital. *Hospital Financial Management* 26 (January 1972):18–21.

Brandon J: Tefra: Impact on hospitals, nurses, physicians and patients. *Health Care Supervisor* 3, no. 3 (April 1985):78–86.

Brooks EE, Madison DL: Primary care practice: Forms of organization. In *Primary*

Care and the Practice of Medicine, Noble, J (ed). Boston, Little, Brown, 1976.

Bosterman R: *The Complete Estate Planning Guide.* New York, McGraw-Hill, 1976.

Caplan A: If there is a will, is there a way? *Law, Medicine and Health Care* 13, no. 1 (February 1985):32–33.

Center for Research in Ambulatory Health Care Administration: *The Organization and Development of a Medical Group Practice.* Cambridge, Mass: Ballinger, 1976.

Deguchi J, Inuji T, Martin D: Measuring provider productivity in ambulatory care. *Journal of Ambulatory Care Management,* November 1984, pp 1–3.

Gorlick SH: *The Whys and Wherefores of Corporate Practice.* Oradell, NJ: Medical Economics, 1976.

Hallman GV, Rosenbloom JS: *Personal Financial Planning.* New York, McGraw-Hill, 1975.

Hardy CC: Do you have the will to save? *Physician's Management* 18 (April 1978):42–49.

Lance JF: There's something new in disability insurance. *Dental Economics* 65 (November 1975):51–60.

Levy M: Can they cancel your disability insurance? *Medical Economics* 47 (July 1970):189–195.

McClanahan WS: *Estate Planning for the Young Professional.* Indianapolis, Ind, Research and Review, 1977.

McConnell C: Cost-containment: A new way of life. *Health Care Supervisor* 3, no. 3 (April 1985):66–77.

McNerney W: Financing ambulatory health care services. *Journal of Ambulatory Care Management,* November 1984, pp 1–3.

Physician's Office Management Reference Book. Kansas City, Mo, American Association of Family Physicians, 1977.

Reynolds JA: Group-M.D. fringe benefits: Where will they stop? *Medical Economics* 49 (October 1972):211–218.

Sloan F: Physician reimbursement: Diagnosis and prescription. *Journal of Ambulatory Care Management,* November 1984, pp 72–85.

Stoeber EA: *Tax and Fringe Benefit Planning for Professional Corporations.* Cincinnati, Ohio, The National Underwriter Company, 1977.

5

Personnel Management

- How are job descriptions and task delegations implemented?
- What are key elements for effective employee relations?
- What constitutes performance appraisal?
- What responsibilities and problems do office supervisors face?

- How are performance problems managed?
- What kinds of feedback build candor among physicians and office personnel?

Perhaps the most perplexing dilemma, outside of patient encounters, is managing office personnel. Practitioners will be confronted with this task and must resolve the ultimate personnel questions. Who is the "right" person? What is the "right" job for each person?

Medical training has seldom, if ever, addressed the knowledge and skills necessary to select, train, and supervise medical office personnel. Therefore, physicians who devote their careers to office practice must acquire these attributes through self-directed efforts.

Personnel management is a key administrative function. Physicians should be reluctant to divorce themselves from the responsibility. There is much to be learned and gained from maintaining direct involvement in personnel supervision. A realistic expectation for a manager of personnel is to accept that supervising skills evolve over time, and errors in judgment and tact should be converted to learning experiences. There is no predetermined differentiated diagnosis or suggested treatment plan. Each office and group setting will be unique. The only

rule of thumb is, work with all employees and, when appropriate, allow them to actively participate in policies and decisions which affect their working conditions.

This chapter presents the dimensions of personnel management which may be applied in a medical practice. Subjects discussed include clinical and business task analysis, job descriptions, supervision, training, staffing positions, and performance problems.

TASK ANALYSIS

When recruiting employees, it is essential that doctors determine the work which their staff will be asked to perform. If duties and assignments are specified, then it will be possible to determine qualifications and training necessary to complete the work. Doctors may develop a personnel task format which could include: (1) clinical functions—physical exam; history taking; therapy; patient education; laboratory and

Table 5.1   Office Task Analysis Chart.

Clinical				
Height, Weight, & BP				
ENT Screening				
Blood/Urine Specimens				
Immunization				
History Taking				
Throat Culture				
EKG				
Blood Tests				
X Rays				
Prescription Refills				
Well–Baby Exams				
Updating Growth Charts				
Chronic Problem Flowsheets				
Recording Lab Results				
Sutures				
(Other)				
(Other)				
(Other)				
Clerical				
Prepare Medical Records				
File Medical Reports				
Maintain Paper Supplies and Forms				
Maintain Office Files				
(Other)				
(Other)				
(Other)				
Secretarial				
Correspondence & Mail				
Physicians' Schedules				
Personal Files				
Articles & References				
Liaison with Organizations/Agencies				
Magazine Subscriptions				
Reception Area				
(Other)				
(Other)				

Table 5.1 *Continued*

Tasks	Individual(s) Responsible	Frequency	Supervision	Discussion of Results (Date)
Patient Contact				
Registration				
Incoming Calls				
Appointments				
Call–Backs				
Daily Charges/Receipts				
Referrals				
Telephone Messages				
(Other)				
(Other)				
(Other)				
Business Functions				
Cash Receipts				
Office				
Mail				
Posting Charges				
Daily Check–Out				
Bank Deposit				
Billing Statements				
Third Party Forms				
Medicare/Medicade				
Inpatient Charges				
Petty Cash				
Collections & Delinquent Accounts				
Inventory Control & Supplies				
Accounts Payable Files				
Check Preparation				
Payroll Checks				
Vacation Schedules				
Time Off Dates				
(Other)				
(Other)				
(Other)				

x-ray; telephone advice; hospital, nursing home, and house calls; and (2) business functions—appointment system and telephone messages; clerical and filing; secretarial and transcription; billing, collections, and insurance form preparation; inventory control; and accounts payable. Task analysis also involves establishing: lines of control and supervising responsibilities; time periods which indicate completion dates; and a method of feedback to present results.

Table 5.1 presents a task analysis chart which may assist practitioners in delegating office procedures. The effectiveness of such a technique will depend on its applicability to each office, preciseness for individual employees, and follow-up and evaluation. Job descriptions should also be included in the task analysis function.

Job descriptions assist practitioners in recruiting, interviewing, and evaluating employees. They are also vehicles for employees to learn the expectations as well as comprehend the ramifications of their jobs. There are at least six features which could be incorporated into a job description:

1. **Title of the Position** Each employee deserves a title which they may communicate to others. Very few people are motivated by labels such as "front office person" or "right-hand employee" or "Ms." or "Mr. Everything." A title should be given to each person which clearly defines nature of the work, such as appointment receptionist, billing and insurance clerk, nursing supervisor, and laboratory technician. Titles do not have to be all-inclusive but they should denote primary roles.

2. **Summary of Position** A brief comment about the work itself is appropriate. This summary may also be used in an advertisement for the position. A statement could read: Staff nurse who conducts history taking, patient education, and performs routine medical and laboratory procedures while assisting doctor with office patients.

3. **Duties Assigned** Each employee should be presented a list of duties which they will be performing. It should be noted if these duties are exclusive or with whom they will be shared. Specific duty list for a financial clerk

could include: monthly billing statements; collection letters and phone calls; medicare, medicaid, private third-party insurance form processing; check preparation and budget reports; inventory reports and purchases; and maintain files and prepare weekly and monthly reports.

4. **Knowledge and Skill Requirements** An essential feature of a job description will be an indicator of ability and/or technical skills necessary. Educational and training credentials may be included as well. Knowledge and skills which are desired should be measurable through observation, reference, or execution. A certified medical assistant should have training and/or experience in a variety of clinical and business tasks. These could include electrocardiogram, business machines, laboratory techniques, appointment scheduling, pegboard bookkeeping, and discussing diet and treatment plans with patients.

5. **Accountability** This element of the job description will be instrumental in determining progress, success, or failure of the employee. People tend to be more productive if they know what is expected and can visualize results. Supervisors will also find that evaluation is enhanced if performance is described in quantitative terms. This could be achieved by preparing daily logs, with weekly and monthly summaries. A receptionist could be accountable for scheduling 40–50 patients daily, processing cash receipts and balancing charges and collections daily, preparing new charts and encounter forms, posting balances to accounts, receiving 100–150 phone calls daily, and screening messages for nurses and doctors.

6. **Supervision** Each employee should have another person who has responsibility for training, directing, and evaluating their work. An employee's immediate supervisor should be indicated in the job description. There should also be some information as to the type and frequency of direction which will be given. Supervision of the office nurse could be described in the following manner: The nursing supervisor will assign duties to the office nurse on a weekly basis. During patient care doctors will provide primary direction. There will be formal evaluation ses-

Table 5.2 Receptionist and Nurse Job Descriptions

Title	Receptionist	Office Nurse
Summary	Greets, schedules, and conducts financial matters with all families and patients.	Responsible for patient flow from reception area until conclusion of office visit.
Duties	Handles appointment schedule, telephone communications, financial transactions, billing, and collections; prepares medical and financial records; performs clerical duties and filing for office systems; interacts with nurse for efficient patient, nurse, and physician scheduling.	Prepares and screens patients; assists doctor throughout exams and procedures; returns phone messages; performs tests, procedures, history taking, and other medical routines under supervision of doctor; interacts with receptionist for efficient patient, nurse, and physician scheduling.
Knowledge and Skills	Has high school diploma plus previous training in business office, preferably health care office practice; has knowledge of financial and clerical systems; skilled in typing and business machines; good at personal and telephone communications; organized and accurate.	RN, LPN, or certified medical assistant needs: previous experience in health care setting, preferably office practice; knowledge of lab tests, diagnostic equipment, and medical procedures and protocols; skills in patient communication and education.
Accountability	Reliable, confidential, prompt. Capable of efficient scheduling of patients, nightly cash-out and posting of charges and receipts, keeping accurate and organized records; is congenial and sensitive attitude toward patients and other staff; is willing to resolve problems and inefficiencies; will compile daily and weekly productivity reports.	Reliable, confidential, prompt. Efficient and thorough in patient care and in completing medical records; can use medical supplies and equipment in a cost-effective manner and analyze diagnostic data, with monthly reports.
Supervision	Reports to office manager and/or medical director; may have limited authority over clerical assistants and part-time staff.	Reports to office manager or head nurse. Also works under direction of physician during patient care responsibilities. May have limited authority over medical assistants and part-time staff.

sions quarterly with nursing supervisor and physician.

Table 5.2 presents job descriptions for nurse and receptionist.

EMPLOYEE RELATIONS

New Employee

Several steps will facilitate entry of a new employee into the practice. Whether this is a new position or an established job which is being filled, care should be taken to recruit, interview, select, and train the most appropriate person. Too often, when one or more of these stages is expedited, a personnel problem evolves. It is a misfortune and expense to both employer and employee to terminate a person within weeks or months of the initial hiring.

Recruitment

When a position becomes available, either through creation of a job or attrition, several methods are available to solicit candidates. First of all, current employees or previous personnel could be considered. Promotion from within is healthy for the practice. If this does occur, then the position to be filled becomes a lower-level job. In addition, the new employee is not as threatening to other staff and is less of a liability to the practice if there is unsatisfactory performance.

New applicants may be recruited through several sources. These include newspaper ads, local medical society references, hospital personnel files, and employment agencies. A typical newspaper ad could read as follows:

Medical receptionist for four-physician practice. Responsible for appointments and schedules, bookkeeping, and medical records. Five years' experience in medical or other professional practice preferred. Send typed resumé and salary history.

If you are seeking applicants for the initial staff of a new practice, it will be imperative to screen several candidates. Resumés may be screened prior to interviewing applicants to prevent meeting with people who are not qualified.

There are several points to review when screening resumés: responsibility in previous jobs; length of time since last full-time work; supervision; degree of flexibility in work; amount of money expected. Previewing resumés will help determine which people merit interviews and who are top candidates.

Interviewing

When several candidates (at least five) have been preselected, then interviews should be arranged. A suggested format would be to arrange all interviews within a one- or two-day period, allowing 30 minutes per interview, with 10 to 15 minutes between candidates. Applicants should be asked to complete a brief application form before the interview. Figure 5.1 is a typical employment application.

When planning for the all-important selection interview, the following guidelines may help develop a productive atmosphere.

Prepare for the Interview. A job description and personnel policies should be reviewed. Questions should be formulated from these items and the applicant's resumé. Candidates could also be asked to respond to a few situations which they may face in the position.

Develop Proper Climate. The applicant may be set at ease with a few general and cordial opening remarks. You may discern spontaneity by allowing the candidate to initiate the encounter. If the person is nervous, then there should be an effort to relieve anxiety by allowing the other person to speak in general terms.

Get Applicant to Talk. Use open-ended questions and probe general statements by the applicant. Seek clarification, i.e., "tell me what a typical day was like on your previous job?" "What specific things caused you problems, and when and how often did they occur?" Ask

for clarification of such statements as "I really like to work!"; "I enjoy being with patients!"; "I am not working for the money!"

Control the Interview. Utilize a structured format of questions, probes, and different topics to move the interview and seek information. Let the applicant know the interview plan. Avoid dominating the session with anecdotes and a history of the practice or self.

Listen and Observe. If the candidate is speaking, then it will be easier to listen and observe. Watch for nonverbal signs and side stepping when such topics arise as irregular work hours, performance standards, supervision, and patient care demands.

Record Pertinent Information. Taking notes during and immediately after the interview will help in assessing candidates. After several candidates it may be difficult to recall pertinent data.

Close the Interview. When there has been a suitable exchange of information and the interview has accomplished its purpose, terminate the encounter. A closing statement could be: "Is there any other important information I should be aware of before we conclude this interview?" or "During these last few minutes, what else is important for me to know about you?"

Figure 5.2 provides a list of questions to use as a guide in interviewing applicants. The importance of the position and qualifications of the candidate will determine the extent of use of the guide.

Discussion of Interview Guide.

1. What prompts you to consider leaving your present job?

This question may indicate driving ambition or chronic dissatisfaction. The response should indicate logic and realistic appraisal of career goals. The answer should not reflect a sour grapes attitude toward a past position or employer.

2. Describe for me, if you will, a typical day on your present or last job.

Figure 5.1   Employment Application Form

___

Name _____   Social Security No. _____

Address _____   Telephone Number_____

Date of Birth_____

Person to be notified in case of emergency _____
                                             (Name)   (Address)   (Telephone)

Employment History
(Most Recent Job First)

Company/Institution	Dates	Position	Salary/Wage	Supervision

Education Background
(Most Recent First)

Institution	Dates	Training/Major	Degree/Diploma	Advisor

Type of Position Desired? _____

Special Skills_____

Career Interests_____

Membership in professional organizations _____

_____

Achievements/Awards _____

_____

Professional references _____
                        (Name)   Address)   (Phone)   (Position)

                        _____
                        (Name)   (Address)   (Phone)   (Position)

Signature _____   Date _____

Work History
1. What prompts you to consider leaving your present job?
2. Describe for me, if you will, a typical day on your present or last job?
3. What particular part of your job did you like best?
4. How did you like working for your last employer?
5. How does the job for which you are applying relate to what you have done in the past?
6. If you could have changed things in your last job what would you have changed first?

Education
7. Why did you (did you not) go to college?
8. Why did you choose your major? Would you choose the same major today? Why?
9. What subjects in school were the hardest for you to master? What subjects were the easiest for you?

The Family
10. Is your family in good health? If there are any problems, who and what is involved?

Attitudes & Self Concept
11. Which of your previous bosses did you like most? Why?
12. Were you satisfied with the progress you made in your last job? Why?
13. What do you think has contributed most to the successes you have had?
14. What hobbies do you have? How do you spend your spare time?

Health
15. Do you have any health problems which could impede your work performance?

Sensitivity
16. What situations annoy you most?
17. What is your interpretation of success?
18. Why did you go into the type of work in which you have spent most of your time?

Self Evaluation
19. What might cause you to fail on the job we are discussing?
20. If you get this job, where do you see yourself in the future?
21. What additional information do you think that I should have about you?
22. Why do you want to work for our particular office? What do you know about our profession?
23. What do you consider to be your major strengths and weaknesses?

Figure 5.2 Interview Guide

The exaggerator or boaster will attempt to squeeze into a typical day's activity the functioning of an entire year. Relationships between individual and superior and/or peers will also reveal status within the organization and will verify responsibilities outlined on the application form.

3. What particular part of your job did you like best?
Analyze the response to see if it fits in with what duties might be in your office. If the job liked least will be present in the new job to a large degree, inquire as to how this will be dealt with.

4. How did you like working for your last employer?
Does the individual show respect and/or knowledge of past employer's problems, or is there an immature attitude toward normal practice inadequacies?

5. How does the job for which you are applying relate to what you have done in the past?
Each candidate will naturally try to slant experience to fit needs of the new job. It is the interviewer's task to sort out these skills acquired on past jobs and relate them to possible use in the new position. In the event that there are no related skills, the practice should view the individual as a trainee, regardless of age.

6. If you could have changed things in your last position, what would you have changed first?
This question may provide insight into the applicant's analytical skills. Discussion could include how to make recommendations and strive for improvements.

Education

7. Why did you (did you not) go to college?
Responses may indicate desires to further career and preferences for enhancing education and training.

8. Why did you choose your major or special field? Would you choose this again?
This may indicate which additional studies will be pursued to change careers. However, a positive response with self-satisfaction for the ma-

jor chosen may indicate a satisfied and well-adjusted individual.

9. What subjects in school were most difficult for you?
What subjects in school were the easiest for you?

An individual should not be placed on a job requiring skills where scholastic achievement in related subjects was admittedly low.

The Family

10. Is your family in good health? If there are any problems, who and what is involved?

A sick child or a chronically ill spouse may frequently cause absenteeism, as well as become a financial burden to the individual. A job problem may be in the offing if a candidate is in poor health.

Attitudes and Self Concept

11. Which of your previous bosses did you like most? Why?

It is quite human to respond to good treatment; be cautious of the person who discusses favorites. The candidate may respond only to acceptance but not to constructive criticism.

12. Were you satisfied with the progress you made in your last job? Why?

If the individual was satisfied, it could mean a mature appraisal of the situation. If not, was someone else blamed? If blame is placed on another, determine if it is biased reaction or realistic.

13. What do you think has contributed most to successes you have had?

It is true that "no man is an island" and no one has ever been successful completely because of oneself. Education, relatives, economic conditions, and many other variables enter into any success.

14. What hobbies do you have? How do you spend your spare time?

The answer here can corroborate the answer to extracurricular interests. It can also indicate whether the candidate is people-centered or self-focused.

Health

15. Do you have any health problems which would impede your work performance?

This question should determine interests in personal health and whether health maintenance is followed. In addition, the response to this question will enable the interviewer to find out if the applicant has a chronic condition which may require regular attention. Further, it may indicate a situation which would incur a financial drain upon the individual. Too much concern about finances and/or health can certainly affect work performance.

Sensitivity

16. What situations annoy you most?

This question may indicate a lack of tolerance for getting along with certain kinds of people. It may, in fact, exhibit a prejudice which could be extremely unfortunate in working with certain office personnel, patients, and physicians.

17. What is your interpretation of success?

If the answer is out of proportion to reasonable expectations, the person may never be satisfied and may affect motivation of other office personnel.

18. Why did you go into the type of work in which you have spent most of your time?

This question may indicate motivation, dedication, and commitment to both the health care profession and specific areas of expertise.

Self-Evaluation

19. What might cause you to fail on the job we are discussing?

If you detect a good deal of anxiety and if it is stronger than the reasons for anticipating success, attitude must be seriously questioned.

20. If you get this job, where do you see yourself in the future?

A sense of future and career can be discussed even at the lowest level of skill or competence. One should look for realistic answers to this question, although enthusiastic ambition is certainly more desirable than no ambition at all.

21. What additional information do you think that I should have about you?

The person may have been saving a bit of information for the last. At this point, for example, you might find out that your applicant has a unique talent or interest or has a desire for an innovative facet of medical practice.

22. Why do you want to work for our practice? What do you know about the health care profession?

These two questions usually go together. Has there already developed an identification with your practice or profession or is this just a shotgun approach to getting a job?

23. What do you consider to be your major strengths and weaknesses?

Responses should be judged on candor and insight. How objective are strengths presented and to what degree have weaknesses been converted to opportunities for growth. It may also be helpful to seek information about how strengths and weaknesses have been discovered or determined.

Selection

Most office positions require skills which can be evaluated or tested. A typed resumé, handwritten application, verbal communication, and personal demeanor during the interview may help assess skills. Spontaneous responses to problems and office situations may indicate levels of maturity and decision making. A typing test or a transcription test may also provide selection data.

Several factors which could be incorporated into final selection of a candidate include: use of office personnel in the interviewing process; objectifying selection by listing strengths and weaknesses of each applicant; second interviews for the top two or three candidates; checking employment references and seeking information from previous supervisors; discussion of wages, benefits, and future compensation; presentation of office manual and job description; establishment of a probationary period of one to three months; and a general agreement among partners about the candidate.

Contracting

Whether or not there is a formal employment contract, a contractual process should be initi-

ated. Key elements in this process would be mutual understanding, with verbal and written communication of performance expectations; commitment by employer to develop an orientation and training program tailored to employee's needs; commitment by employee to share anxieties, frustrations, as well as satisfactions of the new experience; and definite dates for progress reports and evaluation.

Training

Initial work experiences often cause new employees to feel insecure and intimidated. This is usually coupled with feelings of envy, confusion, and threat by existing office staff. There should be every effort to recognize needs of new and experienced employees and address these during training.

Performance File

During the first days of employment, a formal interview should be arranged between the new staff member and his or her immediate supervisor. This session could include: discussion of job description with particular emphasis upon skills and attitudes and early results expected; presentation of office manual and personnel policies with review of such issues as dress code, working hours, benefit stipulations, office routines and schedules; discussion of supervision and office relationships; and methods for evaluating performance and mutual feedback opportunities. The essence of this session should be written and placed in a personal file to which the employee has access.

The performance file should also contain employee's resumé, application, and job description. Throughout employment it will be imperative to document performance, both positive and negative. Doctors and supervisors should make special effort to recognize work of their staff and record significant events. Documentation will serve as a useful tool for decisions regarding merit increases, bonuses, promotions, as well as actions such as warnings, probation, and termination. It will be essential to have such data if there is a rebuttal from an employee regarding negative feedback or disciplinary action. To avoid undesirable publicity and long hours of guesswork, objectify and document each critical incident. Just as accurate medical records are the key to quality health care, conclusive employment records are an aid to effective employer-employee relationships.

Training Activities

Depending upon time constraints and work demands, a variety of activities should be considered for the training period. These could include:

1. Several days of observation of primary tasks and related tasks which affect the position
2. A learn-by-doing time with daily and weekly feedback
3. Learning resources and materials for at-work and take-home reference
4. Job rotations in work areas which precede and follow the work of the new employee
5. Schedule review sessions with employees' needs and performance being discussed
6. Time for the new employee to assess the practice and relationships
7. A written statement by the new employee which indicates goals, expectations, strengths, and areas for growth

It will be important to set a date for training to end. A reasonable time would be three to six months. Caution should be exercised not to end training too soon or prolong it because the employee is not meeting expectations.

Training activities may take a toll upon office staff, supervisor, doctors, and patients unless a plan is developed. This plan could use outside resources, such as local telephone company, hospital personnel, and community-based education programs. In addition, all office staff may participate in orienting new employees. Both approaches will broaden employees' perspective and enhance appreciation of the scope of the practice. Table 5.3 is an overview of a training plan for an office nurse.

Performance Appraisal

The recruitment, selection, and training of employees are the foundation of personnel management. Within the first three months, a performance appraisal system should be instituted

Table 5.3 Training Plan for Office Nurse

Weeks 1–2	• Meet with supervisor • Observe nursing routines, appointment receptionist, and laboratory technologist • Review medical records and telephone messages • Work with doctors during routine patient visits • Meet with supervisor
Weeks 3–4	• Observe business functions and assist in filing laboratory and medical reports • Begin patient work-ups, screening routines, and laboratory procedures • Attend hospital/community/education programs on patient education, CPR, X ray, medical ethics, etc. • Meet with supervisor
Weeks 5–6	• Rotate through all office functions, at least ½ day with each employee • Work with all doctors, at least 1 day • Attend medical conferences in hospital • Meet with supervisor
Weeks 7–8	• Perform daily work routines as written in job description • Present formal write-up on goals, expectations, strengths, and areas of growth • Meet with supervisor
Weeks 9–12	• Revisit activities and functions in weeks 1–4 • Perform daily work routines • Develop special interests agenda; i.e., patient education, counseling chronic disease patients, etc. • Conclude training phase with formal interview

Training activities should facilitate the early development of the new employee. Be careful that they do not wear down the person or create an unrealistic image of the forthcoming responsibilities.

as the personnel "maintenance" function. Performance appraisal is the heart of personnel management because it serves as a support system for both the management of the organization and the employees. It is the mechanism by which supervisors inform their subordinates of job expectations, accomplishments, changes in responsibilities, and areas for improvement. It provides employees the opportunity to discuss their satisfactions and dissatisfactions and to explore issues regarding future roles and responsibilities.

The essence of performance appraisal is the comparison of actual performance with prestated goals and job expectations. A performance appraisal cannot begin until the employee has been on the job a period of time, working under a clear set of guidelines and responsibilities. The first appraisal should probably occur within a few months, to ensure that the employee has a clear understanding of the job and that the employee's skills do match the demands of the work. Before the end of the first year, a formal evaluation of the employee's work, followed by an appraisal interview, should be conducted. Integral to the performance appraisal system is an employee's performance file. The file should be established during the selection process and thereafter serves as a performance documentation folder.

Self-Appraisal

Prior to each appraisal interview, employees should be asked to appraise their own performance. This process helps to set the stage and indicates that employee views and needs will be incorporated into the appraisal. The following are some questions which may guide an employee's thinking about performance, progress, and plans for the future.

What do you consider to be the most important abilities which your job requires?

What are some aspects of your job that you enjoy? Do not enjoy?

In what ways does your supervisor help you in your work?

In what aspects of your work do you need additional training?

What have been your major accomplishments this year?

What changes would you recommend to increase your effectiveness?

Do you have any suggestions that could help improve the organization?

Are all your capabilities being used in this position?

Are you interested in assuming more responsibilities?

What are your long-range plans? What type of work or position would you like to have five years from now?

These questions should be posed to the employee before the interview, and, if possible, written responses should be obtained. The in-formation given on the self-appraisal could be used to open discussion during the interview.

The Appraisal Interview

Mahler (1976) offers six suggestions for conducting the performance interview: (1) coach on results, (2) get down to cases, (3) determine causes, (4) make it a two-way process, (5) set up an action plan, (6) provide motivation.

Coach on Results: Have employees state their understanding of the goals and expectations and define the results. Determine how the results met the prestated objectives. If a variance occurred then decide if the deviation was outside an acceptable limit. The key is to attack the variance and not the person.

Get Down to Cases. Avoid generalizations and undocumented references. Identify specific responsibilities and performance. Cite data. Provide examples or incidents. Whether giving positive or critical feedback, the employee wants to know precisely what issues are being discussed.

Determine Causes. When variances or discrepancies are noted, then the focus should be on the causes, so that problem solving can begin. Employees should be asked to identify possible causes. Do not dwell on the past, but move to suggestions to improve the situation.

Make the Appraisal Two-Way. A joint problem-solving process requires a two-way dialogue. Using the self-appraisal responses and asking nonjudgmental questions may ensure that the employee's opinions are being considered. When any actions are proposed, it will be important to hear the employee's point of view.

Set Up an Action Plan. Deciding on an action plan moves the discussion from past to future. An action plan should include very specific suggestions, no more than one or two per issue, and a method for follow-up. All action plans and follow-up methods should be written into the summary report of the interview.

Provide Motivation. At the conclusion of the interview the supervisor should stress the employee's strengths and the benefits the employee will receive by achieving the de-

Figure 5.3

<u>EMPLOYEE PERFORMANCE REVIEW</u>

(Complete in duplicate. One copy to employee, one for personnel records.)

NAME _____ DATE OF REVIEW _____

JOB TITLE _____ FULL TIME/PART TIME _____

<u>BACKGROUND INFORMATION</u> (from personnel records)

Length of employment _____ Date of last review _____

Current pay rate or step-in-grade _____

Summary of attendance record _____

_____

<u>EMPLOYEE INFORMATION</u> (to be completed by employee)

List skills acquired or upgraded since last review _____

_____

Applicable continuing education _____

_____

What do you consider your contributions to this office? _____

_____

Comments _____

_____

<u>OBSERVATIONS OF EMPLOYEE</u>   OBSERVATIONS MADE BY _____

Attitude, ability to work with others _____

_____

Observed employee strengths/weaknesses on job _____

_____

Comments _____

_____

_____

Form 9875 Colwell Co., Champaign, Illinois

Figure 5.3 *Continued*

SKILLS REVIEW: Review Conducted By: _____

(List to be taken from   **CODE:**   NI = needs improvement   A = acceptable
job description)   I = improved   O = outstanding

SKILL	CODE		SKILL	CODE

COMMENTS ON SKILLS REVIEW & EVALUATION: _____

_____

_____

RECOMMENDED ACTION: _____

_____

EVALUATION REVIEWED BY:

_____   _____   _____
          employee's signature   date   reviewer's signature

sired results. Emphasis should be placed on progress, achievements, improvement, and success. The attitude and behavior of the supervisor will influence how the employee leaves the appraisal interview.

Figure 5.3 is an example of an employee performance review form which could be completed and distributed to the employee at the conclusion of the interview.

Office Supervision

Supervision is inherent in the execution of a productive organization. When people are assigned duties and responsibilities with definable outcomes, then supervision is necessary. There are several functions which supervision must serve—selection and training, coordinating work routines, performance assessment and evaluation, intraoffice communications, and result analysis and reporting.

The office supervisor must possess credentials as both a health care practitioner and manager of people. These qualifications may be obtained either through formal training or experience. Respect will occur only if expertise is apparent to those being directed. Authority can be granted, but trust and respect must be earned and maintained.

Specific responsibilities which could be assumed by an office supervisor include: scheduling and prioritizing all employees' work assignments and daily routines; maintaining employment records, vacations, benefits, sick leave, etc.; establishing inventory control and ordering supplies; conducting staff meetings, coordinating doctors' schedules with paramedical staff; preparing administrative and financial reports of daily productivity, eg, patient visits, office collection rate, billing and insurance logs; reviewing budgets and expense statements; conducting individual performance appraisal sessions and maintaining personnel files; developing liaison relationships with medical, business, and community organizations; and designing patient-flow and paper-flow systems.

Office supervisors will face several challenges. They must avoid the pitfalls of "protecting the doctors" and thus rewarding physicians' negative behaviors by overlooking inefficien-

Title—Office Supervisor

Summary of Position
Directs the work of all paramedical staff, consisting of nursing, business, clerical, and secretarial staff. Participates in planning and decision-making with medical director.

Duties
Initiates recruiting and selection of new personnel; trains and retrains staff; establishes task assignments and prioritizes workload; conducts semi-annual performance appraisal sessions with each employee; moderates weekly and monthly staff meetings; participates in each work area on a periodic basis; presents a monthly administrative analysis of patient volume, financial productivity, and expenditures; maintains inventory of all supplies and equipment and prepares a replenish plan with vendors; oversees billing and collections and corresponds with each delinquent account; recommends accounts to be written off or turned over to collection agency; meets with patients who request to discuss policies, financial problems, or dissatisfaction with services; maintains all payroll and employment records of personnel.

Knowledge and Skills
Minimum five years in medical/health care facility, preferably physician's office with some supervisory experience. Bachelor's or Associate degree desired.

Requires skills in 1) selecting and training nursing and business staff; 2) organizing and evaluating work assignments; 3) financial analysis and reporting; 4) communication with patients, physicians, and community agencies; 5) capability to fill in at any job in the practice.

Accountability
Responsible for implementing policies and procedures in the office manual; identifying problems and meeting with practitioners to determine appropriate strategies; monthly reports to entire physician group, and weekly meetings with Medical Director; reports will include collection ratio—total and in-office, third party payback periods, expenses—actual vs. budget, demographic data, and other pertinent information for analysis and decision-making; recommends salary increments and bonuses for office staff.

Supervision
Immediate supervisor is Medical director, who is a selected representative of doctors. Must meet with approval of all doctors to receive increases in compensation and to continue in good standing as an employee of the practice.

Figure 5.4 Office Supervisor Job Description

cies, which may be unknown. They must also be wary of office staff who are constantly referring to patients as the problem. Patients are clients and must always be in the forefront of service. Patients will want a voice and deserve to be heard. The practice will also become prey to pharmaceutical sales reps, medical supply dealers, insurance and investment representatives, community agencies, governmental officials, and other well-meaning figures. An effective means for meeting these challenges is anticipation and preparation. Office policy statements for interoffice activities is as important as the intraoffice manual.

Figure 5.4 presents a detailed job description for an office supervisor. Middle-management positions are instrumental for organizational growth. Chapter 6 contains several sections which have application to those with supervisory responsibilities.

STAFFING POSITIONS

Several critical positions require full- or part-time employees. These include receptionist, nurse, secretary, business clerk, laboratory technician. Depending on practice size and volume, one or more people may be needed in these positions.

Reception

Office receptionists will be involved in several practice functions encompassing specific areas of responsibility: patient contact, finance, scheduling, medical records, and clerical work.

Patient contact occurs through face-to-face and telephone communications. Both types of encounters are demanding and necessitate specific skills. When patients visit the office, they deserve cordiality and sensitivity. Many bring emotional concerns with their physical ills, and thus the entire practice may become a therapeutic agent. Telephone conversations require a willingness to listen and convey a supportive tone. During all patient interaction, receptionists must recognize and respond to anxiety without overreacting. In addition, there will be many times when they must be willing to con-

sole, guide, comfort, and reassure in a sensitive and understanding manner.

Financial responsibilities of the receptionist will include asking for and receiving payment for services, recording transactions, daily accountability of funds, bank deposits and receipts, posting and tabulating ledgers, and other miscellaneous money management. Qualities necessary are honesty, accuracy, thoroughness, and dedication.

Scheduling is one of the most frustrating tasks of a receptionist. Appointments begin the patient flow system and will dictate efficiency and perhaps even quality of care. Time use for doctors, nurses, and other staff can be maximized by efficient scheduling. Every physician and staff member should have a daily schedule. The receptionist should be central to this process so that at least one person is knowledgeable of time commitments and constraints.

Medical records are the lifeblood of the practice. This information system must be developed and maintained with the utmost organization. It should be accessible by many, controlled by a few.

Clerical and filing duties will be instrumental for office efficiency. There will be periods of high volume and demanding workloads. It is imperative that forms, records, and other office systems are in order. They should be assessible for all personnel with a comprehensible coding or interpretation system.

Nursing

Nursing functions may include several features, such as screening examinations, history taking, drawing specimens, laboratory analysis, conducting diagnostic tests, acute care of trauma, nutrition and diet therapy, assistance in minor surgery and other treatment procedures, and various forms of patient education and counseling.

Nursing responsibilities may be assigned to RNs, LPNs, certified medical assistants, physician's assistants, or trained medical assistants. The mix of full-time and part-time staff will depend upon patient volume, type of health care problems, and preferences of physicians.

Clinical responsibilities will involve preparation of patients during office visits and assistance to family members before, during, and after doctor visits. There will be a variety of technical procedures including injections, first aid, emergency treatments, collection and handling of specimens, EKG and x-ray procedures, sterilization of instruments, and maintaining diagnostic equipment. In addition, nursing staff will be responsible for restocking supplies and instruments which are required for routine and special procedures. They should possess a general knowledge of microbiology—smears, cultures, immunology—and pharmacology—drug reactions, medication dosages, counteracting drugs, cardiopulmonary resuscitation, neurological exam, allergy injections and skin tests, spinometry, and vision and hearing tests.

When the physician is comfortable delegating and supervising, there will be many roles the nurse may assume. Patients are often receptive to nurse interaction and are accepting of the expansion of responsibilities under physicians' directions. Domains open for nursing involvement include hospital, nursing home, patient's home, community agencies, schools, chronic disease education and follow-up, pre and postnatal care, well-child examinations, and individual and group counseling. Nursing serves a support role to patients, physicians, and other staff members. Thus, there must be a high degree of ethical behavior, with extreme caution to respect confidentiality and privacy of the doctor-patient relationship.

Business

A business staff position may be necessary as the practice increases in patient and financial volume. A full-time or part-time position could be considered when there is substantial daily or weekly workloads which have significant impact upon cash flow.

Many physicians are deceived in thinking that receptionists or nurses can perform all business aspects. Business skills and knowledge are distinct, and receptionists and nurses may not have the same motivation to complete these tasks as a person with specialized training.

Responsibilities which may be delegated to a business staff person could include inventory control, third-party forms, workers' compensa-tion, medicare and medicaid procedures and statements, collection phone calls and letters, accounts receivable and delinquent accounts, follow-up on no-shows, evaluating automated systems, updating fee structure, preparing checks for payments of invoices, and maintaining an expense and budget report. This last function could provide regular productivity summaries and financial reports.

Expertise includes knowledge of bookkeeping systems and financial analysis, ability to work with accountants and other money-management consultants, and management of relationships with financial and governmental institutions. Attitudes which will be important include tact, organization, thoroughness, and accuracy.

Productivity reports which should be an integral part of business analysis include: daily collections and patient volume; daily reports of receipts from office, billing, and third parties, weekly reports of no-shows, insurance forms, collection calls, and letters; monthly charges and receipts—outpatient, inpatient, and other categories; patient volume by physician; expenses by major classification salaries; benefits, office supplies, medical supplies, utilities, and overhead; and average receipts and costs per patient visit.

Secretarial

A practice with two or more doctors and more than five paramedical staff may need secretarial assistance. This function will be responsible for correspondence, transcription, scheduling, filing, and arranging travel and other professional commitments. If one or more of the doctors has a leadership position in the hospital or a community agency, then secretarial assistance will be extremely valuable and may even be funded by the respective institution. Secretarial responsibilities should be integrated into all aspects of the practice so that this role does not appear separate from other office staff.

Secretarial work activities include: maintaining a calendar of activities and meetings for nonpatient care events for each doctor and the practice in general; receiving all incoming communication and correspondence, and effectively dispensing such; typing letters, papers, reports for medical, administrative, and educational matters; initiating all travel arrangements from transportation and hotel reservations to itinerary and preparatory and follow-up correspondence; and implementing a filing and classification system for all documents and records of the practice. Since most of the physician and staff time will be centered around patient care, the secretarial position will need to maintain the organizational system in a friendly and cooperative atmosphere.

Laboratory

A group practice may generate a large enough volume of medical procedures and tests to justify a laboratory specialist. This person could offer: better quality control; patient, staff, and physician education; and maintenance of the costly equipment. If the office practice is performing a high volume of lab tests, x-rays, and other medical procedures, then care should be taken to employ a certified staff and to closely adhere to professional standards and regulations.

PERFORMANCE PROBLEMS

Performance problems are inherent in personnel management, no matter what the nature of the business. Three personnel issues which affect office productivity are: (1) establishing a hierarchy of authority and supervision which facilitates work relationships; (2) determining whether a performance discrepancy is the individual's responsibility or a symptom of a broader problem; and (3) disciplining and terminating an employee without destroying morale and breaking down trust.

Authority and Supervision

Office efficiency and working relationships are often adversely affected by either nonexistent or unclear delegation of responsibility and supervision. Physicians as a group have been characterized as obsessive, compulsive with high control needs. These qualities are valuable when completing tasks as individuals. However, when faced with motivation of patients and office staff, these traits are counterproductive.

Practitioners must select people whom they will trust and then alter their role as sole performer to trainer and facilitator. Many performance problems may be eliminated by choosing the right supervisory person and matching capabilities with work expectations and/or preparing a thorough program for orientation and training, so that the supervisor and staff are aware of responsibilities and desired results.

The middle-management personnel of an organization is crucial, since they interface with both staff and physicians. They must have respect from subordinates and confidence of superiors. If a supervisory staff is employed, it will be imperative to keep this group well-informed and provide adequate authority to execute decisions. Areas of responsibility which require appropriate delegation of authority include: determining individual staff members' work schedules; training new employees; implementing predetermined practice policies; ordering supplies; resolving staff working relationship conflicts; communicating new policies and procedures and assessing reactions; and interfacing with selected individuals outside the practice, i.e., drug representatives, sales reps, and community officials.

When these responsibilities have been delegated, a feedback and report system can be established so that physicians are informed of performance and results. Potential situations which may indicate a breakdown in delegation and/or supervision are: (1) office manager's inability to direct work because physicians are circumventing procedures regarding schedule changes, personal practice preferences, or dissatisfactions; (2) backlogs of work are mounting in the business and clerical area because there has not been delegation to one primary individual for results; and (3) patients' complaints are not being resolved because no one appears willing to provide recommendations.

Effective managers of office practice must become skillful at seeing initial happenings and reactions and obtaining background information before arriving at decisions or solutions.

Physicians must also be prepared to accept some of the responsibility for causing the problems and be willing to acknowledge their inadequacies, if appropriate.

Performance Discrepancy

When a staff member is performing in a manner which is either unproductive or counterproductive, an assessment of the discrepancy should begin. Mager and Pipe (1973) suggest consideration of two basic performance issues: Is it skill deficiency or attitudinal deficiency? If the problem can be directed to one of these two categories, then a plan may be prepared.

Skill Deficiency. Skill deficiencies may occur when there has been inadequate training or if the work has been recently changed or modified. There may not have been an appropriate match of the employee's talents to the demands of the job, or the employee may have been overly optimistic of his or her capabilities. Key questions to be raised in assessing the skill deficiency would be: Is retraining a possibility? How often is the skill needed? Can the work be modified? Can the individual perform at desired expectations?

If it appears that skill deficiency can be resolved, then a plan may be developed. Discuss work requirements and expectations with the employee and seek mutual understanding of results. Arrange for additional training with particular emphasis upon needed skills. Provide immediate feedback when this skill is performed. Document this assessment process in the event that suggested improvements do not result.

Attitudinal Deficiency. If it appears that the staff member has the ability to perform satisfactorily and training was adequate, then the problem may be attitudinal. This is a more involved performance discrepancy and requires thorough investigation.

Attitudinal problems may be assessed by posing the following questions. Are consequences for poor performance being enforced? Is good performance being punished? Is nonperformance being rewarded? Does performance really matter—how much positive reinforcement? Examples may help illustrate these points. Good performance is often punished by giving the extra work and additional responsibilities to high achievers and thus rewarding staff or physicians who have not assumed their commitments. Nonperformers may be rewarded in the case of the receptionist who keeps the schedules light so that the work day will not be hectic or physicians who will not complain about problem patients. Positive reinforcement may break down if physicians or office supervisors do not personally acknowledge good work.

If the attitudinal deficiency becomes paramount then the following format could be considered: obtain information from several sources; reconsider consequences of performance and nonperformance; cordially discuss situation with employee; develop a specific plan for accomplishing results; document interviews because there is a high probability of repetition and/or further discrepancies.

Discipline and Termination

One of the most difficult situations which managers and supervisors face is the disciplining of subordinates. There is no patented approach for this process. Each situation and employee is unique. Preparation can only be undertaken in a preventive sense or through a well-organized and -maintained performance appraisal system.

Discipline. Assuming that an appropriate process was established to determine the nature of the performance discrepancy, and that it appears there is little recourse but to begin a disciplinary procedure, the following should be considered.

Accumulate all available data in written form and present it personally. Conduct a formal interview and state the disciplinary steps which will be taken. This could involve days, weeks, or months to change behavior or learn the appropriate skills. Establish a series of progress points within the time frame. Prepare a written statement from this meeting and have the employee sign it. It may even be appropriate to have the employee write up his or her reactions to the session and a plan for change. Specific elements of the disciplinary procedure should be confidential, except where it directly affects another staff member. At the specified intervals, follow-up sessions should be conducted and formally documented in the same format as previously described.

Termination. When termination appears imminent, then the probationary period should be concluded. If skill deficiency is the ultimate cause of termination, then there should be documentation of the qualities and talents which were *not* satisfactorily demonstrated. Employees could be encouraged to seek employment opportunities where their qualifications could be better utilized. It is not uncommon for employees to come to an understanding that the demands and the multifaceted duties of a busy medical practice exceed their capabilities.

If an attitudinal deficiency is causing the performance discrepancy, then termination may be considered, with arbitrators available should sessions become emotional. Attitudinal issues will often be contaminated by denial and rationalization. There may be adequate skills to complete the tasks, but interpersonal relations and work conditions of other employees are adversely affected.

CONCLUSION

Personnel management is both a discipline within the academic realm of business administration and a departmental function within industry and government. The purpose of this chapter was to highlight the essential elements so that practicing physicians may understand their responsibilities as personnel managers. This aspect of medical practice management does not have to remain a perplexing dilemma if office practitioners and their supervisors will undertake to: (1) plan and commit themselves to personnel policies; (2) approach each employee as a separate member of the organization, possessing motivation and growth needs; and (3) delegate responsibilities and remain available for feedback and evaluation of results.

Physicians will find trained specialists and extensive references available as they execute personnel management responsibilities. Such issues as recruiting, training, selecting a supervisor, performance appraisal, discipline, and termination may benefit from consultation.

The results of effective personnel management will be obvious. Morale will be high, patients will comment upon the positive atmosphere in the office, work will be completed regardless of the seasonal demands, and, most important, physicians and office personnel will have ample time to devote to family and personal interests.

References

A physician's problem that's strictly personnel. *Physician's Management,* May 1978, pp 21–25.

Avoid these pitfalls in hiring discrimination. *Physician's Management,* March 1977, pp 43–48.

Balinsky B: *The Selection Interview: Essentials for Management.* New Rochelle, NY, Martin M. Bruce, 1962.

Broadwell M: *The Supervisor as Instructor.* Reading, Mass, Addison-Wesley, 1970.

Bucks A: Performance appraisal: Evaluating the evaluation. *Health Care Supervisor* 3, no. 4 (July 1985): pp. 17–30.

Center for Research in Ambulatory Health Care: *Organization and Development of a Medical Group Practice.* Cambridge, Mass., 1976.

Kach PA: The how and why of job descriptions. *Medical Record News,* October 1973, pp 38–40.

Leaverton LE: Personnel policies for the medical office. *Journal of Iowa Medical Society,* December 1969, pp 1119–1120.

Levoy RP: 14 keys to close harmony with your staff. *Group Practice,* March 1973, pp 7–10.

McConnell C: Finding the new supervisor: Inside or outside? *Health Care Supervisor* 3, no. 1 (October 1984): pp. 69–79.

Mager RF, Pipe P: *Analyzing Performance Problems, or You Really Oughta Wanna.* Belmont, Calif, Lear Siegler, Fearon Publishers, 1973.

Missildine H: Planned interviews key to successful hiring. *Physician's Management,* August 1973, pp 70–76.

Simpson D: The performance appraisal interview: Putting it all together. *Health Care Supervisor* 3, no. 2 (January 1985): pp. 63–76.

Smith HP, Brouwer PJ: *Performance Appraisal and Human Development*. Reading, Mass, Addison-Wesley, 1977.

Taylor RB: A certified medical assistant: The best all-round aide you can hire. *Physician's Management,* April 1977, pp 62–64.

Thompson J: The professional way to dismiss an employee. *Physician's Management,* May 1978, pp 27–30.

6

Leadership in Medical Practice

- **What are the formal and informal elements of an organization?**
- **How do core dimensions of motivation apply to the supervision of office personnel?**
- **What style of leadership do you possess? What detracts from effective leadership?**

- **What are the essentials of efficient use of time?**
- **How can one prepare to manage change and conflict?**
- **What are the unique aspects of leadership of professionals?**

Physicians have achieved many successes prior to their emergence into the private practice domain. Throughout medical school and residency training they have exemplified shrewd judgments and keen decision making. They have studied and worked with learned and skillful teachers. However, the realization that this preparation may not completely suffice will become evident. The roles of manager and leader are bestowed upon the physician regardless of personal preferences. Thus a new body of knowledge and array of skills must be included in the physician's armamenterium of talents.

Management is both a science and art. The scientific base is rapidly developing as research into the organizational and human relations aspects provides a fund of information which explains, analyzes, and even predicts the process of working with and through others toward the accomplishments of predetermined goals and objectives. The art of management, which is characterized by the ability to execute the knowledge and motivate people, has been pre-

sented through the successes of leaders in various organizations and institutions.

This chapter draws upon traditional and contemporary views of management and leadership, with particular emphasis toward an application for medical practice. Both physicians and their supervisors may benefit from this discourse. Subjects which are addressed include: organizational structure, motivation, management models, practice leadership functions, time management, and change and conflict. These issues are presented to enable physicians and supervisors to better understand the workings of their respective practices and perhaps develop strategies for more effective problem solving and decision making.

ORGANIZATIONAL STRUCTURE AND DYNAMICS

Office practitioners will be faced with the challenge of organizing and administrating in the same fashion as leaders in the industrial world.

Managerial expertise may be attained by understanding basic principles of organizational theory and applying these to the medical practice.

Classical authors described the formal features of organization based upon a bureaucratic framework, whereas contemporary organizational research has identified the informal dimension. The formal structure is described in organization charts, policy manuals, job descriptions, and work schedules. The informal organization has its impact at an interpersonal level and often influences quality of performance within the formal system. In comparing medical practices which may have a similar number of physicians and staff and comparable facilities and patient care responsibilities, it is not uncommon to find that office milieu may be decidedly different because of the informal organization.

Formal Organization

Argyris's (1957) analysis depicts the relative differences between the formal and informal workings of an organization. Characteristics of the formal organization are described in the following paragraphs.

Specialization. This characteristic is often referred to as division of labor. Tasks which are essential for patient care, ie, nursing, laboratory, and x-ray, and business operations, ie, reception, billing, and clerical, are delineated so that one individual has primary responsibility for their accomplishment. The advantage is that office personnel may become expert in their respective work and will feel responsible for performance. Concentrating efforts on a limited endeavor will increase quality and quantity of output.

Hierarchy. A second characteristic which is formalized in organizations is the chain of command. Positions of authority and responsibility are arranged in a hierarchy of importance. Authority emanates from the top and is justified because of expert knowledge, status, or credentials. It is posited that organizational efficiency will result if authority and responsibility is established on a vertical plane. Physicians and more highly trained paramedical staff are asked

to assume their appropriate roles as managers of the office organization.

Uniformity. Another characteristic involves the implementation of policies and standards in a consistent manner. The practice must have a high degree of predictability so that physicians, staff, and patients may understand the purpose and function appropriately. This concept could be applied by developing patient care protocols, employee policies, and financial guidelines.

Unity of Command. Each participant in the organization should be responsible to, and receive directions from, a supervisor. This principle is especially important when training, performance appraisal, and disciplinary actions are taking place. Employees deserve direct communication and feedback. Regardless of the size of the practice, all staff members should have an immediate supervisor who understands their work and assists them directly. In addition, when decisions or policies are made, it is imperative that the immediate supervisor be informed and allowed to implement them.

Span of Control. Administrative effectiveness is increased if a leader's span of control is limited to a few subordinates: fewer than six is preferable. This will provide for the establishment of working subgroups and shorter lines of communication. If possible these subgroups could be developed within office functions, ie, clerical staff, nursing, secretarial.

Delegation. An essential organizational precept is that authority should equal responsibility. This implies that when a colleague or employee is delegated a responsibility, then the appropriate level of authority should be granted to accomplish the task. Authority delegation occurs when the subordinate has some control over financial resources or other personnel and can represent the organization in a decision-making situation.

Practicing physicians will build a formal organization by developing policies and procedures, establishing levels of supervision, and implementing practice routines and tasks. These structural components will not ensure organizational effectiveness, but management cannot begin without them.

Informal Organization

The formal aspects of organization proved quite reliable for explaining and predicting success during the earliest years of our economy. Traditional institutions were normally autocratic, and employees were content in a more subservient role. However, as societies' needs changed, competition for both material and human resources intensified, and another element of organizational systems became quite evident. The behavioral and interpersonal feature was discovered, and the informal organization evolved from the social interaction among personnel.

Flippo (1970) presents the essentials for an informal organization: small group process, unofficial leaders, gratification of members' needs, and a grapevine of communication that reaches throughout the organization. Longest (1976) further describes this phenomenon by stating that membership in the informal organization strongly influences performance and relationships and that consequences of the informal network may be positive as well as negative. Leaders need not fear the interpersonal element, but they must recognize it and appreciate its impact upon the organization.

Impact of the informal work group upon a medical practice may be seen when a new person is added to staff or when a change in supervision occurs. If the informal organization is cooperative and not threatened, then efficiency is maintained. However, if even the least of changes is resisted or appears inappropriately disruptive, then an informal organization may become a barrier. Other indications that an informal organization may be at odds with the authority may be seen in the following ways: little or no candid discussion in office meetings, reluctance of staff to become self-directed or engaged in planning or problem solving, rebuttals that the work was not clearly defined or that "no one told us," higher turnover at the supervisory level than staff level, and an inordinate amount of time interpreting policies and procedures. Each of these issues may be justified on occasion. However, if the result is disruptive and nonproductive happenings, then the interpersonal dimension must be investigated.

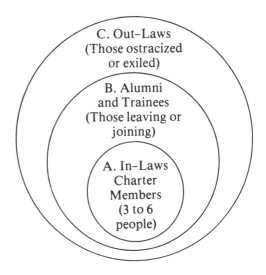

A. Primary Members

B. Auxiliary Members

C. Nonmembers

Figure 6.1 Levels of Membership in Informal Organization

Regardless of the design or sophistication of the formal structure, the informal organization will most probably have the greatest influence upon the ultimate success of the practice. Figure 6.1 diagrams three levels of membership found in the informal organization.

MOTIVATION

A most difficult managerial task is to foster a high level of motivation among office personnel. The newness of any work will cease, and mundane features will become inevitable. Maintaining morale and productivity will be the challenge for physicians and their office supervisors.

Considerable literature has been directed toward motivation and interpersonal strategies which enhance working conditions. Theories of several authors are presented here to increase awareness of motivational concepts and their application for the medical office practice.

Job Enrichment

Hackman and Oldham (1974) analyzed the concept of job enrichment. Their research uncovered six core dimensions which may enhance work satisfaction. Figure 6.2 shows the integration of these core job dimensions with psychological states and outcome results.

Skill Variety. Utilization of different skills will have an impact upon motivation. People accrue a variety of interests and capabilities, and they are normally very receptive to expansion of responsibilities. This motivational element does not imply that work should be constantly shifted or that expertise should not be fostered. However, when a set of tasks has been executed skillfully then the employee may be offered opportunity to take on new projects and responsibilities. Nursing tasks may be expanded to include brief history taking, preliminary examinations, and participation in follow-up care of chronically ill patients. A receptionist may become involved in patient education.

Task Identity. When an employee has developed an understanding of responsibility in medical practice, the need to undertake an identifiable task from start to finish will surface. We have often heard our children say, "Let *me* try it now!" When staff indicate such readiness, it is appropriate to provide them the opportunity to assume responsibility for initiation and completion of a routine or a set of tasks. For example, nurses may wish to greet patients in the reception area, begin preliminary screening and assist during physician encounters, then return with patients to the receptionist. Business staff may become proficient at working with accounts from the initial charge, through billing and insurance form preparation, to collection of payments. These start-to-finish tasks also provide data for subsequent problem solving.

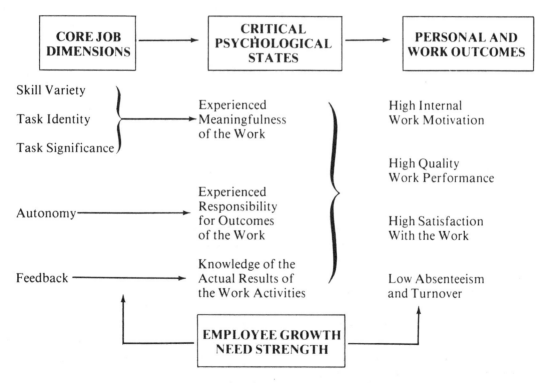

Figure 6.2 The Relationships Among the Core Job Dimensions, the Critical Psychological States, and On-the-Job Outcomes *Source*: Hackman & Oldman, "A New Strategy for Job Enrichment," Technical Report #3, Department of Administrative Science, Yale University, May, 1974.

Task Significance. Medical practice offers the challenge of working in a setting which directly affects the quality of life. All staff members deserve an opportunity to sense the importance of their work upon the lives of others. Physicians can incorporate this dimension by sharing results of treatment plans and allowing staff more involvement in patient care. If staff are active in patient care and the realities of practice, then their work experience will be meaningful.

Autonomy. Along with a certain childlike joy in getting to "try it" comes a universal wish for competence and autonomy for the chance to "do it all by myself." Even in a system of health care where caution and extensive checks and balances exist, there will be opportunity to allow freedom of decision and discretion in work determination. Responsibility cannot be learned, it must be given. Independence may be provided for a nurse by delegating direct patient care, patient education, and recommendation for therapeutic plans. Business staff may be given freedom to arrange special payment plans for families with financial problems. Physicians will not be abdicating their authority if they follow up delegation through progress reports.

Feedback. Assessment of job performance and a sense of achievement may be conveyed to employees both in the visible results of their work and in evaluations provided by others, especially by supervisors and physicians. Staff should be offered many opportunities to see the outcome of their efforts whether they work directly with patients or with some other aspect of the practice. Nursing staff might be asked to perform laboratory and diagnostic tests which they will present to the physician for verification. A receptionist may assume responsibility for balancing charges and receipts daily and mailing all statements monthly. Formal and informal feedback can be provided during group meetings or individual performance reviews.

Relationships. Most staff will have contacts with patients, physicians, and other staff. This may not be a motivational element unless there is a breakdown in one of these relationships. Physician and staff relationships may be strengthened by joint activities and shared re-

sponsibilities. Individual and group sessions with patients and families may also be a stimulus to staff motivation.

Table 6.1 outlines applications of motivational principles.

Hierarchy of Needs

Abraham Maslow (1954) a renowned behavioral psychologist, expanded upon earlier theories of motivation. He arranged his theory of human needs in a hierarchy. That is to say, the appearance of one need usually rests upon the prior satisfaction of another. According to Maslow, "Man is a perpetually wanting animal. . . ." The hierarchy of human needs, as depicted by Maslow, is presented in Figure 6.3.

Biological Needs. Basic needs must be satisfied before others. For many of us biological needs are satisfied without even thinking about them. A receptionist in a comfortably heated, properly lit, well-ventilated office has many of these needs satisfied without even being aware of them. However, when these needs are not met—if the room is smoke-filled or the employee is experiencing hunger or thirst—motivation will be directed toward resolution of basic needs. Patient satisfaction will be secondary if staff are physically or psychologically deprived.

Security Needs. Safety, familiar surroundings, and people among whom we can feel comfortable will help satisfy security needs. Regardless of what may appear to be a continual desire for freedom, the majority have a need for stability, predictability, and organization. Office practice may provide many securities by means of a well-functioning system, adequate pay and benefits, and a consistent work routine.

Social Needs. People normally enjoy the association of others. Intensity of socialization may vary, but a sense of affection and friendship is needed by all. Elderly patients often consider a visit to the doctor a social occasion. Physicians and staff should be appreciative of this need. Social needs of office personnel may also be provided for within an atmosphere of congeniality and sensitivity. The practice

Table 6.1 Motivation Principles and Applications

Principles	Application
Responsibility and personal achievement.	Removing some controls while retaining accountability. Allowing receptionist to balance nightly fees and submit bank deposit.
Responsibility and recognition.	Increasing accountability for own work. Having each employee report their usage of supplies and equipment and recommending increases or modifications.
Responsibility, achievement, and recognition.	Giving a person a complete natural unit or module. Nurses control nursing station and lab, receptionists oversee reception, clerical, and business areas.
Responsibility, achievement, and recognition.	Granting additional authority and freedom in work activity. Encouraging staff to establish their own schedules and time constraints. Nurses scheduling ECG's, urine and blood tests, etc. Receptionists allowed to work patients into schedule without checking with doctor or nurse.
Internal recognition.	Making periodic reports directly available to personnel rather than to supervisor only. Financial statements, collection ratios, and expenditure reports could be presented directly to physicians at monthly staff meetings.
Responsibility, growth, and advancement.	Assigning individuals specific or specialized tasks enabling them to become experts. Training nursing personnel to administer tests and injections, as well as conducting patient education to individuals and groups. Sending receptionist to continuing education program to revise medical record system.

should also have an area where staff may relax and retreat from the hectic office pace.

Esteem Needs.   When social acceptance is attained, then respect, recognition, and approval will present themselves as needs. Most people do not publicize this need, but they certainly respond to its satisfaction. Care should be taken not to placate or give superficial praise. Words alone may not provide gratification for patients and staff. Physicians should acknowledge staff performance in formal meetings and with tangi-

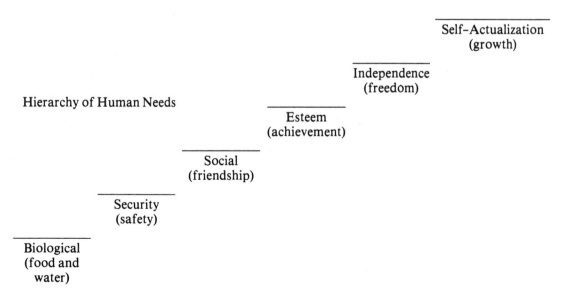

Figure 6.3 Maslow's Hierarchy of Needs

ble offerings. Certificates and plaques are appropriate and have a lasting impact.

Independence Needs. "Free to be you and me!" the song goes. This cluster of needs motivates us to accept responsibility, develop competence and maturity. In the office, independence may be achieved by permitting employees involvement in decision making, policy setting, and use of resources. Free expression of ideas about scheduling, office design and routines, and collection policies may fulfill the staff member's need for independence.

Self-Actualization. Maslow believed that very few truly attain this level or remain in this state for very long. People may possess a few elements of growth which can be nurtured. This may involve a sense of charity, a seeking for new truths, a willingness to modify deficiencies or an unceasing drive for ethical and moral standards. Qualities which Maslow observed in his studies of notables may serve to illustrate self-actualization. They include: perception of reality; acceptance of self, others, and nature; spontaneity; detachment and a sense of privacy; freshness of appreciation; seeking peak experiences; democratic character; and enjoyment of other's successes. When these motivational elements appear, they indicate a high-quality individual who merits praiseworthy attention.

In summation, Maslow believed personal needs overlap. They vary in intensity among individuals and can be fulfilled in many ways. Needs which may have been dormant can be reactivated by events or individuals. The meaning and condition of motivation are as individualized and personalized as a person's name or face. Thus, if our leadership role requires motivation of people, we must develop keen observational and listening skills. We must probe for understanding and thoughtfully analyze what we see, hear, and know.

Satisfiers and Dissatisfiers

The nature of meaningful work was a primary concern to Frederick Herzberg (1966), a noted industrial psychologist. His behavioral studies were depicted as "motivation-hygiene theory." His research design was based upon two very basic employment questions: "Can you describe, in detail, when you felt exceptionally good about your job?" and "Can you describe, in detail, when you felt exceptionally bad about your job?"

Analyses showed that good feelings related to job experiences. These were content factors. Bad feelings were most often related to surrounding or peripheral aspects of the work and were characterized as context factors.

Satisfiers. Content factors which resulted in satisfying work experiences are as follows: achievement, recognition, work itself, responsibility, advancement, and growth. Satisfiers are termed "motivations," since they effectively stimulate employees to greater performance and productivity. Achievement refers to the satisfaction of completing a job, solving problems, and seeing results. Recognition is in terms of a job well done. Work itself is the context of job, routines, challenges, and degree of difficulty. Responsibility and authority refer to employees' control over the job and the work of others. Advancement is upward mobility, including status, money, and authority. Growth involves learning new skills and expanding work significance.

Dissatisfiers. The context or environmental factors causing dissatisfaction include: company policy and administration, supervision, working conditions, interpersonal relations, salary, status, job security, and personal life. Dissatisfiers are the hygiene factors. These are considered deficit needs, as their importance is felt only in their absence. Company policy and administration reflected feelings of adequacy or inadequacy in organization and management, such as lines of communication or determination of authority figures. Supervision refers to the competency or technical ability of supervision, such as willingness to teach or to delegate, and fairness of treatment. Working conditions include quantity of work, facilities, and resources. Interpersonal relations include relationships with supervisors, peers, and subordinates. Salary includes all types of compensation. Status is restricted to employees' feelings about their jobs. Job security may be determined by objective signs such as longevity, tenure, and organizational stability. Personal life relates only to factors at work, such as changing location, working late hours, or taking work home.

Applications to Medical Practice. Physicians should be aware of the disparity between motivation and hygiene factors. Personnel are often rewarded with financial bonuses, gifts, uniform allowances, time off, and modern equipment and facilities. These are hygiene factors which, once given, may not satisfy further. In addition, if they are not given on a regular basis or are removed, they may become sources of dissatisfaction. If physicians are truly interested in staff motivation, then they should consider motivations which affect staff at a personal-need level. Office staff are subordinate to physicians, but this secondary status does not have to detract from feelings of achievement and self-esteem. Receptionists, nurses, and business personnel are important entities and are capable of planning and evaluating, as well as implementing. Incorporating them into these functions will be a true stimulus to increased productivity. There is no intention to demean the distribution of gifts and fringe benefits but only to keep these rewards in perspective. They should not be given as a prelude to future performance but as gratification for past endeavors.

Coaching and Counseling

During the normal course of employment, there will be several incidents which necessitate a direct two-way dialogue between supervisor and subordinate. These counseling sessions may be scheduled as six-month or yearly performance reviews, or they may occur spontaneously in response to a critical situation. A tone of seriousness should prevail whether the session is to be positive or negative. Physicians and supervisors are seldom prepared for this role, and as a result these encounters become either punitive or "gripe" sessions. A more common happening is that they occur beyond the time corrective action may be therapeutic.

Obstacles and Dilemmas

There are very few patented strategies. Coaching and counseling each encounter will require a flexible interviewing style and situational management approach.

Obstacles to effective coaching may arise when the staff members resist change or deny that a problem exists. It will be imperative to have all the facts at hand and be firm, yet conscious of the individual's unwillingness to accept failure or a negative evaluation. Another source of difficulty may be in physicians' misuse of power and authority. There are few problems which are one-sided. Physicians and supervisors could do some soul-searching to assess how they may have contributed to the problem.

A dilemma may enter into the process. This involves a subordinate's inability to view behavior with sufficient candor and objectivity. Thus the supervisor must impose personal ideas and opinions during coaching sessions. If a concrete plan is mutually accepted and it contains the motivational elements previously discussed, then the dilemma may be resolved.

Guidelines

Guidelines for an effective coaching session include: asking staff to analyze their own performance; maintaining two-way communications—each speaks and listens equally; planning for each session and submitting in writing both objectives and conclusions; expecting and allowing for disagreement; realizing that total agreement is unattainable and working to establish achievable expectations; determining a timetable for follow-up with mutually accepted plans for implementation.

Keys to Motivating

Achieving motivational skills requires taking risks, testing new approaches, seeking feedback, and evaluating the results. Physicians have the capability to listen, respond sensitively, lead discussions, resolve conflicts, and offer constructive critique. Previous training and experiences have touched upon all of these attributes. Leading people and managing an office practice involves application of these same attributes, but on a different level. Feinberg (1969, 1975) offers physicians several keynotes for motivating staff. See Figure 6.4.

MANAGEMENT MODELS

Learning and skill development are enhanced if the subject matter can be developed into a cognitive framework. This will enable the learner to visualize concepts and perhaps develop a more thorough comprehension. Through scrutiny of researchers and practitioners, management theory has been abstracted and conceptualized into models. Presented here are four of these models and their applications. These should, first, enable physicians to become aware of their personal style of directing and behaving; second, enable those with leadership responsibilities to gain insight into the behavior and motivations of others; and third, suggest strategies which may facilitate decision making and problem solving.

Establish consistent standards and communicate them:
If an individual is being evaluated according to a fair standard, then there is an understanding of what is expected. If policies are modified, it is essential to communicate this in advance.

Be aware of your biases and prejudices:
Are you aware of your prejudices? If you manage based upon biases, your associates will perceive them and know you as a supervisor who is influenced more by opinion than fact.

Let people know where they stand:
The positives and negatives regarding an employee's work which you have perceived should be presented objectively in a performance review.

Give praise when appropriate:
Praise is like seasoning—a little bit at appropriate times and places is better than a heavy dose at one time. It is especially helpful to praise someone at the height of anxiety.

Care about employee's feelings:
Lack of communication with employees about their feelings is summed up succinctly: "Sticks and stones can break my bones . . . words can sting . . . but silence breaks the heart."

Build group trust:
This is closely allied to caring for employees. Recognize goals and needs of fellow workers and, when possible, involve individual goals and needs with group goals and needs. One of the better methods to motivate people is to enable and facilitate achievement of one's fullest potential. Group trust evolves from the trust each individual has in the manager and other group members.

Exhibit personal dedication:
The best motivation is a leader personally committed to excellence and self-respect. People enjoy working for a leader who exhibits positive qualities: honesty, sincerity, understanding, pride, compassion, dedication, and concern.

Be tactful with employees:
Tact is evidenced by courtesy, a sense of balance, an appreciation of others' views. It has been said that Thomas Jefferson, with all his brilliance, always made others feel at ease. He seldom sought to overshadow or astound and was amazingly considerate.

Be willing to learn from others:
Know your limitations. Realize that you may not have all of the information and knowledge which could be helpful. A teacher must be his or her own #1 student. A great speaker must first be a skilled listener.

Stay flexible:
Be sensitive to the possibility of change, especially when ideas or pressures rise from below. Winston Churchill said "To improve is to change, so to be perfect is to have changed often."

Allow freedom of expression:
Each employee ought to have the right to make his or her own job more interesting. Each individual has some urge for independence and need to demonstrate competence. Assuming your subordinates display reasonable maturity and competence, allow them to do things their way when appropriate.

Encourage ingenuity and creativity:
Challenge your subordinates by encouraging them to question existing systems and propose innovations. Remember, your subordinates are the ones who are closest to the workings of your programs and policies and they may have valid suggestions for progressive change.

Figure 6.4 Motivation of Others

Leadership Personalities

Gerald Bell (1973) developed a theory of leadership personality following eight years of research which included case studies of over 3,000 individuals. He gives credit to several people as an influence and inspiration to his work, including Chris Argyris, Carl Rogers, Abraham Maslow, and David McCelland. Bell came to the conclusion that we were born with a natural urge, a biogenetic heritage to be achievers. He also discovered other needs which have resulted from impressionable experiences.

By the time we are a few years old, we have been exposed to experiences which may have thrust upon us rewards for being dominant, orderly, and rigid. Perhaps parents were our models for these traits. In the face of hostilities or adversaries, we have learned to rebel or attack. We have been hurt and have learned how to avoid discomfort. Also, we have received kindness and love, and we have been rewarded for pleasing others. And finally, our need to perform may have been reinforced by the funny things said and done which were encouraged by people we respected. Thus, Bell identified six personality traits which may influence leadership—commanding, attacking, avoiding, pleasing, performing, and achieving. Extreme definitions of each of these personality types are outlined below. Very few fit into the extremes, but each person has a style or tendencies which may be categorized into one or two of these personalities.

The Need to Command. The commander needs to control each situation; dominate every group; and live an orderly, systematic life. Ambiguity and uncertainty are disliked. The world is seen in clear-cut categories, and new situations are approached in a dogmatic and stubborn manner.

The Need to Attack. The attacker needs to release hostilities without accepting responsibility or dependence on others. Tear down a plan but offer no solutions. Being an authority rebel, the attacker loves to argue and debate. Tactics included are sarcasm, cynicism, and negativism.

The Need to Avoid. The avoider fears failure. The goal in life is to hide. Self-confidence is lacking, and preference is for assignments that are stable and routine. Usually very few risks are taken, and low goals are set.

The Need to Please. The pleaser needs approval and acceptance. Acceptance is sought from all associates by being kind and generous and by going along with others because building friendships is the top priority. Assignments which involve dealing with people on an easy, sociable basis are preferred.

The Need to Perform. The performer needs to gain prestige and recognition. There is continual striving for respectability and properness. Accordingly, the performer changes values to go along with the most advantageous position and is very difficult to pin down. Tasks are chosen which maximize image and prestige, regardless of whether the task is worthwhile.

The Need to Achieve. The achiever needs to maximize potential, to reach the highest level of personal competence to become self-fulfilled. Work is challenging, yet toward realistic goals. Feedback is accepted about results, and creative and new methods are often explored to reach objectives.

Worst-Fit Situations

Each of the personality styles will be inappropriate if certain conditions exist. The following are worst-fit situations for each style:

Commander
- Complex and unpredictable situations
- Constantly changing environment

Attacker
- Pleaser situations
- Close interpersonal contact—public relations and listening

Avoider
- Performer settings
- Public exposure
- Situations calling for extrovert behavior

Pleaser
- Attacker environment
- Competition and aggressiveness
- Conflicts and tough problem solving

Performer
- Avoiding situations
- Repetitive tasks
- Rigid structure

Achiever
- Commander environments
- Extensive rules and regulations
- Extreme conformity

Best-Fit Situations

Each personality will be particularly effective if exercised in a compatible environment. The following are best-fit situations for each style:

Commander
- Clear-cut tasks
- Orderly and precise organization
- Stable environment

Attacker
- Hostile environment
- Critical evaluation and discovery of weaknesses
- Loose structure
- Self-directed pursuits

Avoider
- Repetitive jobs
- Well-defined organization
- Low-risk assignments

Pleaser
- Loose organization
- Time and freedom to be around people who are friendly

Performer
- Prestige and visibility available
- Political and social situations available
- Public relations and promotions

Achiever
- Challenge of uncertainty provided
- High degree of discretion called for
- Opportunities to assert self and supply personal approach

Growth

Regardless of one's primary or secondary personality, there may be future situations which will require different approaches. Each physician leader should appreciate the need for growth and seek out opportunities to increase team building and motivational skills. The following are suggestions for growth for each style.

Commander
- Learn to feel submissive and equal to others
- Try to see both sides
- Become less organized and more spontaneous
- Get involved in unstructured situations

Attacker
- Agree with others
- Take broader responsibilities
- Provide constructive analysis of others
- Depend on others
- Relate to "nonattackers"

Avoider
- Build self-confidence
- Take risks
- Do things *now*
- Seek honest feedback
- Face conflicts
- Seek out achievers as models

Pleaser
- Voice disagreements
- Take the initiative
- Develop convictions
- Confront conflicts
- Set higher goals

Performer
- Slow down and reflect more
- Honestly look at self
- Do not show off
- Establish more genuine relationships
- Seek candid feedback

Achiever
- Learn patience
- Learn self-reliance
- Try being spontaneous and natural
- Explore and seek new experiences
- Sharpen perception of reality
- Establish close, genuine relationships
- Establish realistic goals and ideas

Dimensional Management

Buzzotta, Lefton, and Sherberg (1972) developed a systematic approach for understanding managerial behavior. Their theory is an extension of Blake and Morton's Managerial Grid

(1964). These organizational psychologists described behavior along two dimensions:

Dominance _____ Submission
Hostility _____ Warmth

They believed that each person will behave somewhere between dominance and submission and somewhere between hostility and warmth. The point along each dimension is variable by situation and level of comfort, but each physician, staff member, patient, etc, has a predominant mode of acting which will cluster at some location.

An extremely dominant person will have a drive to take the lead in face-to-face relationships. Dominant people are active, "take-charge" types who display self-confidence, forcefulness, ambition, and a strong desire for independence. They are attracted to situations in which they can exert control.

Extreme submission involves a willingness to accept leadership and guidance by others. Frequently plagued by self-doubt, submissive people fear new initiatives and have a strong need to conform. They are willing followers but very reluctant leaders.

Extremely hostile people take the attitude that other people don't really count for much. Hostile people are distant, self-centered, and cold; they are often insensitive and unresponsive to the needs, feelings, and ideas of others.

Very warm personalities exhibit concern for others based on a belief that they count as much as themselves. Warm people are outgoing, aware of and sensitive to other people's needs, feelings, and ideas. Concerned about themselves, they are nevertheless responsive to other people's needs.

All physicians occupy a position somewhere on each dimension. Thus, to understand a managerial behavior, we must consider both dimensions simultaneously. The easiest way to do this is to intersect the dimensions.

As Figure 6.5 shows, managerial behavior can be described by the quadrant into which it falls when both dimensions are considered. This does not mean all physicians behave in four and only four ways. Actually, there are as many different behaviors as there are physicians. But these behaviors can be grouped, for analysis and understanding in one of the four quadrants.

Q_1 *Dominant Hostile* (Power Strategy) Medical practice provides ultimate gratification Decisions are made at the top Personal success is priority motivation	Q_4 *Dominant Warm* (Growth Strategy) Success is equated to both quality patient care and office efficiency Three levels of needs: self, others, and professional Mutual acceptance of responsibility
Q_2 *Submissive Hostile* (Survival Strategy) Accept minimum responsibilities Colleagues and staff cannot be trusted Patient education is not worth the effort	Q_3 *Submissive Warm* (Sociability Strategy) Patients and staff will comply if they like the physicians Friendships will ensure productivity Decisions are best when they make people happy

Figure 6.5 Dimensional Management Model

Dominant-Hostile Q₁

This behavioral style is characterized by an individual who is hard-working, short-tempered, and overly critical of others. A basic need could be for independence and is motivated by status and self-esteem. Assumptions about others include: colleagues are threats, and deception is appropriate; patients are not capable of taking responsibility and must be directed; and staff require decisive leadership and tight control. If a physician is faced with the dominant-hostile behavior in others, the following strategies may be facilitative:

- Allow negative emotions to ventilate.
- Do not become involved in arguments.
- Recognize control needs.
- Probe broad assertions and curt remarks.
- Remain objective and factual.
- Summarize key thoughts and look for mutual agreements.

Submissive-Hostile Q₂

This behavioral style is characterized by safety and security needs. An individual exemplifying this behavior is easily threatened and will avoid most conflict situations. Assumptions about others include: colleagues are intimidating and interaction should be minimal; patients are uncooperative and unappreciative and deserve little attention or effort; and staff are trouble-makers and cannot be trusted. If a physician is faced with submissive-hostile behavior in others the following strategies may be facilitative:

- Behave reassuringly.
- Recognize reticence to change.
- Avoid moving in too fast and talking too much.
- Establish trust.
- Guide gently but firmly.
- Mention benefits to satisfy security needs.
- Confront resistance and passivity, as last resort.

Submissive-Warm Q₃

This behavioral style is characterized by sociability, friendship, and a need for approval. Individuals with this trait are frequently in conversations and enjoy keeping discussions lighthearted. Assumptions about others: Colleagues deserve 100% support, and fellowship will prevent problems; patients will respond if they like their doctor; and staff will be loyal if they are having fun and are treated as equals. If a physician is faced with the submissive-warm behavior in others the following strategies may be facilitative:

- Recognize social needs.
- Allow meandering without losing direction.
- Probe the quick assertions.
- Bring unspoken concerns to surface.
- Avid exploiting submissiveness.
- Help organize thoughts and actions.

Dominant-Warm Q₄

This behavioral style is characterized by an interest and concern for others while recognizing the importance of achieving organizational goals. Assumptions about others include: Colleagues are resources and partners in problem solving; patients should be involved in health care decisions, and compliance will result from doctor-patient rapport; staff will be motivated if their work is challenging and the physicians provide effective direction and two-way communication. The Q₄ believes conflict contributes to learning, creativity, and innovation. Strategies which the Q₄ employs to execute participative management include the following:

- Develop subordinates to assume delegated responsibilities.
- Build teams as working subgroups.
- Confront dissension and indecision at its earliest stage.
- Redirect hostility toward problem solving.
- Identify resources and consultants.
- Anticipate change and build receptivity to innovation.

The Q₄ approach understands that decisions will produce greater commitment if the ideas are generated from the people who have to implement them. This is not a denunciation of responsibility, but an intelligent use of organizational resources.

Leadership Style

Hersey and Blanchard (1974) used two traditional types of leadership behavior to develop their model. They designed a four-dimensional model and an assessment questionnaire based on the concepts of task and relationship.

Task behavior is defined as the extent to which a leader is likely to organize and define the roles of group members. It is further characterized by endeavoring to establish well-defined patterns of organization, channels of communication, and methods for getting jobs accomplished.

Relationship behavior is the extent to which a leader is likely to maintain or foster personal relationships within the work environment. It is characterized by socioemotional support, friendship, and mutual trust.

By combining the high and low ranges of task and relationship behavior, a four-dimensional model Figure 6.6, is developed to view leadership behavior. This model shows the implication of combining task and relationship behaviors.

Leadership style is the consistent patterns of behavior which are perceived by others when a physician is influencing the activities of staff, patients, or colleagues. A predominant style evolves from successful experiences and through observations of role models. Second-ary styles may also be developed as alternative behaviors. A physician may choose an "actively leading" style when beginning a practice, and then, when the practice is under way, shift into "working along with" and "structure and responsibility" style with colleagues and staff. A "hands-off" style may be appropriate in specific situations to allow a staff member time to carry out a delegated task. The high task and high responsibility style is probably the most effective position for the majority of management situations.

Style adaptability is the degree to which a leader adapts to the demands of a given situation. A physician with a narrow style range can be effective if the practice remains static. Flexibility will be necessary when the practice is undergoing change, and colleagues, staff, and patients require frequent communication. The style range which has the highest degree of adaptability is high task and high relationship.

The leadership-style assessment model provides insight into personal behavior and further conceptualizes situational management. While it is useful to have awareness about leadership style, it is even more important to know how consistent this perception is with how one's behavior is perceived by others. If self-perception is similar to the perceptions of patients, staff, and colleagues, then the probability of success is greater.

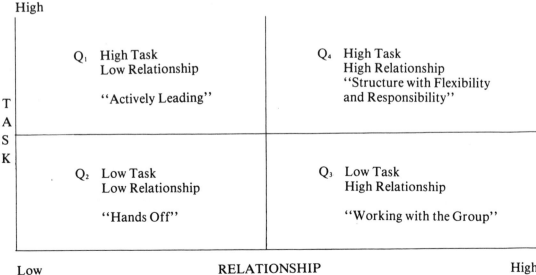

Figure 6.6 Task and Relationship Dimensional Model

Effectiveness Dimension

Reddin (1977) presents an excellent synthesis of leadership theories. Similar to previous authors, Reddin describes behavior from four perspectives. The assumption is that any of the four types could be effective depending upon the situation.

The effectiveness dimension is built upon the two general methods of leadership behavior—task orientation and relationship orientation. From these two methods, Reddin proposes four behavior types: integrated, dedicated, related, and separated. Within these four categories he further describes an effective and ineffective dimension which is seen in the style of leadership.

Dedicated behavior is characterized by a high task and low relationship orientation. The *ineffective* dimension of this behavior would be described as autocratic, with a style that is overly critical, threatening, dogmatic, and aggressive. The *effective* dimension of the dedicated behavior would describe a benevolent autocrat, with a style that is decisive, energetic, industrious, and evaluative.

Separated behavior is characterized by a low task and low relationship orientation. The *ineffective* dimension of this behavior would describe a deserter, with a style that is passive,

uncommitted, hindering, and uninvolved. The *effective* dimension of the separated behavior would be seen as bureaucratic, with a leadership style that is rational, controlled, and regulation-oriented.

Related behavior is characterized by a high relationship orientation. The *ineffective* dimension would describe a socializer, with a style that is dependent, yielding, compliant, and helpless. The *effective* dimension of the related behavior would describe a developer, with a leadership style that is trusting, supportive, sensitive, and understanding.

Integrated behavior is characterized by a high task and high relationship orientation. The *ineffective* dimension would describe a compromiser, with a style that is unpredictable, inconsistent, and indecisive. The *effective* dimension for the integrated behavior would be seen in an executive with a leadership style that is adaptive, team-oriented, situational, and motivating.

The effectiveness dimension approach emphasizes adaptive and situational behavior. It further concludes that anyone may perform leadership functions if they are placed in the appropriate environment. This appears to dispel the myth that leaders are born.

A composite of the four-dimensional leadership models with the effectiveness dimension is pictured in Figure 6.7.

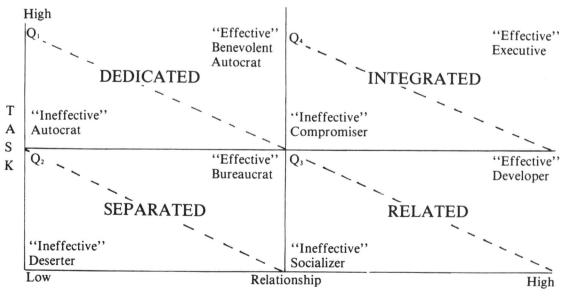

Figure 6.7 Four-Dimensional Effectiveness

TIME MANAGEMENT

Perhaps the most evasive resource to incorporate into a practice is time. Patients, staff, and colleagues are all victims of mismanaged time. Resolving this dilemma will require an office system which is organized and uses delegation as a management principle. Mackenzie (1972) and Lakein (1973) have presented time management as an area of knowledge which physicians could study and apply to the hectic pace of their professional and personal life.

A common statement voiced by physicians and staff is "We try so hard but where does the time go?" There is little doubt that misuse of time and the resulting inefficiency is perplexing. It is present in many offices as evidenced when patients are kept waiting, paper work is backlogged, test results are not filed, and home life begins to suffer the consequences. Anger, guilt, and defensiveness are common. Physicians, staff, and family members are both persecutors and victims in an endless cycle of frustration.

Office personnel are normally quite candid about physician inability to manage time. They report several specific issues which may be classified as time wasters: not adhering to scheduled appointments and meeting times; accepting interruptions irrespective of obligations to patients or staff; inadequate or unclear written directions to nurses and receptionists, necessitating follow-up questions and clarification; insistence on "stat" lab work and diagnostic tests for patient and physician convenience, regardless of office demands; and inability to terminate personal encounters with patients, staff, and colleagues. Time is also lost through an unclear or nonexistent priority system, overcommitment of energy and resources, indecision and inability to delegate, and a reliance upon crisis management and interim solutions. Figure 6.8 presents the major time wasters and time savers in medical practice.

Managing time is one of the keys to managing the stress inherent in the demanding role of physician. If physicians and other professionals are to control their multifaceted and often conflicting responsibilities and still have time to enjoy their personal lives, they must develop a time-management plan that contains one or more of the following five strategies: (1) self

Time Wasters
Physicians maintain an "individualized" style of practice
Unclear job descriptions and reporting relationships
Interruptions during office hours
Orders are all considered "stat"
No protocols for telephone messages and appointments
Frequent socializing by physicians and staff
Excessive responsibilities outside of the practice
Infrequent, or non-existent, office meetings

Time Savers
Daily briefing sessions with physicians and staff
Office policy manual
Patient information documents
Monthly staff meeting
Computerized billing system
Utilization of part-time employees for peak times
Pre-printed forms for appointments, telephone message, and other regularly used documents

Figure 6.8 Time Wasters and Time Savers in Medical Practice

management, (2) qualitative analysis, (3) organizational approach, (4) delegation and decision making, and (5) conducting meetings. Each of these areas should be explored to determine which is most relevant to the individual and the situation that require time-management assistance.

Self Management

The first, and most important, perspective is self management. The individual must begin with an assessment of life and career goals and then identify personal strengths, assets, and areas of improvement that will influence the attainment of goals. The essential components of a self-management (or life-management) plan would include: *long-range goals* (one to five years); *short-range goals* (less than a year); *objectives* that are measurable and attainable; *individuals* and *resources needed* to accomplish objectives; *progress reports* on a quarterly and yearly basis to measure achievements: and *evaluation* to revise plans if necessary. A self-management plan should be compiled into a workbook that can be reviewed periodically. This workbook could become a chronology of the individual's life and serve as an invaluable reference when important personal and career decisions are made.

Qualitative Analysis

A second perspective of time management is to focus on the nature of events and activities. This qualitative approach for organizing time includes such factors as duration, density, location, succession, grouping, and vividness. Bebace, Beattie, and Catlin (1983) described these six dimensions and their application to professionals as follows. *Duration* is the length of time of an event, including preparation and aftermath. A patient visit or hospital meeting may last twenty minutes or one hour, but the duration of the activity often begins before the stated time and lasts well beyond the actual adjournment. Unless the full amount of time is planned for, both the stated event and the events before and after may be adversely affected. *Density* is the number of events that are scheduled with a given time frame. Depending on the nature of the task or situation, some tasks should be reserved for a large amount of separate time, such as a counseling session or preparing for a presentation, while other tasks can be arranged in rapid succession, such as phone messages, reviewing the mail, and signing medical records. *Location* is the temporal or physical position of an event. Scheduling an activity in the morning or at the end of day or week may lead to a more successful result. In addition the site or physical surroundings may influence the quality of the experience. *Succession* concerns the order of occurrence of events. The sequence of work or meetings should be carefully planned to allow for the appropriate amount of preparation and execution time. It may be unrealistic to schedule a series of patient visits after a highly emotional event. *Grouping* involves the clustering of similar or related events with a given span of time. Even though professionals pride themselves on their ability to perform many and varied activities, organizing events in a pattern may improve efficiency for self and others. *Vividness* is the degree to which an event stands out from other events. Some people and situations have a pervasive effect. Once again it will be important not to underestimate the impact of highly significant occurrences upon the other events in close proximity.

Organizational Approach

A third approach to time management is organizational. If professionals and organizations adhere to the principles of planning, orientation, consolidation, and communication, then both the physicians and the practice as a whole will work more efficiently. *Planning* time should be allocated to all major tasks and events. Establishing a priority list that ranks activities by importance is recommended to determine which activities should be attempted first, second, and third. Updating plans and priorities will be necessary as situations and resources change. *Orientation* involves previews, training sessions, informational meetings, and advance discussion of expectations and requirements. Written goals, job descriptions, tours, policy manuals, and pilot tests, dry runs, and other types of preliminary events are examples of orientation. *Consolidation* means to economize time and space by grouping events and/or people. Some tasks may be more efficiently performed in a centralized system, such as clerical work, billing, medical records, and administrative paperwork. It may also be necessary to merge two or more jobs into one as the organization expands or automates the financial and clinical functions. *Communication* with key individuals requires meetings to inform, monitor, and evaluate. Previewing or debriefing the day or week may avoid misunderstandings and repeated mistakes. When retention and accuracy are essential, written communications should be used. Group meetings may also be more effective and efficient than conducting a series of one-to-one sessions.

Delegation and Decision Making

Delegation is an instrumental tool for time management. Delegating to subordinates is a calculated risk! However, if physicians and supervisors accept that gains will overcome losses, then subordinates will become more proficient in accepting responsibilities.

Barriers which impede delegation are: preference for doing, instead of managing; uncertainty regarding the how, what, or when of tasks; comfort with confusion and trivia; and unwillingness to develop subordinates for fear that they may surpass the supervisor in certain skill areas.

Keynotes for time-effective delegation are: selecting and training of qualified subordinates; mutually determined tasks and outcomes; establishing timetables for progress reports and results; and delegating responsibilities in a vertical order.

Decision making is an extension of delegation and will be equally important in maximizing the use of time. The following seven rules on decision making should be very helpful to physicians who are interested in mastering the difficult art of making important decisions in a time-efficient manner.

1. **Make decisions one at a time.** Do not try to make decisions on a whole package of problems. Even though one decision bears on another, make them one at a time.
2. **Make policy decisions first.** If you have a whole bag of decisions, divide them into two types: *policy,* this is the long-range philosophy of running your practice or your life; and *operational,* day-to-day activities. Make the policy decisions first.
3. **Make important decisions first.** Line up all the decisions (policy and operational) in order of priority and take the time to make decisions about the most important matters. It often happens that by making the big decisions first, many small ones disappear.
4. **Set a decision date on your calendar.** Select a day to make a specific decision. Until that day let your mind play with the problem, unworried. Collect opinions and facts, but do not worry. When the day comes for the decision, make it, but not before.
5. **Separate the decision from your concern about announcing the decision.** Make the decision as if no one would ever know who made it. Too many decisions are influenced by concern about announcing it.
6. **Assume you are to make some wrong decisions.** Those who are too concerned that

they be absolutely right tend to procrastinate. It takes a few wrong decisions to learn how to make right ones.
7. **Learn not to make decisions too early.** If the situation is important allow enough time to give the decision ample thought. Then, once you decide, make the decision work.

Conducting Meetings

Meetings are a major time consumer. Physicians will be called upon to participate and lead committees and groups. Communications in a group setting is more time-efficient than a series of individual meetings. However, to ensure satisfying results a structure should be established and participants' roles defined.

Meetings will help group process and provide opportunities to present progress reports and receive input and feedback. Physicians and staff enjoy the experience of hearing from others, and discussing their opinions and views before an audience. In addition, the group meeting may determine what degree of consensus exists for an issue under consideration.

Guidelines. The following guidelines may be instrumental in achieving positive results through meetings.

Before
• Explore alternatives to meeting.
• Limit your attendance.
• Keep the participants to a minimum.
• Choose an appropriate time and place.
• Define the purpose.
• Distribute the agenda in advance.
• Time-limit the meeting and the agenda.

During
• Start on time.
• Stick to the agenda.
• Control interruptions.
• Accomplish your purpose.
• Restate conclusions and assignments.
• Adjourn the meeting as scheduled.
• Use a meeting evaluation checklist as an occasional spot check.

After
• Expedite the preparation of the minutes.
• Ensure that progress reports are made and decisions executed.

• Survey all committees, investigating whether their objectives have been achieved and if not when.

Group Building. There are several roles which leaders may perform to facilitate group process and move the meeting to an appropriate conclusion:

The initiator suggests new or different ideas for discussion and approaches to problems.
The opinion giver states pertinent beliefs about discussion and others' suggestions.
The elaborator builds on suggestions of others.
The clarifier gives relevant examples; offers rationales; probes for meaning and understanding; restates problems.
The tester raises questions to test out whether group is ready to come to a decision.
The summarizer reviews discussion, pulls it together.

LEADERSHIP OF PROFESSIONALS

Leadership research commenced in the late 1940s at Ohio State University, University of Michigan, and Harvard. The preceding description of management models resulted from these early studies which found that leaders tend to operate in one of four ways: autocratic, benevolent autocratic, consultative, or participative. The major contribution of this theory was the idea that a range of styles exists as opposed to the "great man theory" or "leaders are born not made." During the 1950s and 1960s, the human relations movement had a major influence on leadership theory. Leadership was viewed not only as the "management of tasks and functions" but also as the "management of people." A further evolution of leadership theory occurred in the late 1960s with the advent of the contingency or situational model of leadership. This approach emphasizes the need for leaders to first diagnose the needs of the subordinates and the organizational situation before they choose their leadership style. Some situations will require the leader to take a very active "hands-on" style, and other situations may necessitate that the leader delegate and allow others to take the initiative. In recent years, the study of leadership has expanded into the realm of professional organizations. Professionals have been moving out of the solo practice mode, into large-scale organizations, such as health centers, educational institutions, and research and development companies. As professionals become a larger percentage of the corporate work forces, a new managerial challenge was born.

Characteristics of Professionals

One important research finding was that professionals who work in organizations are different from the nonprofessional workers (Kerr, Von Glinow, Schrieshiem, 1977). Characteristics that distinguish professionals and thus influence how they can be led, are classified as follows; expertise, ethics, collegial maintenance of standards, autonomy, commitment to calling, and identification with profession.

The *expertise* which is possessed by a professional is seen as the product of a prolonged period of education and training. This knowledge and skill base brings with it a desire for special recognition. In some instances the professional possesses such unique abilities that she or he may have no peer within the organization. Professionals are socialized to a code of *ethics* which governs their work and relationships—Physicians have the Hippocratic Oath. Ethical principles often supercede professional and organizational norms. *Collegial maintenance of standards* means that professionals choose to set and enforce their own methods of conduct and behavior. They believe that they and they alone have the knowledge and understanding to judge and control the quality of their performance. Because of the extensive, and costly, education required to receive their credentials, they expect a very high degree of *autonomy*. This means self-control over goals, decision making, expression of ideas, access to information, and most importantly involvement in decisions which affect them. Professionals demonstrate a *commitment to profession* and their specialized field of expertise which often may put them in conflict with their role as an organizational member.

These characteristics are of particular importance when professionals work in a group or within a larger system. Drucker (1976) enumerated the following differences between professionals and nonprofessionals as organizational members. Professionals are typically viewed by others in the organization as being more concerned with their own interests, eg, patients and pet projects, than in working as a team to solve organizational problems or to follow standard routines. Professionals are often dissatisfied with the pragmatic approach, and are intolerant of authority figures and bureaucratic policies. Professionals are less loyal to their employing organization and are quick to criticize and rebel. Professionals place more emphasis on freedom of expression and quality of work life than on financial rewards. Professionals will accept expertise-based authority rather than legislated authority. Professionals will place personal and professional values over organizational goals and objectives.

Managing Professionals

The number and impact of professionals in organizations has created a new challenge for organizational leaders. Since professionals have a different orientation to organizational procedures, authority, and reward systems, those who have responsibility for managing professionals, or who have administrative roles in professional organizations, must recognize the uniqueness of this environment and utilize a more "collaborative" approach in their management style. McCall (1981) offers the most cogent description of the qualities needed for effective supervision in a professional organization. They are technical competence, controlled freedom, acting as a metronome, and fostering challenging work. *Technical competence* is required because of the professionals' need for associating with other professionals and their preference for authority based upon expertise in their chosen field. Preferably the manager of professionals would be of similar background and credentials as the group. The management of professionals involves recognizing ideas emerging within the group, defining significant problems and issues, and providing technical support or advice as needed. If the manager is not of the same level of expertise or a member of the profession, it will be important to demonstrate a high level of knowledge and skill regarding administrative responsibilities. *Controlled freedom* requires the manager to consider a give-and-take communication style, especially in decisions affecting the individuals or the group. Allowing the group to influence plans and future actions will be incumbent upon the manager. Emphasizing goals and objectives will be important; however, care should be taken not to explicitly define the means of reaching them. *Leader as metronome* implies a more subtle form of leadership and direction. If changes occur or priorities need to be redefined, it will be more important to manage the "process" than the actual issues. The process involves keeping people informed, moving in a thoughtful manner, and allowing the individuals responsible for implementation to set their own pace within reasonable limits. *Work challenge* is seen as the ability to instill excitement and a sense of importance in the work environment. Leaders must recognize the demands and constraints on the system and, if necessary, support the realignment of responsibilities so that the members do not feel they are being given new tasks to fit into an already full schedule. Emphasis should remain on the quality of the work not the quantity. A common flaw in professionals' work ethic is that they can "do it all." Thus a manager of professionals will be called upon to function more as an *orchestrator* than a commanding general.

PRACTICE LEADERSHIP FUNCTIONS

Office practice is becoming a diverse and complex health care organization. Patients are increasing their visits to physicians' offices. Third parties are now reimbursing a portion of the cost for outpatient diagnostic and treatment procedures. Paramedical training is highly sophisticated, and practitioners may choose a certified medical assistant, nurse practitioner, medical and laboratory technologist, or physician's assistant in addition to the traditional registered nurse (RN), licensed practical nurse (LPN), and the medical assistant. The average practice size is increasing in regards to both number of physicians and staff. Thus, to effectively administrate office practice, it will be necessary to develop appropriate leadership functions throughout the organization. This section will highlight several roles: medical director, practice manager, office supervisor, and administrative assistant.

Medical Director

When the practice includes three or more physicians within an office setting, a formalization of the medical director role could be a consideration. This function is probably executed in solos and partnerships by informal methods, with frequent communication among physician and office staff. However, as the number of personnel increases and time and work constraints prevail, it will be necessary to structure the authority system and flow of communication.

There are several qualifications to consider in choosing the physicians who will assume the medical director role. These qualities include: flexible leadership style which enables one physician to adequately represent the physician group while directing activities of paramedical staff and implementing practice policies; experience in office practice which provides a perspective of past and current events necessary to plan and organize; demonstrated competence in patient care and staff relationships so that confidence and trust may be established; capability for managerial development; and willingness to accept and implement the changes and sophistication of the medical profession generally and office practice specifically.

A medical director must be a leader in the following areas:

1. Quality control of all professional activities of physician and paramedical staff, including peer review, medical audits, analysis and validation of record systems, and periodic assessment of staff competencies
2. Professional relationships that maintain information flow to and from colleagues in hospital and specialty practices
3. Intraoffice relations, especially between fellow physicians and staff

4. Professional affiliations, including hospital, local, and state medical societies; educational institutions; and community agencies
5. Office policies and daily routines such as appointment systems, scheduling, financial controls, and patient flow
6. Practice analysis and innovations to maintain the highest quality of care and most efficient office systems
7. Medical ethics, legal, and moral obligations in the presence of legislative investigations and consumerism

There may be a variety of situations which will frustrate the medical director. A comic strip quote, which is now becoming an organizational adage, applies here: "The enemy is us!" Many problems a director may face will either be self-imposed or will arise within the physician group. Self-imposed problems include compulsive and/or expedient actions which lack reliable information and planning; aloofness from physician and/or staff which deters understanding of core issues; vacillating advocacy from physicians to staff to patients much to the dismay of all three groups; inability to confront problems in their earliest stages; reluctance to delegate responsibilities; and inability to develop subordinates to assume supervisory roles. Peer group will also be a potential problem area. Difficulties may develop when physicians will not relinquish decision making and require input in all practice routines and procedures. Staff may attempt to undermine the medical director by seeking opinions from other physicians or asking if the other physicians agree with the medical director.

Regardless of potential problems, the medical director role is a viable alternative for medical practices, and it should be given careful consideration. Medical directors may facilitate time management; planning for growth and expansion; effective staff, patient, and community relations; they should relieve other physicians from the demands of formal leadership responsibilities.

Another leadership role that has occurred since the rapid growth of HMOs is the medical director position for the corporate prepaid plans either full-time or part-time. Figure 6.9 is a job description for such a position.

The Medical Director must be a practicing physician who is well respected by the community physicians as a person, as a physician and as a clinician. The Medical Director must assume the role of patient advocate by assuring that subscribers receive high quality care at a convenient and accessible location for a reasonable price.

The Medical Director must evaluate the quality of physicians recruited into the plan. Physicians should be recruited from a widely spaced geographic area to meet the growth needs of the plan and so that they will be readily available to the patients.

The Medical Director must work with the Marketing and Finance divisions to coordinate services and programs. The Medical Director also works closely with all departments of the health plan to be sure the Corporation receives a fair return on its investment.

The Medical Director must work with the participating physicians to see that they are adequately compensated and that they are satisfied with their relationship with the plan. The goal is to secure a "partnership" relationship with local physicians so that they are working with the organization to ensure that providers, patients and the health plan receive maximum benefits.

The Medical Director must work with the patients and providers to see that hospital days and cost of inpatient services are appropriate, as well as the use of referrals, urgent care, and ancillary procedures.

Some of the specific duties of the Medical Director are: Organizing a recruiting plan; evaluating and approving physicians to work under contract; conducting regular meetings with participating physicians; promptly resolving problems between physicians and the plan; representing the plan to the medical and employer communities; conducting quality of care audits; supporting a system of financial and utilization accountability; and ensuring cost effective care through consultant relations, negotiations with ancillary services, and obtaining volume discounts.

Figure 6.9 HMO Medical Director Job Description

Practice Manager

Certain practice conditions may require a practice manager. Intricate business systems are being adapted to medical settings, and office finances require specialized expertise and frequent management intervention. It is unlikely that a medical director, who will also have patient care obligations, can personally direct all management and supervisory functions.

Prior to considering a practice manager position or selecting candidates, physicians should agree to the responsibilities which they will delegate. The following are tasks which may be included in the practice manager job description:

1. Recruitment, selection, and training of all nursing and business personnel
2. Direction of all financial functions and reports practice statistics monthly to physician group
3. Regular meetings with financial and legal consultants; advice and recommendations on business management decisions
4. Implementation of all financial, medical, and clerical procedures which are included in the office manual
5. Proposals on all investments and expenditures relative to office practice, and other professional matters which have financial implications.

Since few physicians have taken direction or worked in a colleagual environment with nonphysicians, the impact of a nonphysician member of the management structure should not be underestimated. In choosing an individual for practice manager, factors to consider include: leadership style of medical director; philosophy of the practice; management strategies which are currently underway and those needed for the future; formal and informal organization of physician and paramedical staff; and the presence of computerization, professional corporation, nurse clinicians, financial advisors, and legal consultants.

Upon selection and training, the practice manager must receive support and encouragement early in the employment process and be allowed to expand knowledge and skills. Physicians should be willing to accept that the manager will soon become as knowledgeable of many office features as they themselves. When modifications or changes are suggested, these ideas should be viewed as productive and progressive, rather than an accusation that something or someone in the past was at fault. There is no intention or endorsement for abdication of authority—that belongs at the physician level. However, a practice manager could be viewed as an executive who merits participation and input throughout the organization.

Office Supervisor

Regardless of the practice size or the existence of medical director or practice manager, there is need for at least one supervisory person beyond the physician. Even a two-person staff needs someone identified who possesses a higher level of responsibility and competence.

Initially a supervisor could be the most qualified or highly trained person in the office. An important attribute for any supervisory individual is to be recognized as knowledgeable and skillful by fellow workers and physicians. Since there is constant interface between physicians and staff, the supervisor must have the respect of both groups. Most practices will not have the luxury of a supervisory staff who are divorced from practice responsibilities. Thus, this person, whether head nurse, chief receptionist, or business manager, must continually exhibit high performance in her or his respective office assignment.

Major duties of the supervisors will include:

1. Establishing daily and weekly work routines and prioritizing minor conflicts
2. Conducting weekly and monthly meetings with office personnel
3. Training new employees and recommending continuing education for experienced personnel
4. Collecting, tabulating, and/or reporting practice statistics such as patients seen, outpatient and inpatient revenue, insurance forms processed, office and billing collections, and number of lab and diagnostic tests
5. Participating in performance appraisal interviews with physicians and/or practice manager
6. Meeting with patients, individually or in groups, regarding practice policies and patient education.

Administrative Assistant

Practice growth and the professional development of physicians may generate the need for an administrative assistant, often referred to as "executive secretary." A large physician group in a single- or multispecialty practice with a practice manager may have many important responsibilities which could be delegated to a person with executive assistant talents.

Just as for the other key positions, there should be a clear understanding of the scope of the work before selecting the individual. Administrative duties which could be assigned to a person with advanced secretarial and clerical skills include: maintaining the monthly calendar for all practice personnel and activities; scheduling non-patient-care appointments; arranging travel itineraries; typing and filing correspondence to and from the practice; maintaining medical and educational files; communicating to and from medical and hospital committees; preparing monthly and yearly practice reports; participating in office research activities; and serving as a backup person in reception, business, and clerical functions.

An administrative assistant will be exposed to confidential and highly sensitive information and must be mature and loyal. Communication skills, both oral and written, will be imperative. In addition, working hours may be varied and unpredictable. Previous experience, either in a similar setting or comparable work, will be a necessity. This is *not* the position for a newly trained person or a personal friend or relative of a physician or colleague.

CONCLUSION

Leadership skills can be equated to the performances of great orchestra conductors, team victories in sports, and successful fund-raising and political campaigns. The measure of difference is not the knowledge of the situation but the ability to achieve results through the efforts of others.

Management is the scientific base, whereas

leadership is the artwork. Artistic achievements may be attained through practice and adherence to a few fundamental precepts. The first is *discipline*. Evidence supports the fact that people who do not possess self-discipline in all aspects of life and work will be less than successful. Discipline in emotional, professional, family, social, and physical aspects are keynote if one desires to lead others and aspire to become a role model. A second precept is *concentration*. The mastery of any art requires thinking, planning, anticipating, and a general sense of perception and deliberation. A third precept is *patience*. If one is seeking quick results, one seldom learns an art. Our competitive and achievement-oriented society fosters exactly the opposite. People think they lose something unless they do things quickly; yet they do not know what to do with time gained except squander it. A final condition of learning any art is *concern*. If the art is not of supreme importance, the learner will never master it.

Drawing upon the teachings of notable humanists C. Rogers, E. Berne, and A. Maslow, I propose six ingredients for leadership success.

1. **Live in the Here and Now.** A person whose mind and body are in unison knows what is happening and understands feelings and beliefs surrounding events.
2. **Recognize Yourself.** We often set goals for ourselves, but how often do we reflect upon achievement and say "Nice job, Self!" As one develops inner strength, the ability to motivate others will be enhanced.
3. **Know Your Limitations.** Be aware when you reach your highest level of competence. Learn how to sidestep incompetence. Blindspots and inadequacies will always be present. The effective person knows how to recognize these or has established support systems to provide necessary assistance.
4. **Enjoy People and Accept Differences.** If a relationship is entered into through professional, social, family, or other factors, then consider investing in the strengths of others and minimize the focus upon their deficiencies. It is easy to terminate uncomfortable relationships, however, the challenge is to revive an unstable or disenchanting association.

5. **Set Your Own Goals.** Frustrations can be minimized if objectives are clear and attainable. Abraham Lincoln said, "If I am aware of where I am going, I have a better idea as to how I can get there." If we achieve our personal goals, we may be less interested in what others are doing or what others say about us.
6. **Take Responsibility for Your Own Feelings and Actions.** There is only one person totally responsible for your behavior—*you!* However, we often hear: "*They* make me feel so bad!" "I can't do anything right when *they* are around" "I just can't take *them* anymore" "*Nobody* can understand me—the dummies!" "He or she makes me angry/sad/upset. If you will accept the premise that each person is ultimately responsible for his or her own feelings and actions, then no one can determine your behavior.

References

Argyris C: *Personality and Organization*. New York, Harper and Row, 1957.

Bebace R, Beattie K, Catline R: Psychological aspects of the problem of time in practice management. *Continuing Education for Family Physicians* 18, no. 3 (1983): 293–298

Bell GD: *The Achievers*. Chapel Hill, NC, Preston-Hill, 1973.

Berne, E. *What do you say after you say hello?* Grove Press, NY 1972

Blake R, Morton J: *The Managerial Grid*. Houston, Tex, Gulf Publishing, 1964.

Buzzotta VR, Lefton RE, Sherberg M: *Effective Selling Through Psychology*. New York, Wiley Interscience, 1972.

Drucker P: Professionals in organizations, in A. Filley, R. House, S. Kerr (eds) *Managerial Process and Organizational Behaviors*. Scott, Foresman, Glenview, Ill. 1976.

Feinberg MR, Tandesky R, Tarrant JJ: *The New Psychology for Managing People*. Englewood Cliffs, NJ: Prentice-Hall, 1975.

Flippo EB: *Management: A Behavioral Approach,* ed 2. Boston, Allyn and Bacon, 1970.

Hackman JR, et al: A new strategy for job enrichment. Technical Report no. 3, Department of Administrative Services, Yale University, May 1974.

Hardy C: The role of medical director in group practice. Presentation, Annual Conference of Medical Group Management Association, Cleveland, Ohio; September 19–22, 1971.

Hersey P, Blanchard KH: So you want to know your leadership style? *Training and Development Journal,* February 1974, pp 22–37.

Herzberg F: *Work and the Nature of Man.* Cleveland, Ohio, World Publishing, 1966.

Kerr S, Von Glinow M, Schriesheim J: Issues in the study of professionals in organizations: The case of scientists and engineers. *Organizational Behavior and Human Performance* 18 (1977):135–146.

Lakein A: *How to Get Control of Your Time and Your Life.* Signet, 1973.

Longest BB: Management Practices for the Health Professional. Reston, Va, Reston Publishing, 1976.

McCall M: *Leadership and the Professional.*

Technical Report, Greensboro, NC, Center for Creative Leadership, 1981.

McCelland D: Toward a theory of motive acquisition. *American Psychology* 20 (1965):321–333.

Mackenzie A: *The Time Trap.* New York, Anacom, 1972.

Maslow A: *Motivation and Personality.* New York, Harper and Row, 1954.

Morano V: Time management from victim to victor. *Health Care Supervisor* 3, no. 1 (1984):1–12.

Nirengberg JS: *Getting Through to People.* Englewood Cliffs, NJ, Prentice-Hall, 1963.

Numerof R: *Manager as conflict negotiator. Health Care Supervisor* 3, no. 3 (1985): 1–15.

Reddin WJ: An integration of leader-behavior. *Typologies Group and Organizational Studies* 2, no. 3 (September 1977):282–295.

Rogers, C: On Becoming a Person, Boston, Houghton, 1961.

7

Office Systems and Communications

Management of medical organizations is complicated by the multiple demands of medical and business routines. It is unlikely that running a medical practice will become less complex, given the rapid changes underway in both the financing and delivery of health services. The successful implementation of clinical and business functions of the organization will depend on the incorporation of a variety of office systems and communications procedures. Office systems should be designed for patient scheduling, health care records, and practice analysis. These systems should be formalized by written guidelines so that they can be maintained by office personnel and monitored by supervisors and physicians. One of the most important systems needed in a medical practice is automation, and Chapter 8 is devoted solely to the computerization of medical practices. *Communication procedures* must be developed for the office personnel, patients, and those individuals the practice communicates with outside the office. Telephone systems, office staff meetings, patient satisfaction, and patient education

are four important communication areas within the practice. A manual of office procedures is the essential practice communications' document.

OFFICE SYSTEMS

Patient Scheduling

Patient scheduling is central to the overall operation of the medical practice. Time efficiency, patient satisfaction, and staff morale are all influenced by patient scheduling. A patient-scheduling system should begin with a written set of policies and instructions and be implemented by the use of a well-designed appointment book.

Scheduling Policies

Office policies for patient scheduling could include the following:

Physicians' weekly office hours are planned two months in advance.

Several periods are available each day for emergency visits.

All routine-care visits require a prearranged appointment.

Each patient is asked the "reason for the visit."

Patients who are more than 30 minutes late may be asked to reschedule the visit unless unforeseeable circumstances occurred.

Patients who bring more than one family member for a visit are charged for each individual seen.

Early morning and noon hour are preferred times for lab tests and nurse visits.

No-shows are documented in patients' records and may be called by the receptionist.

When the patient scheduling system has been implemented, an evaluation should determine if changes are needed. Each staff meeting should include comments from the receptionists and nurses about the schedule. Patient feedback should also be monitored to assess how patients perceive convenience and accessibility of the practice.

When scheduling policies are established, receptionists should be given specific instructions regarding physician preferences for patient-care routines. Factors to consider in these instructions are:

Selection of specified half-days for particular types of patients or problems, such as counseling, prenatal care, and diabetics

Scheduled time with ancillary staff for health screening, follow-up assessments, patient education, and wellness programs

Predetermined time for routine lab and x-ray procedures

Monthly schedule for staff meetings and other non-patient-care activities.

A published list of time allotments should be available for staff and patients. Figure 7.1 offers an example of appointment time allotments for a primary care practice.

Appointment Book

The appointment system is a contract among the patients, physicians, and the practice. All parties involved should honor this time schedule. *Patients' time is just as valuable as physicians, and every attempt should be made to stay on schedule.* Many variables can affect the appointment system, such as parking, time of day, number of physicians in the office, availability of treatment rooms, and proximity of the office to the hospital. Patient satisfaction and ultimately financial return may be negatively affected if scheduling problems occur.

The appointment book should be the singular responsibility of the receptionist, under the supervision of the office manager. Physicians and other staff personnel should not enter or delete appointments without the approval of the receptionist or supervisor. The book should be designed and maintained for: patient entry into the practice, staff and physician work schedules, and scheduling of ancillary services. An appointment scheduling format is shown in Figure 7.2.

Bookkeeping

The cash management process in a medical practice requires a systematic bookkeeping method for tracking the inflow and outflow of money. Regardless of whether the practice is automated or uses manual procedures, bookkeeping routines will be needed for receivables, fees, payables, and third-party payments.

Receivables. Cash receipts and accounts receivable provide the practice the cash to pay for expenses, salaries, and expansion of services. Some of the bookkeeping features for monitoring the receivables are: daily log of office, hospital, and nursing home visits, charges, and receipts; daily record of cash collections and additions to account balances; aging patients' accounts by the number of days since the last payment; monthly mailing of billing statements, weekly processing of third-party claims; and, most important, the close supervision of the office personnel who handle money and who produce the financial reports.

Fees. A comprehensive schedule of professional fees for office visits, procedures, tests, and other practice charges should be kept up to date and made available for physicians, staff, and patients. Along with the fee schedule, a

Type of Visit	Physician Time (Minutes)	Nurse Time (Minutes)
Physical Exam (New Patient)	30	15
Physical Exam (Established Patient)	15	10
Office Visit—New Problem	15	5
Office Visit—Follow-up	10	5
Pap Smear & Pelvic Exam	20	15
Well-Child Exam	10	10
Work-in — Acute Care	10	--
Prenatal Visits	10	10

Other Scheduling Instructions:

Provide for at least two work-in's per half day

Hourly periods should not contain more than one pelvic exam or complete physical

Nonemergency diagnostic testing and blood drawing between 8-9 am

Saturday appointments for acute care, only (no visits scheduled prior to Friday pm)

Figure 7.1 Appointment Time Allotments

rationale should be developed and adhered to. Charges could be determined on a per-minute basis, percentage over the actual costs of the tests, and a set fee for non-patient-care procedures such as insurance form preparation, year-end financial statements, legal advice and depositions, and other special requests requiring physicians and staff time. If fees are determined in advance and publicized, then physicians may be less reluctant to discuss charges. It also allows those seeking the health services to know ahead of time what the cost will be and to decide if they still want the services. A relative value scale published by the Health Care Financing Administration is included in the appendix (Appendix 4, Figure 11).

Payables. Another important cash management feature for the bookkeeping system is accounts payable. This is the outflow of money, ie, the payments made to maintain the practice operations. Expenses are paid for payroll, office supplies, equipment, rent, utilities, insurance, and taxes. Just as receivables require an audit system, payables will also necessitate a similar control process. Check registers may be purchased or designed which record payments on a tabulation sheet to categorize monthly expenses. A file of paid and unpaid invoices should be maintained along with the cancelled checks. The medical director and office manager should meet monthly to review all payments and cosign the checks.

Third-Party Payments. Third-party payers are becoming a major source of reimbursement for health services. Patients pay for about 25% of medical services directly; the remaining portion comes from private insurance companies, Medicare or Medicaid, or prepayment plans. Several routines can be instituted to expedite payments from third parties:

Use a universal claim form to file all insurance payments.

A. Physician Schedule

_____   _____
(Physician)   (Date)

Time	Patient Name/Phone #	Chart #	Patient's Comments[1]	Visit Codes[2]
9:00				
—				
—				
—				
—				
10:00				
—				
—				
—				
11:00				
—				
—				
—				
12:00				

[2]Visit Codes (utilize number of codes needed)

1. New Patient—New Family
2. New Patient—Established Family
3. Established Patient
4. Employment/Insurance Physical Only
5. Other (Explanation–i.e., patient's relatives, visitors)

WI – Work–in
PE – Physical Exam
ER – Emergency
P   – Personal Reason
C   –11 Counseling
ROV– Return Office Visit
P&P – Pap & Pelvic
WC – Well–Child
EX – Extended Procedure

[1]_(Indicate "no-show" with NS_
in Patient's Comments column)

B. Nurse Schedule

_____   _____
(Nurse)   (Date)

Figure 7.2 Appointment Scheduling Formats

Design an office encounter form that can suffice for third-party reimbursement; information required is diagnosis, date of onset, physician's signature, address, and tax identification number.

Encourage patients to review their coverage and payment policies in advance of the services or procedures performed.

Maintain a close relationship between practice staff and representatives of third parties.

Keep current guidelines of third-party organizations in the office.

Maintain a monthly report of third-party charges, receipts, and claims.

Medicare and Medicaid reimbursement plans have several unique features which will require close scrutiny by the practice. _Medicare_ is a federal program intended to reimburse medical costs for the elderly and for those people who are eligible for social security benefits due to disability. Part A coverage provides for hospital care. Part B is optional and requires the patient to pay a monthly premium plus a deductible, approximately 20%. Medicare payments can be made to the beneficiary or directly to the provider. If the practice takes direct payment, then it must consider the reimbursement as payment in full for the charges. There is increasing pressure upon physicians to "accept assignment" for their services and to limit their reimbursement to only the portion the government pays. If this becomes a standard, then Medicare payments may result in a 20% to 25% discount of the normal charges. *Medicaid* was established to ensure that indigent patients have access to quality medical services. To obtain federal participation in a Medicaid program, each state must provide certain services to citizens classified as needy. North Carolina's Medicaid program is county-administered and state-supervised. Counties determine Medicaid eligibility, and the state authorizes services to be covered and ensures proper payment to health providers. The following are mandatory services for Medicaid recipients in North Carolina: physician care, inpatient and outpatient services, early and periodic screening, diagnosis and treatment, skilled nursing care, laboratory and x-ray, home health services, and family planning. Physicians and office staff should stay in contact with county and state officials to determine criteria for patient and family eligibility.

Health Care Records

Physicians and other health care providers will be responsible for documentation of personal and medical data for the thousands of patients they will treat. Family and medical history, symptoms and problems, medications, allergies, and other health issues will need to be recorded and maintained for future reference. A thorough system of health information plays a crucial role in such features of medical care as comprehensiveness, continuity, and prevention. The group practice model requires a complete and readily accessible medical record.

Components. Various types of information may be included in the medical record, but the data included generally fall into five categories: patient and family information, medical history, progress notes, lab reports and medication records, and various flow sheets. Included with the *patient and family information* should be such administrative facts as chart number, name, birth date, address, phone number, employer, medical insurance status, and similar information about family members. A copy of this information should be maintained in the record. Patients should be asked at each visit if any of this information has changed. *Medical history* should include allergies, immunizations, review of systems, occupational hazards, and other pertinent information to aid in current or future care. A standardized questionnaire may be a valuable tool, especially if it is easy to complete and can be tabulated and recorded directly into the record by the nurse. *Progress notes* represent what remains of the traditional patient record. A chronological account of patient activity is a useful guide if it includes such information as signs and symptoms, physical findings, lab results, subjective impressions, diagnoses, and treatment plans. Abnormal findings should be highlighted for quick reference. *Flow sheets* can be used to follow the course of a particular medical problem or the patient's health status. Physical findings and lab results as well as other pertinent data can be recorded in columnar form so that the patient's progress can be reviewed as one reads left to right. Flow sheets are particularly useful to chart child development, to monitor chronic diseases, and during prenatal care. Appendix 7 includes examples of these various components of medical records.

Filing and Storage. Handling medical records is another important consideration. Records may be filed alphabetically by patient name or numerically by chart number. Numerical filing with a cross-index will be required for automated systems. Color coding or marking each chart by the year of the encounter will be helpful when purging files. Open shelving is the preferred method of storage, because it provides access by several people. Separating active and inactive patient files will also conserve space. Microfilming may be necessary, since physicians are required to maintain patient records for at least seven years.

Special Concerns. The question of who should have access to the medical records is frequently of concern. The medical record is the legal property of the physician and/or the practice. However, the patient has the right to any and all information in the record. Another important consideration is the filing of telephone messages and other patient encounters that may not have necessitated an office visit.

All patient contacts should be documented in the medical record, especially those involving medications, treatment plans, referrals, and other clinically related encounters. The practice staff can design a non-office-visit form to record these types of contacts in the chart.

Practice Analysis

The viability of the medical practice will depend upon many organizational factors, not the least of which is the management information system. Productivity information will be essential to analyze current activities, identify problems at their earliest stage, and pinpoint specific areas in which to institute solutions. The three major areas to incorporate into a "practice information system" are patient flow, financial management, and demographic and diagnostic profiles. Computerized systems are programmed to provide individual physicians and the practice with a comprehensive practice management information system. The larger and more complex the organization, the more appropriate will be the implementation of automated data retrieval and analysis.

Patient Flow. The features of patient flow which merit reporting and analysis include: number of patients seen in the office, hospital, nursing home, and other settings; number of new patients and families; number of telephone calls, during the day and after hours; cancellations and no-shows; and any other classifications that will be useful for analyzing practice management and health care trends.

Financial Management. Office finances require close scrutiny for obvious reasons. It is not enough to file income tax forms and receive quarterly statements from the accountants. A daily, weekly, and monthly financial picture must be maintained. Financial reporting should include charges and receipts, collection rates, expenses versus budget, and cash flow analysis. Individual providers should be presented with their separate productivity analyses, along with the total practice's productivity.

Demographic and Diagnostic Profiles. Age, sex, illness, and disease will vary within the patient population, by provider and perhaps seasonally. By analyzing this information the practice may be able to determine the need for different types of services and equipment and the potential demand upon the practice at a particular time of year. This information also allows physicians to conduct research within their practice. An example of a practice analysis report that could be provided for individual physicians and the total practice is seen in Figure 7.3.

COMMUNICATIONS

Medical practices operate within an intricate network of people and systems. Even though physicians and other health professionals may be highly qualified in their field, their effectiveness will also depend upon a wide range of communication procedures and skills. Initial attention should be directed to the intraoffice communications, such as that among patients, office personnel, and colleagues. Telephone systems, staff relations and meetings, and patient education are some of the more formal intraoffice communications procedures. External communications will be needed to build and secure relations with the hospital, community agencies, third-party organizations, and other public and private institutions.

Intraoffice

Even though physicians spend considerable time communicating verbally to patients and staff, they should also incorporate written-communication documents into their clinical care and office management.

Patients

Surveys of patients have uncovered a variety of common complaints about physicians and their communication styles. Some of the most frequently mentioned statements were:

Doctors are more interested in my illness than in me as a person.
Doctors are constantly behind schedule and sel-

FINANCIAL ANALYSIS			DIAGNOSTIC ANALYSIS		
Charges	Monthly	Year to Date	Major Category	Quarterly	Year to Date
I. Professional Services			Prophylactic		
Initial office visit			Cardiac, vascular		
Nurse visit			Respiratory		
Routine office visit			Allergic, endo, metabolic		
Extended office visit			Mental		
Physical exams			Genito-urinary		
			Signs, symptoms		
II. OB-GYN			Disorder — bone and		
Pelvic exam			joint		
Prenatal care			Digestive		
Post partum exam			Nervous system		
III. Office Procedures			Skin, cellular		
ECG			Accidents		
Sigmoidoscopy			Infectious disease		
Eye exam			Other		
Hearing test					
Cryosurgery			Major Diagnosis		
IV. Inj. & Immunization			1. Hypertension		
			2. Other symptoms		
V. Laboratory			3. URI		
Urine			4. Anxiety		
Pregnancy test			5. Pelvic exam		
Pap smear			6. Depression		
Glucose			7. Pap smear		
Hematocrit			8. Well-child exam		
Throat culture			9. Diabetes mellitus		
			10. Obesity		
VI. Hospital Care			11. Congestive heart failure		
Admission work-up			12. Physical, special		
Routine care			13. Bronchitis		
			14. Cystitis		
VII. Other			15. Emphysema		
Counseling	_____	_____	16. Family relations	_____	_____
Total charges			**Sub-total**		
Payments					
Insurance					
Cash payment					
Money order					
Personal check					
Attorney payment	_____	_____			
Total payments					
Collection ratio = $ payments/$ charges					

DEMOGRAPHIC ANALYSIS

Sex	Month	Year to Date	Marital Status	Month	Year to Date
Male			Single		
Female	_____	_____	Married		
Totals			Separated/divorced		
			Widowed	_____	_____
Age—			**Totals**		
0-12 yrs					
13-19 yrs			**Family Care**		
20-39 yrs			Entire family		
40-60 yrs			Part of family		
61 yrs & over	_____	_____	Individual only	_____	_____
Totals			**Totals**		

Census
   Rural   Urban
   Suburban   Inner City

Figure 7.3 Practice Productivity Analysis. (Reprinted by permission from Aluise JJ, 1977. The Physician as Manager, 'What' and 'How' of Practice Management Education. *Journal of Family Practice* 4(2). Appleton-Century-Crofts.)

dom recognize that my time is just as important as theirs.

Office staff seldom take patients seriously; they give us very little respect.

Doctors do not take time to explain the treatment plan or the fees.

Doctors and staff do not always respect patients' need for privacy.

It appears that there may be a communications gap between the medical profession and its consumers. Both physicians and office personnel should make a concerted effort to bridge this gap. One of the ways to determine if the practice is meeting its patients' needs is to survey patients on a regular basis. Figure 7.4 is an example of a patient satisfaction survey that can be completed by patients when they visit the practice or can be administered by telephone or mail.

As was discussed in the chapter on marketing, a variety of patient communication materials can be distributed to keep the information flow open between the practice and its patients. The *letter to new patients* provides a personal communique from the physicians to the new members of the practice. If the practice has added a new physician or made other major changes, it is important to convey this information to all patients as quickly as possible with additional patient letters or bulletins. The *patient information booklet* is a more substantial document that can be used with new and existing patients. It may also be worthwhile to consider a *patient newsletter* that could include features on the office personnel, new developments in the practice, policy changes, and a section on patient education. The most important message in the communications process is not the content as much as it is the intention of the practice to reach out and keep the patients informed.

Office communications should not be construed as merely administrative and managerial. They can also apply to the doctor-patient encounters, in the form of patient education. Ideally, written materials and brief instruction sheets would be used to reinforce the verbal directions. The information to be covered by patient education should be relevant to the common problems and procedures of the practice. For a primary care practice a suggested list of topics could be as follows:

Preventive Medicine. Such as nutrition, immunizations, safety, substance abuse, occupational health hazards, self-exams, and regular checkups

Common Acute Disorders. Such as colds, flu, ear infections, veneral diseases, wounds and fractures, and other seasonal or geographic problems

Chronic Diseases. Such as diabetes, hypertension, arthritis, ulcers, allergies, asthma, and congestive heart failure.

Home Nursing Care. Such as taking temperatures, collecting urine specimens, providing first aid and cardiopulmonary resuscitation, and caring for the disabled

Problems Related to Life Stage. Such as child development, menstruation, menopause, pregnancy, marriage, family planning, contraception, and care of the elderly.

Appendix 7 presents a list of printed patient education materials and the addresses for ordering them. Materials can also be obtained from school supply houses, public health departments, hospitals, and the local school system. Physicians may prefer to design educational and instructional handouts. Examples of some patient education materials that were prepared by physicians and other health professionals are also included in the appendix.

Telephone

The most crucial communications instrument in the medical office is the telephone. The telephone transmits information about schedules, emergencies, and a variety of other inquiries and messages. With the increasing emphasis upon prepayment and decreased use of health services, the concept of "telephone medicine" may soon become a principal method of physician-patient communications.

The key to a good telephone management system is the office personnel. In practices with two or more physicians, it may be necessary to designate one or two people as *telephone receptionist*. The person could be located in the front office with access to appointment schedules and medical records. The advantages of a primary telephone receptionist are twofold—such a receptionist provides relief from telephone interruptions for other staff while they check people in and out and do other clerical duties, and pa-

To Our Patients:

The physicians and staff of our practice are interested in your opinions about the services we provide. Please take a few minutes and answer the following questions. This information will be very helpful to us as we continue to serve you and your families health care needs.

Is this your first visit to the practice?   Yes _____   No _____

What factors influenced your decision to choose our practice?
       Friend or family member _____
       Patient of the practice _____
       Referral from another physician _____   Who was the physician? _____
       Telephone listing _____
       Other _____

Were you able to obtain an appointment with a reasonable time?   Yes _____   No _____
       If not, how long did it take? _____

Are the office hours convenient?   Yes _____   No _____
       If not, what would be more suitable? _____

Were you treated courteously by the office personnel?   Yes _____   No _____
       If not, please explain _____

Did you find the reception area comfortable?   Yes _____   No _____
       If not, do you have any suggestions? _____

Were you satisfied with the time it took to see the doctor?   Yes _____   No _____
       If not, approximately how long did you have to wait? _____

Were you satisfied with the medical services you received?   Yes _____   No _____
       If not, please explain _____

Were you treated courteously by physicians?   Yes _____   No _____
       If not, please explain _____

What other suggestions do you have to help us provide better health services?

                                                                            THANK YOU FOR YOUR COOPERATION,

Figure 7.4   Patient Satisfaction Survey

tients begin to relate to just one person and thus are more willing to allow screening questions about the urgency of their problems. Figure 7.5 presents a set of telephone protocols which is a handy guide for training telephone receptionists.

The *nursing staff* and *other health professionals* soon become the next step in the telephone answering schema. Clinical personnel can provide very adequate information and support via the telephone in such areas as medication questions, lab and diagnostic test results, calls to pharmacists, referrals to other physicians and community agencies, and nonurgent messages from the hospital or other professionals. Some practices have instituted a *telephone call period* in which physicians, psychologists, nurse practitioners, nutritionists, and other health professionals are available to respond to patient inquiries at no additional cost.

Office Staff

Just as patients require a variety of communications procedures, officer personnel deserve an information exchange with the physicians and practic supervisors that is characterized by an open, two-way process. An important starting point in organizational communications is to solicit ideas and suggestions about the operation of the practice from the personnel. Figure 7.6 is an example of a staff opinion survey that could be administered to office personnel. This information can be useful in evaluating the current clinical and management system and in considering changes for the future.

Once the organization develops mechanisms to ''listen'' to its employees, then it can begin to formalize office communications. Two tangible methods of communication within the practice are: (1) an office procedures manual that spells out the policies and expectations of the organization, and (2) a regular staff meeting between employees and the supervisors and physicians to discuss issues of importance and to problem-solve. An *office procedures manual* ensures that all employees have access to a common set of policies and procedures. Figure 7.7 provides a comprehensive outline for a medical practice office manual. Responsibility for designing and updating this communications document goes to the office supervisor and medical director. All employees should have access to this document or should be given a modified version pertinent to their areas of responsibility.

Since the most dynamic form of communication occurs in face-to-face encounters, another important dimension of office communication will be the *staff meeting*. These meetings are an invaluable means of obtaining staff input and presenting first-hand information to the employees. Staff meetings require planning and management skills. The following *guidelines* may be helpful for those who have the responsibility for leading these meetings:

Schedule meetings on a regular basis, at least monthly.

Arrange the meeting time and place to ensure the highest attendance possible.

Plan and distribute the agenda in advance.

Vary the agenda to include administrative, clinical, personnel, and other relevant topics.

Use some meetings for staff development—the monthly office meeting is an excellent opportunity for physicians and other health professionals to provide staff education, presenting new clinical methods and management innovations.

Each meeting should have a written summary that outlines major discussion points, plans, decisions, and future agenda items.

Physicians

Since the group practice model is becoming the most common form of practice, physician-to-physician communications is of great importance. Even though administrative meetings are often disdained, physicians should set aside a regular meeting time with their partners. A format similar to the office staff meeting could be followed. Features of the *physician meeting* include preparing the agenda for the staff meet-

Figure 7.5   Telephone Protocols

Appointment Schedules
Who is your physician?
When do you wish to see the doctor?
What symptoms have you had?
How long have they persisted?
Your procedures will require (X) minutes.
Your appointment is (Date) (Time)
Please come 15 minutes early.
The visit will cost approximately ($) and we appreciate payment at the time of the visit.

Receptionists' Reference List

	Time	Cost
Initial/Complete Physical Exam	30 min.	$50
Routine OV	20 min.	$15
Acute OV	10 min.	$10
Well Baby	15 min.	$12
Counseling	45 min.	$35
OB—Initial	30 min.	$350
—Prenatal	15 min.	

Figure 7.5 *Continued*

Screening New Patients*
Who referred you to the practice?
What type of physician were you previously seeing?
How many family members will be enrolling in the practice?
How will you finance your health care?
All office calls are on a cash basis.
Initial visits are ($X), routine visits will be ($X).

Adult Acute Illness
When did the pain begin?
What symptoms are you experiencing?
When did you last see a physician?
Are you taking any medication?
Can you come directly to the office?
Doctor will return call at (time), please be available.
Pharmacy—name, address, phone?

Pediatric Acute Illness
What are the child's symptoms?
If fever, how high?
Medications?
What has child been eating?
Vomiting? Diarrhea?

(ATTACH MESSAGES TO PATIENTS' CHARTS AND INFORM NURSES/
PHYSICIANS)

Emergency Calls
Name, address, phone number?
Is anyone with you?
Bleeding? Broken bone?
Can you come to office/hospital?

(CONTACT NURSE/PHYSICIAN IMMEDIATELY WITH PATIENT STILL ON LINE)

Personal Calls
May I ask who is calling?
The doctor is seeing patients, where can you be reached? When?
May I tell the doctor the reason for the call?
Doctor will return your call at (time).

*These questions may be valuable when the practice is selectively adding new patients.

ing; reviewing financial reports; meeting with financial and legal consultants; and setting time schedules for clinical and personal committment. These meetings should also have written summaries.

Interoffice

The physicians' office practice does not operate in a vacuum. It is involved in an intricate network of health care systems within the community. Physicians and other health professionals will become affiliated with a hospital, community agencies, third-party payment companies, educational institutions, and other organizations. Before joining or working with outside organizations, physicians should understand the purpose and function of each affiliation and the time and financial implications of membership.

The physicians and supervisors of the practice are interested in the opinions of our personnel about how the practice can function more effectively. Please take a few minutes to answer the following questions.

ALL RESPONSES ARE ANONYMOUS.

Which of the following areas of the practice do you believe need to be improved?

Appointments ____	Telephone System ____	Business Office ____
Billing ____	Insurance Claims ____	Receptionist area ____
Waiting room ____	Medical Records ____	Nurses station ____
Laboratory ____	_____	_____
	Other	Other

COMMENTS _____

Which of the following practice functions do you believe need to be improved?

Patient Education ____	Physicians' Schedules ____
Office Meetings ____	Staff Evaluations ____
Staff Schedules ____	_____
_____	Other
Other	

COMMENTS _____

Do you receive enough information to adequately perform your work?   Yes ____   No ____
   If not, please explain _____

Do you believe the supervision you receive is adequate?   Yes ____   No ____
   If not, please explain _____

What other ideas do you have to improve your job? To improve the practice?

                                                    THANK YOU FOR YOUR COOPERATION

Figure 7.6 Staff Opinion Survey

Figure 7.7 Office Procedures Manual Outline

This office procedures manual has been prepared to assist both physicians and office staff in understanding the organization and operations of the practice.

It is a guidebook to the workings of our medical office. This document will aid office personnel in understanding the scope of our practice, both inside and outside the office. Personnel policies are also included and should be reviewed carefully so that misunderstandings do not occur. Each employee will find that their responsibilities are outlined. This communication is intended to facilitate an awareness of the office tasks which will be necessary to insure the highest quality patient care at the most economic cost.

Introduction and Description of the Practice

Section 1: Patient and Community Relations
   A.   Philosophy of the Practice—Family and Patient Care
   B.   Patient Satisfaction
   C.   Ethics, Confidentiality, and Sensitivity
   D.   Representing the Practice in the Community

Section 2: Personnel Policies
   A.   Job Descriptions
   B.   Employment Stipulations
      1.   Daily/Weekly Hours
      2.   Vacations, Holidays, Work Leaves

Figure 7.7 *Continued*

        3. Compensation
        4. Fringe Benefits
        5. Probation
        6. Termination
    C. Supervision
        1. Training and Retraining
        2. Performance Appraisal
    D. Performance Standards
        1. Quality and Quantity of Work
        2. Breadth of Responsibilities and Skills
        3. Initiative and Cooperation
    E. Personnel Policy Statement Per Employee
    F. Organizational Chart
        1. Authority and Supervision
        2. Practice Functions—Medical, Business, Lab, etc.

Section 3: Financial Operations
    A. Budget and Expenditures
        1. Personnel Salaries and Benefits
        2. Medical and Office Supplies
        3. Facilities—Rent, Leases, etc.
        4. Services—Housekeeping, Accounting, Maintenance
        5. Utilities and Telephone
        6. Travel
        7. Miscellaneous
    B. Daily Cash Receipts
        1. In-Office, Billing, and Third Party
        2. Accounting System and Audits
        3. Daily, Weekly, Monthly Reporting
    C. Billing and Collections
        1. Monthly Statements
        2. Credit and Collection Policy
        3. Collection Agency
    D. Insurance and Third Party
        1. Medicare and Medicaid
        2. Blue Cross/Blue Shield
        3. Workman's Compensation
        4. Filing Requirements and Records
    E. Petty Cash
    F. Inventory and Supplies
        1. Equipment
        2. Inventory Controls—On Hand, Order Dates and Reordering
        3. Supplies and Reordering—Unit Costs, Quantity Discounts
           a. Medical—Exam Room, Paper, Instruments, Surgical
           b. Laboratory—Reagents, Solutions, Test Materials, Specimen Collections
           c. Medications and Drugs
           d. Business and Reception Offices
    G. Fees and Charges
    H. Financial Records and Reports
    I. Taxes
        1. Payroll
        2. Income
        3. Property

Figure 7.7 *Continued*

Section 4: Office Tasks
    A. Appointment Scheduling
        1. Time Allotments
        2. Routine and Emergency Visits
        3. Recall
        4. No–Shows and Cancellations
    B. Filing
        1. Financial Documents
        2. Medical Records
        3. Correspondence
        4. Personnel Policies
        5. Educational Materials
        6. Miscellaneous
    C. Reception
        1. Reception Room and Office Decorum
        2. Registration Forms
        3. Preparation of Medical/Financial Forms
        4. Verification of Demographic Information
    D. Telephone
        1. Messages—Doctor/Nurse Return
        2. After Hours Calls
        3. Prescription Refills
        4. Lab Results

Section 5: Medical Protocol
    A. Patient Preparation
        1. Vital Signs and History Taking
        2. Examinations
        3. Lab Values
    B. Screening Procedures
    C. Medical Records
    D. Exam Room Preparations
    E. Administering Tests and Injections
    F. Assisting Physician
    G. Laboratory Skills
    H. Emergency Care—Trauma and CPR
    I. Sterilization
    J. Counseling and Patient Education
    K. Communicating to Pharmacies
    L. Restock Supplies

NOTE: Colwell Co., 201 Kenyan Road, Champaign, IL offers an office manual guidebook for the medical office practice.

Hospital. Hospital administrators and medical staff colleagues will have a variety of expectations for the office-based practitioner. Administrators will be concerned about admissions and bed capacity, use of hospital services, participation in fund-raising task forces, and close working relations with the medical community. Medical professionals will be asked to assist in peer review of quality care and cost containment, house staff teaching, continuing medical education, and various departmental and hospitalwide committees. Satisfying all requests for participation will be impossible. Before accepting any outside responsibilities, the following criteria should be considered:

Does this commitment have a definite time
    commitment?

Table 7.1 Community Reference File

Agency	Purpose	Persons to Contact	Phone #
Aged Programs			
Alcoholics Anonymous	Support and counseling		
Alcohol Rehabilitation Center	Detox. and rehab.		
Ambulance Service	Emergency med. transportation		
Child Guidance Center	Child & adolescent counseling		
Childbirth Education	Prenatal classes		
Emergency Room— Hospital			
Family Services	Counseling & financial support		
Fire Department			
Florence Crittenton Home	Programs for unwed mothers		
Goodwill Industries	Employment for the handicapped		
Legal Aid	Legal services for the needy		
Marriage Counselors	Counselors and therapists		
Mental Health Center	Inpatient & outpatient, crisis intervention		
Nursing Homes	Extended medical care, residency, and rehab.		
Planned Parenthood	Screening and examination		
Poison Control Center			
Police Department			
Public Health Dept.	Immunizations, education, disease control		
Rape Crisis Center	Counseling and referral		
Red Cross	Disaster relief, nursing services		
Rescue Squad	Office/home emergency assistance		
Salvation Army	Food, lodging for indigent		
School Systems	Elementary and secondary educ.		
Special Education Programs	Education for retarded and autistic		
Veterans Service Office	Support for benefits and claims		
Welfare and Public Assistance	Financial and legal support		

Are responsibilities clearly defined?
What leadership role is expected?
How does this activity fit into personal and professional interests?
Are the results and expectations realistic?

Ideally, decisions to participate in major hospital and community activities are planned as early as possible.

Community Agencies. Practicing physicians will be a first point of contact for most of the health services of their patients. It is unlikely that any one physician or practice can provide all aspects of the needed health care. Thus, physicians and their office personnel will be di-recting patients and families to the appropriate health-related agencies. Maintaining a file of these organizations will be a valuable tool for referral and consultation. Table 7.1 presents format for a community reference file. If this file is current and available to all office personnel, then a patient can be given a phone number and the name of a contact person.

CONCLUSION

Organizational effectiveness, employee motivation, and financial viability will be maximized if the practice operates systematically and with open communications. Schedules, protocols, flow patterns, forms and charts, medical records, and productivity reports will facilitate a systems approach to office management. Patient scheduling and bookkeeping procedures should be designed so that patients, staff, and physicians function in a predictable and consistent manner. Practice information and statistical reports will enhance the knowledge base of the supervisors and physicians, so that decision making and problem solving can be objective and timely.

The communications channel which flows through a medical practice influences patient care, staff and physician productivity, and time management. Both physicians and staff should share in the formulation of procedures manuals, staff protocols, patient education, and telephone guidelines. Formal methods of communication will not ensure success, but they may allow the practice to operate smoothly.

References

Bartlett E: Accomplishing more with less, using patient education. *Health Care Financial Management,* July 1985, pp 86–95.

Burke D: An integrated medical record system. *Medical Group Management* 30, no. 6 (1983):32–49.

Center for Research in Ambulatory Health Care: *The Organization and Development of a Medical Group Practice,* Cambridge, Mass, 1976, pp 293–315.

Curtis P: The telephone in medical practice. *Journal of Family Practice* 6, no. 4 (1978):897–898.

Do your records really fit your needs? *Patient Care,* June 16, 1976, pp 100–119.

Ehrlich A: *Medical Office Procedures Manual.* Champaign, Ill., Colwell, 1977.

Emberlyn-Torci S, Rowe J: Maintaining medical records. *Medical Group Management* 30, no. 4 (1983):54–57.

Family Health, Inc: *Practice Management Considerations.* Princeton, NJ, Systemedics, Inc, prepared for US Department of Health, Education and Welfare, 1977.

Fox Dr, Battisto TC: Computer input the best way. *Medical Group Management* 21 (September-October 1974):6–12.

Howard WW: *Dental Practice Planning.* St Louis, CV Mosby, 1975.

McConnell C: The supervisor's central role in organizational communication. *Health Care Supervision* 3, no. 2 (January 1985):77–86.

McCormick J: A systematic approach to patient scheduling. *Medical Group Management* 22, no. 4 (May-June 1975):13–17.

Patients reveal 10 most common complaints. *Physician's Management,* February 1978, pp 39–43.

Pope YG: Determinants of medical care utilization: The use of the telephone for reporting symptoms. *Journal of Health and Social Behavior,* June 12, 1971, pp 155–162.

Taylor R: Ten small ways to please patients. *Physician's Management* 54 (April 1978):59–60.

8

Computerization

- How do you determine the need for automation?
- What are the important factors in selecting software and hardware?
- What are the latest developments in computer applications for clinical information, practice management, and medical information databases?
- What are the steps to take when purchasing and installing a computer system?
- How do you evaluate a computer company?
- What needs to be included in a vendor's contract?

The computer has revolutionized the management and clinical functions in medical offices. Regardless of specialty or size of practice, automation is now a viable option. Advantages of computerizing a medical office are well documented. Hardware and software applications can now perform many of the manual office tasks accurately and reliably, allowing physicians and office personnel to concentrate on more important responsibilities. Hardware costs have stabilized at reasonable rates, and computer use has been shown cost-effective for small practices. Applications for a wide range of business and clinical procedures, including appointment scheduling, laboratory reports, and patient education, are successfully in operation. Computerized patient management programs to aid clinical decision making are moving from experimentation stage to the patient care setting.

Despite these many positive features of computers and their declining cost, the implementation of a computer system requires careful investigation. The hardware and software should be designed so that they can easily replace the office's current manual system. Realize however that *a computer system will not cure the problems of a chaotic manual system*. When selecting an automated system, physicians and staff members must rethink business management, patient flow, and clinical procedures so that the new system enhances practice efficiency and maintains the highest-quality patient care. Planning and implementing a computerized system for an existing practice could require nine to twelve months, depending on the difficulty of converting from manual to automated procedures. Be careful not to underestimate the financial investment of automation, since direct and indirect costs could range from $10,000 to $100,000 depending on the size of the system and whether it is a single-user or multiuser system. Regardless of the size of the practice and cost of the system, the steps toward purchasing an automated office system are essentially the same. Any practice contemplating automation would benefit from using a systematic method to evaluate and eventually choose the most appropriate system.

The planning process should include analysis of the facilities, review of the current office and clinical systems, determination of conversion costs, and assessment of personnel requirements. Thorough planning is important to minimize risks in purchasing and installing an office automation system. A systematic approach in making the decision to buy a computer includes a feasibility analysis of a practice followed by a comparative review of computer systems. Physicians considering integrating a computer into their practices must justify its use in terms of cost benefit, assessment of needs, and ultimate value to the operations of the practice. Unless the physicians or the administrator are well-versed in computer systems and have adequate time to plan and oversee the implementation of the computer system, it may be wise to hire a consultant at the very earliest stage of planning.

This chapter presents the essential concepts of computers and their applications for health care organizations. It is not intended to be a comprehensive analysis of medical computer systems, although it offers a broad range of topics and criteria for selecting the most appropriate system. The reader is strongly encouraged to delve more deeply into the subject of computers and their usefulness in medical practices. Several excellent references were consulted for this chapter and are recommended as user-friendly guides to would-be computer consumers. They are: *Computerizing Your Medical Practice,* by Dot Sellars, Medical Economics Company, Oradell, N.J.; *PHYSICIANS' PRIMER ON COMPUTERS,* by Jan Brandejs and Graham Pace, Lexington Books, DC Heath, Lexington, Mass.; *COMPUTERS FOR DOCTORS,* by Laurence Gonzales, Ballantine Books, Cloverdale Press, New York, NY. Several computer journals exclusively devoted for medical applications are also being published. The reference section of this chapter provides a list of several relevant articles from these journals.

NEED FOR AUTOMATION

In her computer guide for physicians and office personnel, Sellars identifies several warning signs that may signal the need for a computer. Organizations contemplating automation may wish to review the following indicators.

Practice Growth. Medical practices are growing into large-scale organizations as they add new health care providers and expand their clinical and business functions. Substantial increases in patient volume and revenue lead to increases in staffing and paperwork and necessitate more efficient work routines. Computers may not bring in new business but they can help organize and manage the growth.

Insurance Burden. Third-party reimbursement has brought with it an abundance of claim forms and payment plans leaving patients and the practice caught in the middle. But, to the great satisfaction of the beleagured office staff who had to face the insurance-form backlog, computer programs are now available to handle the majority of insurance claim preparation.

Collections Declining. Most businesses consider a 3% to 4% loss for bad debts a cost of doing business. When the practice collection rate drops below 95%, the reduced revenue results in lower income to the physicians and staff. Computerized billing procedures keep the financial system operating efficiently and often will result in a higher collection rate from third parties as well as from private patients.

Billing Schedules Unmet. Processing patients' monthly statements and insurance claims is a time-consuming, mundane chore for office personnel. Accuracy and timeliness may become problems when other practice demands take priority. Computer billing programs perform most of the work without any staff involvement and may even operate when the office is closed.

Voluminous Paperwork. Estimates have been made that physicians spend from 20% to 30% of their professional time doing paperwork. Regardless of the specialty or size of practice it is impossible to escape the labor intensive tasks of recording, filing and documenting financial and clinical procedures. A computer system can eliminate most of the manual aspects of these tasks and improve the quality of the business and clinical functions.

Accelerating Expenses. Operating expenses are typically 50% of revenue, and staff salaries account for approximately half of the overhead. If operating expenses are increasing to a higher percentage, especially for personnel, then automation may be an option. Adding new staff members may resolve clerical backlogs in the short run, but it does not address the reason the problem occurred initially. A consultant can be a valuable resource to review the expenses and productivity to determine if automating can help control costs.

Practice in Multiple Locations. As practices expand to satellite offices and affiliations are developed with other organizations, they will need a more sophisticated financial and clinical information system. Because computers are flexible and expandable, they can provide an invaluable source of information for current and future management decisions.

Information-Based Decisions. Health care professionals require a vast amount of information to make business and clinical decisions. Much of the information needed is not easily accessible in manual systems, but computers can now provide almost instantly patient information and detailed productivity reports. Standards of practice may soon require automated systems.

Facility and Space Constraints. Medical practices are constantly in search of space to store medical records, locate personnel, and add new procedures. Computer systems usually occupy less square footage than manual systems do.

SOFTWARE AND HARDWARE

The biggest decision to make in selecting hardware and software is what you want the computer to accomplish. Hardware is the computer itself and the various peripheral devices needed such as printers, monitors, modems and disk drives. Software is to a computer what the records are to a phonograph. It contains the programs that enable the computer to perform business and clinical tasks. The system's output requirements determine the software features needed.

Software

The purchase of a software system will involve several types of decisions. An off-the-shelf system, one that has been predesigned by the manufacturer, can be purchased from a national or local supplier. Some benefits of off-the-shelf software are that it is less expensive, has been tested, and has probably been kept updated. Off-the-shelf programs are available for such applications as billing, word processing, accounting, database management, and general ledgers. In recent years software has also been designed for patient scheduling, medical records, analysis of laboratory tests, and other diagnostic applications. Most practices will probably require some modifications before the physicians will be totally satisfied with the computer applications. If the organization has many unique features and needs, it may require a custom-made system. Evaluating off-the-shelf programs or designing custom-made systems will require expertise and objectivity, which may not be available within the organization. Consultants, especially those who do not represent any particular system, can provide invaluable advice and assistance in both planning and implementing a computer system.

Important things to consider in selecting software are the cost of maintaining the program; ownership and accessibility of the computer source codes; clarity and availability of procedure manuals and other written documents necessary to operate the system: ease of data entry; and the usefulness of the output. Programs should enable data to be entered into the system, either through forms or directly online by office personnel. Evaluate input devices on their compatibility with the organizational work flow and the skills of the personnel. Output, such as reports, statements, and other documents, should be easy to comprehend. An important gauge of output quality is how relevant it is to the management of business and clinical operations.

Hardware

Hardware features of a computer system include the electronic microprocessor, memory, monitor, keyboard, disk drives, printers, and other electronic parts. Memory and storage functions are considered of prime importance for a medical practice because of the large number of patient records and the vast amount of information that is maintained. In determining hardware needs, the consultants and the computer representatives should conduct an extensive review of current patient volume and make projections for the future. Discussions about the value of other applications, such as accessing national databases, conducting clinical research, and developing patient and disease profiles, will also help determine hardware needs.

Medical practices require a large amount of information to be collected and stored. Computers are equipped to record automatically the contents of memory onto disk for storage. This frees space in memory for more data. Tape drives are used when large amounts of information must be stored or submitted to other users, such as insurance companies. Hard disks, which are more durable than floppy disks, are recommended for medical practices. Backup systems will be essential for medical practices as a safeguard against loss of data due to fire, lightning, and other hazards to the automated systems. The two most common hardware systems currently being installed in medical practices are microcomputers and minicomputers.

Microcomputers. The "micro" is the newest computer system developed for managing the small- to medium-size office. Micros generally have limited capability because of their smaller processing unit, memory size, and number of input and output features. Micros can handle word processing and data management. The micros originally were single-user-oriented and performed only one application function at a time. However, multiuser systems are now available that allow more than one function to operate simultaneously. The advantages of a microcomputer are the lower cost, ease of operation, minimal space requirements, and complete control over data. The disadvantages are the relatively slow access time, less disk storage space, and limited selection of software.

Minicomputers. The "mini" is a larger system than the micro and has more memory and disk storage space. Hard disks are usually standard. A minicomputer has a more powerful processing capability with the option to integrate a wide range of input and output devices. It can serve several users concurrently. Minicomputers, which are about the size of a desk, are somewhat larger than micros but are regarded as considerably more versatile. However, with the recent advancements in microcomputers, the distinction between "micro" and "mini" is considerably less. The advantages of minicomputers are easy access, larger storage capacity, multiple simultaneous users, control over data, and the ability to function as a centralized or decentralized system. The disadvantages are that they are more expensive and have high maintenance and repair costs, consume more space, require training of personnel, lack a market for used equipment, and disrupt practice operations when they break down.

HEALTH CARE SYSTEMS

As health care organizations and medical practices evolve into large-scale systems of delivery and financing, they will require advanced management and clinical information services. Considering the highly competitive nature of the medical marketplace, automation will virtually become a necessity. As clinical revenue becomes more stable due to standard fees and contracts, practices must operate efficiently, while offering the same high-quality patient care. Computer applications are at least one major step medical practices can take to meet these economic challenges. The following sections on patient and clinical information, practice management, and national medical information databases describe some of the innovations occurring in health care computerization.

Patient and Clinical Information

The multitude of encounters that take place between a doctor and patient produce a vast amount of information. Computer systems are now collecting and storing demographic, diagnostic, and treatment data for use in individual patient transactions and for clinical research. Concise summaries of patient and family records can be automated and made available to insert in patient records for review in subsequent visits. Clinical judgments and decision making will be greatly enhanced when information is readily available and presented in a systematic format.

The leading automated medical information system is COSTAR (computer-stored ambulatory record). COSTAR was developed by the Laboratory of Computer Science of Massachusetts General Hospital. It was originally funded by the federal government as a project to design a computer system for medical recordkeeping. COSTAR's evolution is unique because it began as a medical information system for improving the quality of medical care. Most other medical computer systems, particularly those available for commercial use, began as financial or business management programs. COSTAR can capture, store, manipulate, and retrieve medical information. Patient information is displayed on video screens to aid in such tasks as scheduling, quality assurance, billing, transferring data, and updating medical databases. COSTAR is also a modular system; it has separate components for registration and scheduling, billing and accounts receivable, medical records, management reporting, security, and integrity. A practice may use one of or all the components. COSTAR has been installed in large and small health care organizations throughout the United States and Canada. The price for a fully operational system is approximately $30,000. A major distributor of COSTAR is Global Health Systems, 1710 Research Blvd, Rockville, Md, 20850.

Several other medical record systems have been developed, but none have attained the marketability of the COSTAR system. Most of these systems are only operational on a limited basis, which may be just in the institution that created them. Associated Radiologists in Saskatoon, Saskatchewan, installed an appointment management module, patient data entry and reference module, accounting module, and statistics module. Abbott Clinic, in Winnipeg, Manitoba, in collaboration with National Cash Register, designed an appointment-scheduling system and accounting system. ARA Systems, in association with Wang Laboratories, designed an administrative and medical information system for the office of Dr. Charles Heistrkamp in Lancaster, Pennsylvania. Arizona Health Plan Data Management System in Phoenix, Arizona, operates an automated medical records system, a modified version of which is being used at the Medical College of South Carolina in Charleston, South Carolina. Cardiovascular Clinic Ambulatory Care in Oklahoma City, Oklahoma, designed and installed a complete financial and medical record system that includes patient scheduling, patient census, patient education, billing, research, and medical records. Clinical Computer Applications at the University of Utah's Department of Biophysics in Salt Lake City, Utah, created a medical decision-making network for such applications as multiphasic screening, admissions, ECG interpretation, pharmacy and adverse drug reactions, history taking, and clinical studies in cardiology and genetics. Medical Information System (MIS 1) operates in a consortium of hospitals in the western United States managed from Technicon Data Center in Los Altos, California. The system includes administrative functions, laboratory, x-ray, pharmacy, EKG, and food services. PROMIS (problem-oriented medical information system) was developed by Dr L. L. Weed at the University of Vermont Medical Center. It began as a federally funded project to design a computerized problem-oriented medical record and is now in use at Doctor's Clinic in Burlington, Vermont, and Baltimore Cancer Research Center in Baltimore, Maryland.

When evaluating an automated clinical-information system, some features to consider designing into your practice's system are:

Physician notes, problem lists, medical summaries
Special instructions, referral messages
Ancillaries, such as vital signs and measurements

Orders for prescriptions, referrals, reports
Laboratory and X-ray interpretations
Health maintenance and risk appraisal
Preventive care protocols
History taking

Computerization of the clinical database and medical record system is still in the experimental stages for many computer companies. Many of the previously mentioned applications, with the exception of COSTAR, were originally designed for one particular organization. However, just as the financial aspects of medical practices have been automated, before long the medical data system will also become a standardized automated feature of the medical practice.

Practice Management

As medical practices grow in size and complexity and require greater management efficiency, scheduling, billing, payroll, accounting, and many other business functions must become fully computerized.

Billing and Collection. Financial management depends on a smoothly functioning billing and collection system. Computer software is available to prepare bills; code diagnoses and procedures for insurance claims; print statements and collection notices; itemize bills by date, service, and physician; cycle billing; analyze accounts receivable; produce multiple third-party payment forms; and compare actual fees to standard fees.

Insurance. Insurance payments represent a large portion of revenue. Reimbursement from third parties requires collecting and coding information and completing various forms. Computerized insurance-claim processing may be the most important reason to automate the financial system. Automation speeds claim submissions, reduces rejection rates, and minimizes office personnel workload.

Accounting. Besides the billing functions, computer systems are now available to perform other business operations such as payroll, accounts payable, deposit slips, W-2 forms, day-

sheets, check writing, and general ledger. As the practice volume increases, these tasks will become overly time consuming if performed manually.

Scheduling. Patient appointments and physician schedules are two functions that can be managed by automation. Appointment books can now be replaced with a system that automatically and neatly schedules, cancels, recalls, retrieves, and prints names, addresses, phone numbers, and purpose of visit or meeting. The cost of implementing an automated scheduling system is probably not justified unless the organization has a large number of physicians and service centers.

Reports. Planning and decision making in both financial and clinical work require accurate and concise information in report form. Regular and special reports can be obtained easily from automated information systems.

Word Processing. Communication systems for medical practices necessitate sophisticated equipment that surpasses the traditional typewriter and dictaphone in both speed and capability. Word processing functions include recording, displaying, editing, filing, and printing such documents as letters, recall notices, yearly statements, medical summaries, and other practice correspondence.

Practice management systems are available from both local and national firms. If the physicians and administrator have limited knowledge and experience regarding computers, then the vendor's reputation and service capability will be important factors to consider when selecting a system. The following is a checklist of key features to incorporate into an automated practice management system:

Easy entry and retrieval of data
Daily journal entries
End-of-day accounting of patients seen by provider
Immediate retrieval of account balances
Daily deposits and posting
Patient appointments
Patient recall system
Record of no-shows and cancellations
Monthly and yearly productivity reports

Productivity reports by provider and cost center
Year-end financial statements for patients
Backup systems

Medical Data Bases

Another innovative feature of computers is their ability to network with other information systems. Computer communications with regional and national databases require a telephone, a computer, a device called a "modem," and a communications program to run the modem. The modem provides the practice with the ability to access information from a variety of sources and to convey information as well. Modems can be the organization's link to sophisticated medical information services.

The American Association for Medical Systems and Informatics (AAMSI) provides access to the two most widely used public information utilities, CompuServ and The Source. AAMSI is located in Suite 4405, East West Highway, Bethesda, Maryland, 20814, and CompuServ is AAMSI's primary outlet. Membership and services are inexpensive and provide physicians with access to a medical information clearing house. The Source is more expensive because it provides users with specialized programs such as drug dosages, blood gases, heart attack risks, and other clinical information for use in daily practice. Journal abstracts are also available through this database.

A more specialized communications system in DIALOG. DIALOG is fundamentally a library. It contains articles, books, lectures, and reports. Users select from 175 databases, such as Index Medicus, MedLine, and MEDLARS. Telephone charges and connection time could be several hundred dollars per hour depending on the database. The address for subscription to DIALOG is 3460 Hillview Avenue, Palo Alto, California, 94304.

The American Medical Association has a medical information system that was designed to enhance physicians' and other health professionals' ability to deliver cost-effective, quality health care. The system is AMA/NET, part of GET TELENET Medical Information Network. AMA/NET offers a wide range of professional resources on clinical and administrative aspects of medical practice. Another feature of the GTE network is MED/MAIL, an electronic mail service, which enables users to send and receive electronic messages and reports. The following services are either currently available from AMA/NET or will soon be available: drug information, disease and diagnostic services, patient management information, educational services, business and professional services, and general medical information and literature.

PURCHASING A COMPUTER

Feasibility Analysis

The initial step when considering automation is to conduct a feasibility study to decide whether a computer system would be beneficial. Although a computer may eventually become an inevitable feature of any well-run practice, it is unlikely that every office would immediately benefit from installing an automated office system. A feasibility study will identify the gaps in the current system where a computer could make an improvement. As discussed previously, such areas include inefficient billing, slow registration of patients, excessive personnel overtime, delayed collections, paper overload, unorganized patient information, delayed filing of third-party claims, and lack of practice analysis reports. Initial investigation into these areas requires physicians to (1) organize a planning group made up of a physician, a member of the business staff, and an outside consultant, (2) conduct a detailed investigation of the practice functions and dynamics that would be affected by the computer system, and (3) explore and compare the operations of automated systems in other medical practices.

Computer Committee

The initial objective of the computer committee is to identify flaws in the existing manual system. A potential blind spot of many computer purchasers is the belief that "once we get the computer, we won't have these problems." If a computer is installed in an office with numerous problems, the only result will be faster and perhaps more complex errors.

After problems have been identified and remedied where possible, the committee should take a look at the remaining inefficiencies and ask: By installing a computer, which of these problems will be alleviated? This inquiry should be followed by an assessment of all office functions to determine which operations could be improved through computerization. Throughout the assessment period, the committee should schedule regular meetings to discuss such topics as available capital resources for the purchase of a computer, financing options, willingness of physicians and personnel to comply with automated procedures, and knowledge and skills of office personnel.

Discussion of these topics and collection of preliminary data take several weeks. At the end of this period, a formal report should be prepared indicating the "computer readiness" of the practice. If the committee concludes that the practice would benefit by automating, a more detailed study is warranted. The consultant should be primarily responsible for the practice analysis to ensure objectivity.

Computer Consultant

The investment in a computer system may be the largest single financial investment the practice makes, with the exception of the purchase of the building. In addition, the impact of a computer system will influence every practice function and every individual who works in the office. The significance of this venture requires a high level of expertise and support. It is unlikely that there people in the practice will have either the time or ability to plan and implement the computer system. A consultant should be hired to perform these roles in conjunction with key members of the practice.

Consultants should be selected for their knowledge and experience in computer systems as well as their understanding of health care systems and medical practices. Ideally, the consultant would review the organization and its needs, assist in the evaluation of vendors, and then work with the practice during implementation. The time commitment could be several months to more than a year. National and state medical societies and universities can be sources of information for computer consulta-

tions. A consultant should be selected only after a review of credentials and references.

Practice Analysis

After the benefits of automating have been recognized, the next step is a detailed study of the practice under the direction of one physician and the office manager or consultant. To avoid biases, the study should precede the evaluation of any specific computer systems. Some of the necessary information will be accessible. Some will require extensive probing. The study should include an evaluation of current billing, scheduling, patient flow, and information systems in addition to a task analysis of personnel. Specific parameters needing examination include the following:

Number of active and inactive patients
Number of patients seen per day
Turnaround time for third-party payments
Collection ratios—office, hospital, billing, third-party
Number of third-party claims processed monthly
Daily and monthly revenue by each physician
Number of outstanding accounts
Amount of time spent on various office functions

To supplement the practice analysis data, other information is needed to determine the complete impact of the computer on the practice. The following questions could be asked: What tasks currently performed by physicians or staff could be standardized? What management reports are needed or preferred? How can the processing of insurance claims be more efficient? Can billing costs be decreased?

Another important source of information during this data-gathering phase is a visit to several other practices using automated systems. During these site visits, information can be obtained on costs, conversion problems, satisfaction of staff, computer applications, personnel requirements, and hardware configurations. As long as the practice is not a test site for a particular company, this information can be extremely useful because it represents an unbiased opinion of the system. A site visit also allows the physician contemplating automation to see the system in operation and observe the procedures and routines that are influenced by computer applications.

Evaluating Companies and Their Systems

Before meeting with computer vendors, prepare a standard list of questions for them. Information should be obtained on hardware and software costs, conversion time, service agreements, training, utility fees, forms preparation, supplies, and other components of the system. Figure 8.1 provides a questionnaire used to evaluate computer systems for a medical practice. This information can be used as a checklist when evaluating vendors or it can be mailed to computer companies interested in selling their system to the practice. Such a questionnaire obligates the vendor to respond in language that the physician understands. It also provides the physician with standard information on each company's system, which facilitates comparisons.

Discussion with vendors should focus on the company's experience in medical office practice and applications of immediate value to the practice. Beware of the vendor who attempts to ''sell the sizzle instead of the steak,'' who flashes fancy screens and printouts but talks little about the practical applicability of the system. Also be suspicious of the vendor who insists on talking in computer jargon (bits and bytes) while saying little about practice management. Such esotericism usually covers a lack of knowledge about computer applications in the field of medicine.

In addition to evaluating the individual vendor, a computer shopper must assess the reputation of the company. A reputable company will employ representatives who not only are knowledgeable concerning computers but also understand the unique needs of physicians within the office practice setting. These characteristics usually require some past experience in systems application within the medical community. A firm should be more than willing to provide a list of references and should arrange a site visit.

After completing an evaluation of the vendors, send a request for proposal to the top two or three companies. Such a proposal should address the unique needs of the practice and should include specific recommendations for hardware and software along with any necessary modifications or enhancements to meet the needs of the practice and physicians. Arrangements for training of physicians and staff members to use the system should be included in the final plan. Service and maintenance costs should be specified along with the parties responsible for each.

The proposal presents recommendations for system implementation, but the contract formally defines the product, services, and conditions of the agreement (see Figure 8.2). Such areas include ownership and use of hardware and software, warranty, service and training, terms of payment, completion of installation, and bankruptcy policies. An attorney and consultant should be involved during the contract negotiations, and competitive bidding should be maintained throughout the contractual process. For final acceptance of a vendor contract, a practice must consider all elements of the transaction, including product, service, reputation, price, contractual obligations, and long-term relationships.

Computerized information and management systems are being installed in hospitals, medical centers, and large group practices at a rapid pace. A key to success has been the administrative organization that is in place or that is established to plan, implement, and manage the computer installation. The installation of computers in ambulatory health centers and small practices has moved much more slowly than in the large health organizations. A possible reason for this lag is that most medical practices are independently owned and operated by physicians. The practice is loosely managed and tends to function with informal procedures and communications. Installing a computerized information system in a medical practice requires adherence to a set of standards and protocols that limits the physicians' individualized style and requires professional and office personnel to work systematically as a team. The first steps in the installation process are to follow the previously outlined feasibility and evaluation

Figure 8.1 Evaluating a Computer System. (Reprinted by permission from Rothenberger LA and Aluise JJ, 1984. Implementing an Automated Financial Management System for Medical Practices. *Journal of Family Practice* 18(5). Appleton-Century-Crofts.)

Vendor's Name   Address/Telephone   Contact Person(s)

Company
1. How long has your company been in operation? _____ years
2. How many staff members do you employ? _____
3. How many practices within a 100-mile radius are currently using your system? _____
References:

Software
Billing
1. Does the system generate an itemized bill at the time of service?
   _____yes   _____no
   If yes, are preprinted forms:
   _____required
   _____not used
   _____optional
2. How long will it take to print 100 statements? _____minutes
3. Can brief messages be printed on preidentified statements?
   _____yes   _____no
   If yes, how many can be printed at one time? _____messages
4. Are accounts automatically stepped through a predetermined collection cycle?
   _____yes   _____no
   If yes,
   Is a message automatically printed?
   _____yes   _____no
   Can the cycle be stopped for special accounts?
   _____yes   _____no
5. How quickly are charge and payment data updated?
   _____immediately
   _____daily
   _____other (specify)

Insurance
1. Which of the following forms can your system generate?
   _____Blue Cross/Blue Shield
   _____Medicaid
   _____Universal HICF
2. Are preprinted forms:
   _____required
   _____optional
3. Does the system print forms in:
   _____batch mode
   _____individually (on demand)
   _____can easily do both
4. Is the insurance information:
   _____stored as demographic data
   _____entered for each individual claim
5. How long does it take to set up and print an insurance form at time of visit? _____minutes
6. Will your system transmit insurance information:
   _____via modem
   _____via diskette
   _____neither

Figure 8.1 *Continued*

Hardware
1. What model system do you recommend for my needs? _____
2. How much memory do you recommend?
   _____K (currently)
   _____K (in 3-5 years)
3. How much disk storage space do you recommend?
   _____MB (currently)
   _____MB (in 3-5 years)
4. How many printers will I need?
   #1 _____(type)   _____(speed)
   #2 _____(type)   _____(speed)
   #3 _____(type)   _____(speed)
5. What type of back-up system do you offer? _____
   How long will it take to back up one day? _____(minutes)
6. Will I need any other peripherals? (please specify)

. . . .

Maintenance
1. Does your company *directly* employ the people who would diagnose and do repairs for the hardware?
   _____yes   _____no   (who does?) _____
2. How long will it routinely take to get a hardware repair person on-site if I need help?
   _____hours/days
3. Does your company *directly* employ the people who would diagnose and do most repairs necessary for the software?
   _____yes   _____no   (who does?)_____
4. How long will it routinely take to get a software repair person on-site if I need help?
   _____hours/days
5. During a one-year time period, how many times can we expect failure?
   (give a range) _____times

Training
1. Is training performed at:
   _____your location
   _____our practice
2. How many hours of training do you offer? _____hours
3. Is follow-up training available?
   _____yes   _____no

Costs
Please approximate the following costs:
_____Hardware (including all interfaces and cables)
_____Software
_____Training
_____Maintenance
Total Costs to Practice

$_____ $_____ $_____ $_____ $_____
   Year 1   Year 2   Year 3   Year 4   Year 5

_____
                              Signature   Date

Clause	Explanation
Definitions	Defines customer, contractor (vendor), agreements, price, premises, tests, completion and acceptance dates.
Premises	Conditions for the preparation and operation of equipment suitable to customer. Delivery and installation requirements.
Information	Responsibility for accuracy and documentation of all pertinent information.
Inspection, testing and acceptance	Equipment conditions, and dates for good working order.
Extension of completion time	Delays in completing contract or omissions of contractual responsibilities.
Delays in completion	Deductions for damages from delay, usually 1% of total contract price for every week's delay, up to 10%
Patents and copywrights	Indemnity against claims, damages, costs, and expenses incurred by the contractor.
Assignment and subletting	Restrictions from assigning, pledging, transferring or subletting by contractor.
Liability for damage	Indemnity against losses or damage due to negligence.
Terms of payment	Payment requirements based upon acceptability of customer, usually within 30 days of receipt in good working order.
Ownership of source codes	Availability of the software programs to the customer.
Warranty	Responsibility of contractor for replacing or repairing defective items, or omissions
Bankruptcy	Right of customer to terminate contract if bankruptcy or liquidation occurs.
Software	All documentation necessary for satisfactory operation.
Maintenance	Conditions for a separate maintenance contract.
Training	Contract shall include instruction of the customer's personnel in use of the system.
Publicity	Contractors shall not advertise or publicly announce the work unless agreed upon by client.
Manuals	Documents necessary for installation, operation maintenance of the system.
Termination	Breach of contract stipulations allowing the parties to terminate the contract.

Figure 8.2 Purchasing a Computer "Model Conditions of a Contract"

steps, which must occur prior to the actual installation stage. The written plan prepared by the computer committee should include:

1. Time line from planning to evaluation—six months to one year after installation
2. Education and training phase for professionals and office personnel
3. Designation of computer coordinator within the practice
4. Yearly budget for expenses
5. Revision of personnel job descriptions
6. Revision of office procedures manual
7. Semiannual management review of the computer system and future applications

Human Aspects

A major concern of the office staff members will be how their jobs will change or perhaps be phased out by the computer. This is a vital discussion topic during the planning and installation phase. Changes and modifications will occur, and some professionals and staff members will have difficulty adjusting to the requirements of an automated system. Some staff turnover and provider dissatisfaction must be anticipated.

Brandejs and Pace (1979) recommend a four-step approach in managing the human as-

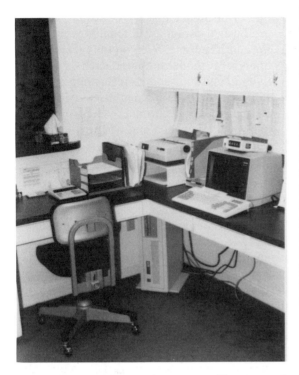

Figure 8.3 An Office Computer. (Courtesy of Washington Family Medical Center, Drs. Thomas Speros and Edward Hill, Washington, North Carolina.)

pects of computers; they call it the "SOAP" method. The first step is the subjective (S): The individual's perceptions of computers and applications should be discussed at informal meet-

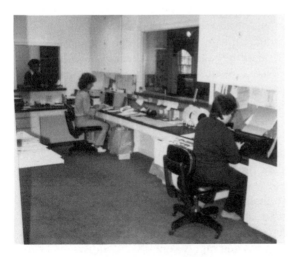

Figure 8.4 Computerized Information and Management System. (Courtesy of Washington Family Medical Center, Drs. Thomas Speros and Edward Hill, Washington, North Carolina.)

ings. Patients could also be included. Forewarnings about the start-up problems with new technology and the need for standardized procedures may minimize the negative reactions. The second step is the objective (O): Criteria should be presented to indicate what features and applications will be incorporated and how the system will operate on a day-to-day basis. Roles and responsibilities must be spelled out in the revised job descriptions. The third step is the assessment (A): Attitudes and opinions of all relevant groups should be obtained at every stage of development. Patient and staff surveys provide valuable information about the acceptability and workability of the system. The fourth step is planning (P): Consideration of all possible contingencies will be essential because the system will have delays, breakdowns, and revisions.

Site Preparation

The facility requirements of the computer system will vary depending on the size and sophistication of the hardware and software. The planning stage should include a review of the physical environment and the desirability of multiple locations for computer input and output. Since many medical practices are becoming multiprovider and multisite organizations, a computer system must have the capacity to meet expansion needs. Architectural, electrical, and mechanical plans should be prepared for both current and proposed facilities. Since the physical arrangements of an office are quite variable, as are the patient-flow patterns, an organization may use its consultant to assist in selecting a system that is compatible with the physicians' and staff members' work routines.

The hardware components will necessitate the most physical changes and modifications. The equipment list for a complete in-house system will probably include: (1) central processing unit (CPU), (2) two or more terminals (CRTs), (3) a dot-matrix printer and a letter-quality printer, and (4) computer desks and tables. Because of the wiring and cables, the electrical system will be most vulnerable to problems. A major caution is *not* to overload electrical circuits. Computers should be assigned to separate circuits, with a battery-powered backup and grounded outlets. Other factors affected by hardware installation are soundproofing, ventilation, cooling, heating, carpeting, and lighting (see Figures 8.3 and 8.4).

Spatial arrangements must take into consideration aesthetics, safety of equipment and personnel, storage of supplies, confidentiality of clinical and financial information, and business and clerical work stations. Insurance policies will need to be revised to protect the more expensive equipment.

Conversion

The conversion from manual operations to computerized systems should be a major topic of discussion throughout the planning and final preparation phases. If the manual system has been in effect for a long time or if the personnel are reluctant to change to new methods for performing business and clinical procedures, the conversion process may be a nightmare.

During the conversion process, a series of procedures must be carried out before the system can operate. A few staff members should be selected to work on the following tasks:

1. **Code Master Files** Determine which procedural and diagnostic codes will be used. Establish codes for providers, revenue, cost centers, insurance companies, and other categories of information important to the practice.
2. **Establish Information Forms** Design registration, financial, and diagnostic information forms. Determine what other information will be collected and the appropriate forms to use or construct.
3. **Convert Patient Accounts** Determine which patient records and what previous information will be transferred into the computer system before and during start-up. Patients with account balances and patients seen in the past two years should take priority.
4. **Billing Procedures** Determine when statements will be sent. Establish how prepayment and third-party claims will be processed. Determine how zero-balances and collection letters or messages will be handled.
5. **Inform Patients** Contact patients about the new procedures. Get patient signatures on

file for insurance-claim processing. Register established patients and family members.
6. **Format Reports** Decide on the type and frequency of standard reports, such as productivity analysis, accounts receivable, age and sex registers and patient lists by various classifications. Determine which special reports will be needed and when.

CONCLUSIONS

The business of medicine is becoming much too complex to be performed by the traditional manual methods. Computerization of the financial management system will soon become standard operating procedures for all medical practices. Regardless of the size or type of practice, computer programs have proven cost-effective for patient registration, daily cash management, billing and collections, insurance claims, productivity reports, and financial statements. Other management applications, such as appointment scheduling, word processing, recall systems, and mailing lists are rapidly being designed for medical practices.

Beside the business and finance of medical practice, computers will have an even greater impact on the clinical side of medicine. Because automation provides physicians and other health professionals almost immediate access to a patient's family and disease profiles, to treatment protocols, to drug interactions, and to other clinical, epidemic, and demographic information that in the past would have taken excessive resources and time to obtain, computers may soon become synonymous with high-quality patient care.

The greatest barrier to general acceptance and widespread use of computers in medicine is communication. Health care professionals and data processing specialists speak different languages and often function in vary different environments. Medicine is a complex, multifaceted field dealing with uncertainty and variability, and data processing operates within rigid constraints and highly repetitive conditions. Therefore physicians and other health professionals must acquire a conceptual understanding of computer science and its application to health care, and data processing experts must work closely with their clients so that the automated systems produce the desired organizational and clinical outcomes.

The future success of computerization will probably be directly related to physicians' willingness to move medical services and health care into the age of sophisticated information systems and automated procedures. Problem solving and decision making will become more systematic, and health care providers will have greater access to a broad base of information. The physician's role will change—not drastically, but it will change. As health care professionals, physicians should welcome the change and recognize the benefits that will accrue to them and their patients.

References

Brandejs J, Pace G: *Physician's Primer on Computers.* Lexington, Mass, Lexington Books, DC Heath, 1979.

Brovino JD: *Computer Applications for Patient Care.* Reading, Mass, Addison-Wesley, 1982.

Fell PJ, Skees WD: *Doctor's Computer Handbook.* Bellmont, Calif, Lifetime Learning Publishers, 1984.

Gonzales L: *Computers for Doctors.* New York, Ballantine Books, Cloverdale Press, 1984.

Katzan H: *Office Automation: A Manager's Guide.* New York, AMACOM Book Division, American Management Association, 1981.

Javitt J: *Computerizing a Medical Office. Byte,* May 1984, pp 171–182.

Kember NF: *An Introduction to Computer Applications in Medicine.* Baltimore, Md, Edward Arnol, 1982.

McConnell C: Video display terminals: a new source of employee problems. *Health Care Supervisor* 3, no. 4 (July 1985):81–88.

McKlung CJ, Guerrieri JA, McClung KA: *Microcomputers for the Medical Profession.* New York, John Wiley and Sons, 1984.

Sambridge E: *Purchasing Computers.* New York, AMACOM Book Division, American Management Association, 1981.

Scharnagl W, Weston G: Selecting and installing an in-house computer system. *Medical Group Management* 30, no. 1 (1983):26–49.

Sellars D: *Computerizing Your Medical Office.* Lexington, Mass, Medical Economics Books, DC Heath, 1979.

Spohr MD: *Physician's Guide to Desk Top Computers.* Reston, Va, Reston Publishing, 1983.

Medical Computer Journals and Reports

Medicomp, 9524-B Lee Highway, Fairfax, Va, 22031 (703) 591-0914.

Physicians and Computers, P and C Publications, 2333 Waukegan Road, Suite 5280, Bannockburn, Il, 60015.

Annual Proceedings of the Symposium on Computer Applications in Medical Care. IEE Computer Society, PO Box 80542, Worldway Postal Center, Los Angeles, Ca, 90080.

9

Professional Relations

- • How does informed consent affect doctor-patient relationships?
- • What are legal aspects of medical records?
- • What are the implications, procedures,

and preventive measures for medical legal proceedings? Malpractice suits?
- • What associations and affiliations are essential to a practicing physician?

Health care places physicians in a highly visible position. They are called upon to be practitioners, representatives, critics, and advocates of their own profession as well as to interface in these capacities with business, governmental, educational, and health-related institutions. The public eye is keen, and the government's reach is close. Public relations and a desirable community image should become foremost in the actions and verbiage of physicians.

This chapter addresses the responsibilities of physicians which evolve from relationships with patients, colleagues, other professionals, and the community. Legal problems are discussed with an emphasis upon medical legal affairs, the physician as witness, and preventive measures. The advantages of affiliation with associations, institutions, and other professionals are presented to provide insight to the array of relationships most physicians will become actively involved in as a result of their practice.

LEGAL ASPECTS OF MEDICAL CARE

Physicians will be entrusted with personal and sensitive information which is deemed confidential. Since physicians are primary health care providers, they are legally accountable for their medical judgments and actions. Practicing in a responsible manner and avoiding legal problems will require: (1) knowledge of medical legal regulations; (2) organization and implementation of efficient and accurate medical records system; and (3) reputation as a practitioner who exemplifies quality patient care. Three medical legal issues which merit attention include informed consent, medical records, and malpractice suits.

Informed Consent

Elements which must exist to impose liability on physicians under the informed consent doctrine are: (1) the existence of the duty to inform, (2) a failure to inform, (3) evidence that if informed, the patient would have chosen a different course of treatment, (4) an injury that resulted from the treatment rendered.

Implied Consent. Consent may be implied by circumstances such as an emergency or disability wherein mental incompetency (due to psychological reasons or drug or alcohol abuse) has incapacitated the patient and time is of the essence. When consent of patient cannot be obtained, it should be obtained from next of kin whenever possible.

Expressed Consent. This is accomplished by disclosure of all material facts necessary for the patient to make an informed decision. The physician's duty to reveal risks and alternatives is measured by what the patient needs to know.

Minors. A medical practitioner should be familiar with the laws affecting medical rights of minors in each respective state. The following general guidelines are subject to individual state variations: (1) Minors under 14 require consent of parent or guardian. If a minor requests treatment only on condition of nondisclosure, the physician must weigh the benefits and risks and document circumstances in the medical record. (2) Minor who are 14 to 18 (or under 21, depending on the state) must give consent as well as parent or guardian.

Special situations in some states where physicians are exempt from liability include: emergencies; patients older than age 18; and in the following categories—venereal disease, pregnancy and contraception, drug abuse, and abortion counseling. In addition, minors in the military service, college, or living apart from parents and over age 14 may consent to medical care.

Form of Consent. Consent may be oral or written. Written consent should be signed by the patient and a witness. Oral consent raises greater problems of credibility. It may be appropriate to have the patient's signature stating that there is full understanding of the treatment alternatives and the risks.

Medical Records

Medical records are privileged or confidential communication between patient and doctor. Disclosure of a medical record is made only with the written permission of a patient to a person designated by the patient.

A legible record showing that a careful diagnosis of the patient's condition was made, that treatment of choice along with alternatives and risks were explained to the patient, and that contains a legible narrative summary provides the best defense to a malpractice claim.

Malpractice cases can be won or lost based upon the medical record. A medical record which is altered after a malpractice suit is filed will be an advantage to the plaintiff. Lost x-rays, missing pages, skimpy notes, and subsequent insertions reflect guilt and neglect. Omissions raise inferences and unanswered questions of negligent care and treatment, all too easily transformed under scrutiny into damaging evidence in the mind of a judge or jury.

Retaining Records. There is no universal statute which requires medical records to be retained. Some lawyers believe that they should be preserved until the malpractice statute of limitations has expired. This may vary from one year to several, depending upon the variations of the statute and its applications. The statute might not even start if a patient is incompetent or until the patient learns of the injury. Originals should be maintained for a considerable period, with duplicates transferred upon request.

Ownership. Medical records are the physician's property. If it is a partnership or professional corporation, the records belong to the organization in the absence of an agreement to the contrary. The term *records* is not limited to the handwritten notes. It includes x-rays, lab reports made by outside institutions, consultants' reports, and other medical correspondence.

Information within the medical record is transferrable to the patient or to anyone else with the patient's consent. However, it would be unwise to part with original documents.

Transferring Records. Copies of all or part of patients' records may be transferred in connection with the patients' therapy. This could be to a colleague, consultant, or even a former teacher whose advice is being sought. This is an implied consent to release information but is limited to disclosure for purposes of therapy. If a medical legal situation is encountered, then written authorization from the patient, executed before a notary public, should be obtained.

Malpractice

John S. Boyden, Jr, MD, LLB has written an excellent article entitled "Malpractice maze: How to get out step by step," in *Legal Aspects of Medical Practice,* May 1978, pp 23–25. Boyden's comments are contained in the following paragraphs.

Initial Contact

The first hint that you are being sued for malpractice is often a letter from your patient's lawyer. Depending on the severity of the patient's complaint, the lawyer will either want to discuss the situation with you or will ask you to notify your insurance company so that a claim settlement discussion can begin.

At this point, some physicians mistakenly assume they can handle the problem themselves. In an attempt to keep the matter from going any further, the naive physician replies to the lawyer's letter, sometimes even agreeing to a meeting. This is a foolhardy course, however, since the physician, in haste to clear up the matter, may inadvertently make disclosures that could be used as evidence at a subsequent trial.

The wisest plan is to turn the letter over to your malpractice insurance carrier immediately. The attorney whom the carrier retains to defend you will either respond to the letter for you or instruct you in the way to reply to it yourself.

Formal Complaint

If the matter is not settled at this point—and it rarely is—litigation will move on to its next phase. You will receive a complaint, detailing

the charges against you, and a summons, bringing you within the jurisdiction of the court until the dispute is resolved.

Because there is a time limit in which to respond to the suit (usually 20 days), your insurance company should be notified as soon as you receive the summons and complaint. The attorney retained by the insurance carrier will file an answer.

As a result of recent legislation, some jurisdictions require a patient's attorney to serve you with a notice of intent to sue before commencing formal litigation. This procedure is intended to provide a brief period of time during which your insurance company can evaluate the case. It is hoped that early settlement of cases can be accomplished at this point without the expense of formal litigation.

When discovery has been completed, the lawyers may attempt to settle the suit out of court through negotiations. Your attorney may also try to have the case dismissed before it reaches trial on any number of legal grounds. Sometimes pretrial conferences before a judge are necessary at this point to focus issues and insure that the trial moves smoothly. It is usually not necessary for you to attend these conferences and negotiations.

Preparing for the Case

To further prepare yourself for the case, learn everything you can about your patient's illness, disabilities, and possible causes for these disabilities. While doing your research, make two lists. The first should include the names of the best local and national experts on the issues in the case. These are the people your attorney may wish to call upon to assist you at your trial. Your attorney can help you define the specific issues in your case.

The second list should include leading articles and texts on the patient's diseases and disabilities. These will enable you to keep track of the most useful references and will also serve as a reading list for your lawyer. Part of the lawyer's preparation for the trial will be to learn as much as possible about key medical issues.

All this sounds like it will take a lot of time. It does. You must be psychologically prepared for a lengthy legal process. You will lose substantial time from your practice during the suit.

This is time for which you may not be compensated. You will also have to learn how to be examined and cross-examined. Your lawyer may question you just as though you were in court to help you feel more comfortable when you have to face the real thing.

You may find that you must risk offending friends and colleagues by refusing to discuss the case freely with them. It is important to avoid discussing the case, because you might make statements that will be conveyed—accidently or otherwise—to the other side. This may sound overly cautious, but I have had just such information brought to me by friends or neighbors of a plaintiff in a malpractice suit.

Trial

Assuming that the case has not been settled or dismissed, the next step is the trial itself. Unlike the prosecution in a criminal trial, the plaintiff's attorney does not have to prove that you are guilty beyond a reasonable doubt. The verdict is based on what is called the burden of proof. The party who presents the greater preponderance of evidence prevails. That is, the jury must decide which side has presented more believable evidence and which witnesses are more convincing.

The plaintiff's attorney does, however, have to prove three points for a verdict against you. She or he must establish that you were negligent, that the client suffered damages, and that there is a causal relationship between your negligence and damages the client sustained.

Proof of negligence is based on three points. First, the plaintiff's attorney must show that you committed—or failed to commit—an act or series of acts. Next, the attorney must call other physicians as expert witnesses to establish a standard of care for your profession in the context of your case. Lastly, he or she must prove that your acts or omissions violated the standard of care established by his expert witnesses.

Proof of negligence in and of itself does not establish that you are liable for the alleged damages. For example, let's say that you drove 100 miles an hour down the main street of your town at rush hour. That would certainly be negligent driving. But if by some miracle you did not harm anyone or anything, then no one would suffer from your negligence. By the same token, proof of negligence in a malpractice suit is not sufficient by itself to establish a case against you.

The plaintiffs' attorneys must also demonstrate that their clients suffered damages. Damages generally fall into two categories: special damages (such as out-of-pocket expenses and the cost of additional medical treatment and loss of income) and general damages. General damages refer to the monetary value assigned to temporary or permanent disability and to pain and suffering.

Proving negligence and damages are essential elements to a plaintiff's case, but they are still not enough to enable the jury to render a verdict against you. The plaintiff's attorney must finally prove that there is a direct causal link between your negligence and the patient's damages.

This final element of the case, called *causation,* is often difficult to prove because the patient's disability and economic loss usually result from more than one causal factor. Abnormal signs or symptoms are frequently the patient's reason for seeing a doctor. Usually subsequent disabilities can be attributed to the progress of the patient's illness rather than to any negligence by the physician. The patient's attorney will try to prove causation (probably with the help of expert witnesses), while your attorney will try to prove that the patient's disabilities are due to other causes.

If the patient's attorney can sustain the burden of proof on all three points—negligence, damages, and causation—then the jury will probably render a verdict against you. Under certain circumstances, judges may revise verdicts, but they are unlikely to do so.

Your attorney may ask the judge to rehear the case or grant a new trial based on the alleged failure of the judge to conduct the first trial within the requirements of the law. The judge will probably refuse, at which case, if you feel the trial was unfair or that the jury's conclusions were unwarranted based on the evidence, you and your attorney may appeal.

Liability Insurance

If you lose on appeal, you will have exhausted all available legal resources, and you must pay the judgment. It is at this point you truly appreciate the value of your malpractice liability insurance. Without insurance, you would be required to pay your own legal fees as well as the judgment. Professional liability insurance entitles you to certain rights and protections. The insurance company must provide you legal defense. Whether the case is won, lost, or settled, it has the duty to defend you vigorously.

Most professional liability insurance contracts contain a provision stating that a settlement cannot be made without the written consent of the physician. However, consent should not be unreasonably withheld, because it may jeopardize your coverage.

You must carry adequate insurance. Check with your insurance agent and local medical society to find out what is considered adequate coverage in your community. Carry at least that amount. Inadequate coverage is a poor bargain, and it puts you at a negotiating disadvantage in the event of a suit.

Legal Caveats

You can help your lawyer in a number of ways. First, as mentioned before, do not respond on your own to a letter from a patient's lawyer. Notify your insurance company first.

Next, be completely honest with your lawyers. Tell them the worst right from the beginning. Lawyer-client privilege prevents your attorneys from being compelled to tell anyone what you have told them, so do not feel that the information will somehow be used against you. On the contrary, your lawyers must know the worst if they are to defend you adequately. One of the greatest dangers to your case is that your lawyers will be surprised by a vital point—something you could have told them beforehand—raised by the opposing attorney.

Of course, some physicians paint such a black picture of themselves that their lawyers must reassure them that they are not as bad as they think they are. Compulsive, conscientious physicians can be their own worst critics. Try to be objective about your case. Do not make it seem worse than it is. But do not conceal vital pieces of evidence from your attorney, hoping they will never come to light. They almost always will. It will be more damaging to you if

your lawyer is not prepared to cope with these "surprises."

One more caveat: don't falsify your records to improve your case. Physicians faced with a malpractice suit sometimes panic and think irrationally. They say to themselves, "I didn't do anything wrong, but these records aren't as clear as they might be. I'll just enter a few things so that the chart will reflect what I really did and thought at that time." The physician would be wise to thoroughly review a subpoenaed record to become familiar with the case and anticipate questions on inquiries.

Physician as Witness

Each profession which serves the public must be prepared to represent itself in the judicial system. The range of cases in which a physician may be asked to testify include personal injury, disputes over life and disability insurance, contracts, trusts, wills, and tax matters.

Preparation to become a witness could begin the first day of practice. Whether the physician represents self or others, it will be essential to establish office policies which respect the rights of others. Medical and clerical records should be designed and maintained so that information is easy to retrieve and accurate. An organized information retrieval system will present an image of professionalism and become a valuable time saver. The following guidelines may be helpful for physicians who are called upon to testify:

1. Contact personal lawyer and discuss the situation.
2. Gather all pertinent information and review it carefully.
3. Request a meeting with the lawyer prior to the date of testimony.
4. Do not release records unless legal authorization is obtained.
5. Document conversations with patients and lawyers and keep a copy in personal file.

Alton (1978) provides advice and suggestions which may help physicians through the arduous and intimidating aspects of legal proceedings. The following material draws from that source.

Cautions

The plaintiff's attorney will attempt to tear down the testimony and will use a variety of cross-examining techniques. Within reason, and at the discretion of the judge, a cross-examiner is permitted to be argumentative and persistent and to lead the witness in order to raise doubt or discover a false statement.

Often an attorney will ask a general or vague question which could possibly apply to the facts of the case involved, push for an answer favorable to the party being represented, and then argue later that the principle established applies to the case in question.

Attorneys often lay traps by leaving vital information out of their questions. Careless answering of such questions will result in an apparent logical syllogism that leads to a damaging incorrect conclusion. Be aware of the quick expert question that can be slipped in among nonexpert questions to catch one off guard. One could be trapped into rendering an expert opinion against oneself or another defendant.

Avoid becoming argumentative and defensive during questioning. This may occur if the issues catch the physician off guard or are construed as an accusation.

Suggestions

The basic principle is that a truthful witness will be able to weather cross-examination. The ability to hold up well under cross-examination does tend to validate the veracity of the testimony. The following paragraphs provide suggestions which may assist physicians during judicial procedures.

Force the questioning attorney to put information necessary to state the question accurately in answerable medical terms. For example, "Counselor, the question cannot be answered properly without knowing more about history and signs and symptoms which the patient is manifesting at the time of the incident."

A good witness must ensure that all necessary information is included in both the question and answer. By responding carefully and qualifying answers to make sure all relevant factors are included, the witness will maintain control of questioning and not be placed in a compromising position.

When a hypothetical question is posed by the interrogation and a physician is asked to "assume" certain facts already in evidence and the witness disagrees with the assumptions, make the answer clear in this fashion: "If everything you asked me to assume were true, which I disagree with (or find very unlikely), my opinion would be . . ." Then present all relevant reasoning and data which led to your opinion.

If the affirmative part of the answer is given first then the lawyer may cut off the qualification. It is important, therefore, to state the qualification first. If you fail to complete your qualifications, make a direct appeal to the judge to be allowed to finish.

Pretrial preparation and familiarity with the relevant medical data involved in the case are essential. In addition, the manner in which questions are fielded and responses are made to the interrogator will be crucial.

An excellent periodical to which all physicians should subscribe is *Legal Aspects of Medical Practice,* published by the American College of Legal Medicine, GMT Medical Information Systems, 777 Third Avenue, New York, NY 10017, (212) 838-7778. The appendix includes a glossary of professional liability terms.

Prevention

The following guidelines could be incorporated into the policy manual of the practice as preventive measures against medical legal problems.

1. Every patient should be treated in accordance with the requirements of good medical practice. Physicians and other health professionals are required to exercise the degree of care, judgment, and skill that is usually exercised by other medical professionals in similar circumstances.

2. No physician or health professional should make a medical judgment, institute a course of medical therapy, or perform a medical procedure which is beyond his or her qualifications. When in doubt, seek consultation.

3. Request x-ray examination whenever a pa-

tient presents a real or suspected bone or joint injury.

4. Do not base an important diagnosis on a clinical impression alone if reliable laboratory diagnostic aids are available.

5. Avoid making an overly optimistic prognosis. Do not promise or guarantee a cure.

6. Do not criticize the handling of a case by another health professional in the presence of a patient or family member.

7. Obtain "informed" written consent for any nonroutine procedure (eg, surgery, blood transfusion, x-ray therapy).

8. Keep proper medical records which clearly show what was done and when it was done. *Do not make any erasures or alterations to the original entry*. Avoid any admission of fault or gratuitous comments regarding the patient's personality (eg, "malingerer," "trouble-maker").

9. Make certain that all diagnostic and therapeutic equipment such as surgical tools, x-ray and diathermy machines, oxygen supplies, heat lamps, and all other equipment used in patient care are safe and in proper working order. Careful attention must be given to the safe storage of supplies of drugs, medications, anesthetic agents, and oxygen. Internal safety-check procedures should be adapted to prevent the obsolescence of pharmaceuticals, accidental mixing of chemical agents, and improper labeling.

10. Exercise tact, consideration, and a professional manner toward the patient and family. Explain what you are doing and why. Remember it is the patient's body that you are treating. When rapport between the medical team and the patient is high, malpractice lawsuits are low.

AFFILIATIONS

Physicians will be asked to represent themselves, their practices and profession, and perhaps their community. Some of these associations will be required, and others may be optional or voluntary. Regardless of the affiliation which a physician may choose to assume, each one should be initiated with a sense of purpose and commitment.

Medical Societies

The American Medical Association (AMA) is the parent body of the medical profession and is a primary association for all physicians. The AMA provides a variety of resources and services either directly or through affiliation with other organizations. In addition, the AMA is an important initial contact for any other national or regional medical organization of interest.

American Academy of Family Physicians (AAFP)

The American Academy of Family Physicians is a national association of doctors of medicine who are engaged in family practice. The academy plays a vital role in all areas of medical education—undergraduate, graduate, and continuing. The AAFP has played a significant role in the establishment of the American Board of Family Practice, the integration of competent family physicians into hospital medical staffs, and the active liaison with American Medical Student Association, encouraging student memberships in the academy. The academy is headquartered in Kansas City, Missouri. It publishes a monthly scientific magazine entitled *American Family Physician,* with a primary care physician and student affiliate member circulation of 125,000. Further information and membership forms can be obtained by writing the Academy at 1740 West 92nd Street, Kansas City, Mo, 64114.

Hospital

Physicians will have several governing bodies. One of these will be the hospital(s) they choose to admit patients to. The hospital is the ultimate medical institution and may reflect on the quality of physicians who engage in its services. Even though medical practices have a high degree of autonomy, community health care standards may be influenced by the hospital.

Physicians will relate to hospitals initially as an applicant for admitting privileges. From this beginning, relationships may evolve into a variety of areas including patient care, education, organizational, and political. Hospital relationships which are instrumental for community practitioners include these with the hospital administrator, chief of medical staff, and heads of departments, especially the emergency room, laboratory, x-ray, and nursing. These relationships should be established as early as possible to ensure knowledge of policies and procedures and effective communication. It is unfortunate to initiate a relationship when a problem or misunderstanding has already occurred.

Hospital bylaws and regulations should be obtained and reviewed, along with other policy statements which will influence patient care or other responsibilities. Specific areas to scrutinize include: committee structure and authority, obligations and restrictions, financial implications, internal decision making, due process, cost containment, and adherence to regional and national standards. Chapter 1 presented a detailed discussion of hospital privileges, medical handbooks, and the application process.

Indications that a hospital is responsive to community physicians may be seen in one or more of the following: selection of a practicing physician as a board member; inclusion of both primary care and subspecialty physicians in planning, recruiting, and decision-making groups; full-time coverage of emergency room; continuing medical education programs convenient for office practitioners; affiliation with medical school and residency programs; and opportunities to use hospital resources and services.

Partners in a group practice could divide the various hospital responsibilities and relationships, while keeping each other informed during regular practice meetings. A solo or two-physician partnership may become either overcommitted by hospital obligations or become isolated because of the obvious time constraints.

CONSULTANTS

The practicing physician will be held personally responsible for many of the financial and legal aspects of the practice. The expertise and skill to execute many of these responsibilities may

not be the forte of the physician. Thus, financial and legal specialists should be consulted to assist the physician. It will be a wise decision to have built a relationship with these resources prior to the immediate need. The relationship between the physician and consultant is highly individualized and should be based on the needs of the physician and the related expertise of the consultant. The only caution to consider is to use consultants but not to become dependent upon them. A rule of thumb might be for the physician to obtain an initial level of knowledge and consider a few alternatives and then call on the consultant to increase the information base and offer additional alternatives or advise in the selection of an appropriate alternative. Physicians should be wary of consultants who present ready-made decisions.

The following discussion is a brief commentary about types of consultants and the degree to which they may be of value. There is not intent to downplay the importance of these consultants, nor to rank one higher than another.

Attorney

An attorney will be a valuable advisor in all aspects of medical practice. Physicians will be asked to originate or sign contracts, leases, agreements, mortgages, loans, and other legal documents. A lawyer may be called upon to design such documents or merely to review and advise. If attorneys are selected initially, they may then guide the physician in other decisions, such as which lending institution, accountant, or advisors should be contacted.

When a physician chooses an attorney, the following should be foremost considerations: Select an attorney who has worked with physicians and has become experienced with the unique facets of medical practice. Consider a group of attorneys who have several areas of expertise, such as real estate, malpractice, contracts, taxes, investments, and professional incorporation. Select an attorney in the local community who is familiar with local resources, institutions, and customs. A personal attorney will be of value legally, in the same way that a personal physician is medically.

Physicians may employ lawyers on a fee-for-service basis or through contractual arrangements for a specified time. Initially, it is advisable to compensate by fee for service or short-term contract (less than six months). Specific issues which require legal guidance and assistance include: articles of incorporation, partnership and employment contracts, wills, mortgages, leases, and medical legal aspects of practice. All these services could be paid when the legal service is rendered. Retainers with lawyers should only be entered into when there is a high degree of trust and confidence and the practice requires continuing legal advice and service.

Regardless of compensation format, physicians should use the same law firm for as many legal functions as possible. This will enable the lawyers to develop a relationship with the physician(s) and to better understand their medical practice. This may ensure more appropriate advice in both routine and emergency situations.

Accountant

Accountants, preferably certified public accountants (CPAs), will provide assistance during the initial stages of practice development and with tax obligations. Similar criteria for selecting an attorney could be applied to choosing an accountant. It would be ideal if the law firm also employed the same CPA.

An accountant experienced in medical practices should establish a workable financial system with built-in controls and audits. In addition, the office supervisor could be trained to tabulate daily and weekly figures and prepare monthly reports for both intake and outflow of cash.

The daily financial system should be developed such that physicians and supervisors are knowledgeable and can perform all functions. Maintaining weekly and monthly reports will be facilitated if each day's cash transactions, charges, and receipts are balanced along with a systematic process of disbursements and check writing. If the practice records are organized and accurate, the accountant will be able to audit the books quickly and at a reasonable expense.

Accountants will be essential for tax advice and preparation of quarterly and yearly returns.

There are several other areas in which they may assist physicians, including computations of payroll taxes, fringe benefits, corporation taxes, retirement plans, auditing financial statements, accounts receivable and collections, and business and personal investment analysis.

Compensation for the accountant should be similar to the lawyer. Each service could be priced with a fixed fee or on a cost-per-hour basis.

Financier

Financial institutions are very receptive to medical practices. Medical practices will generate considerable cash and require a variety of banking services. The local bank will be a valuable financial resource and should be consulted frequently during the various stages of practice development regarding checking and savings accounts, daily deposits, personal and professional lines of credit, safety deposit box, equipment leases, loans, and mortgages.

Both banks and savings and loan associations should be contacted. It would be advisable to use at least one major banking institution and one savings and loan association. A personal contact at each firm should be established with an ongoing association for both personal and professional matters. Bankers normally provide their services at no cost and are quite knowledgeable about both local and national finance. They may be called upon for investment analysis, estate planning, major equipment purchases for the practice, and facility renovation and construction.

Physicians will be inundated by financial dealings and will find having a consultant who can be objective and has no proprietary interest helpful. Bankers will tend to be more conservative, but their advice and counsel will act as a balance to the "sales" approach of the investment marketers.

Management Consultant

The complexities and innovations in medical practice may require physicians to seek more specialized assistance than their legal and financial advisors. Medical management consulting firms are available nationally and regionally to provide a full range of services from filing income tax to computerized billing. Many firms offer monthly and quarterly practice consultations along with their financial systems.

There are several instances which merit consideration of medical management consultants. These include: revising financial and medical record systems, changing the organizational structure of the practice, renovating or constructing a practice, converting to computerized system, and training paramedical staff. Medical management firms offer both services and products, and physicians should not be oversold or become completely reliant upon this service. Their purpose should be to problem-solve, recommend, and remain available for future involvement. Qualified consultants should be willing to train physicians and office staff so that problems may be prevented.

Management firms could be evaluated from several vantage points. They should possess a breadth of expertise and be recognized by colleagues and peers. Services should be offered through a formal contract that specifies types of services, length of time, and reporting methods. The exact cost of services should be known in advance. There should also be a termination clause if it is a long-term contract.

Since the physician is the customer, there should be adequate time to compare services and systems of several firms. If competitive dealings are not encouraged, then physicians should be wary of continuing negotiations.

Insurance Representative

A professional relationship with an insurance agent could be established very early in one's career. This implies not that there are extensive insurance needs but that a working arrangement is secured for future planning and developments.

Associations which reputable agents belong to include National Association of Life Underwriters, American College of Life Underwriters, Association for Advanced Life Underwriting. In addition, there are courses of study which agents can complete to increase knowledge and skills in insurance planning. Both membership in national association and knowledge pertinent to professional career planning should be evaluated prior to establishing a working relationship.

Important attributes of a reputable agent include: (1) flexibility to discuss a variety of programs and alternatives, and (2) a sense of economics to ascertain present financial risk and future return. In addition, an agent interested in a long-term relationship should be willing to establish programs which are compatible with personal and professional goals, regardless of the type or dollar value of insurance sold.

Practice Advisory Board

The use of financial and business consultants may appear to be cumbersome and time consuming. This will be especially true if a physician must communicate individually with accountants, insurance representatives, lawyers, and bankers. Each of these individuals will have an area of expertise to provide at all stages of practice development. To avoid needless meetings and duplicate conversations, it is advisable to establish an administrative board through which these individuals can *pool* their input and assist the physician(s) in decision making and practice planning. This group could meet regularly (bimonthly or quarterly) or could be convened if an urgent matter arose.

A practice advisory board could serve several purposes to a solo physician or group practice. First, they could provide an overseer function to ensure that major decisions, especially financial, were thoroughly discussed and researched. Such issues could include a new building or renovation, new equipment purchases, expansion of financial affairs—insurance, investments, etc, and tax advantages of professional incorporation. Second, this advisory group would be a stimulus for the physician to maintain an organized system of plans and goals, with a report-back mechanism to determine progress and future directions. Third, this group will develop as a more cohesive counsel and gain further insight into the activities and resources of their colleagues. Thus, an accountant and lawyer can effectively plan the ultimate pension profit-sharing program, and the lawyer, insurance representative, and banker can develop a complete estate plan. Finally, the physician and advisory group may ultimately become a further resource to the community in regard to health care planning, community services, and recruitment of other professionals and organizations.

A few cautions should be considered in developing such an organizational entity: Select individuals who have either worked together in the past or appear willing to formulate such a group. Maintain control and direction—don't delegate important responsibilities or decisions which belong with the physician. And finally, keep an appropriate degree of *openness* to this activity to alleviate any notion of ulterior motives or collusions. This can be avoided by documenting all meetings and maintaining thorough records.

CONCLUSION

The legalistic and public relations features of a medical practice may be as important as the full range of medical knowledge and skills. Physicians and their office staff will be entrusted with confidential and privileged information. Honor, trust, and respect must be a keynote throughout the health care system.

Just as preventive medicine is presented to patients, so must physicians prevent problems which infringe upon the legal and moral rights of patients and colleagues. Malpractice has significant implications to the medical profession and the individual careers of physicians. It is imperative to understand the medical legal issues which affect medicine. To learn of these ramifications after the fact will be a risky venture.

Medical professional relations encompass many organizations and institutions. Physicians will seek support from their medical society, hospital, and community, and in most cases there will be reciprocal arrangements. Regardless of the association or undertaking, physicians should clearly understand the purpose and function of the affiliation and should participate in a highly committed and respectful manner.

References

Alton WG: How to keep a plaintiff's attorney honest. *Medical Economics,* 18 September 1978, pp 121–132.

Boyden JS: Malpractice maze: How to get out step by step. *Legal Aspects of Medical Practice,* May 1978, pp 23–25.

Coyne P: Ethics and the AMA. *Private Practice,* June 1978, pp 63–72.

Hagner J: What's behind malpractice insurance? *Legal Aspects of Medical Practice,* March 1978, pp 35–38.

Hertz S: "Legal aspects of medical care affecting tort liability." Unpublished paper, US Department of Health, Education and Welfare, 3, August 1978.

Holley C: Guidelines for treatment of malpractice claims reduces diversity. *Healthcare Financial Management,* September 1985, pp 58–67.

Hollowell EE: No insurance no privileges! *Legal Aspects of Medical Practice,* April 1978, pp 17–19.

How can a doctor fight denial of staff privileges? *Journal of Legal Medicine* 5, no. 10 (1977):33–37.

Marsh F: Health care cost containment and the duty to treat. *Journal of Legal Medicine* 6, no. 2 (June 1985):157–190.

Rothbart P: Liability of corporate physicians in conducting pre-employment and annual physical examinations. *Journal of Legal Medicine* 6, no. 4 (December 1985):477–488.

Shoenberger A: Medical malpractice injury. *Journal of Legal Medicine* 6, no. 1 (March 1985):51–84.

Tovey J: Medical records: A legal update. *Private Practice,* January 1978, pp 79–85.

Wilson M: Exclusive arrangements between hospitals and physicians. *Journal of Legal Medicine* 6, no. 3 (September 1985):373–390.

Zaremski M, Weibel F: There is no answer to the medical malpractice crisis. *Journal of Legal Medicine* 6, no. 2 (June 1985):265–266.

Appendix 1
Computers in Medical Practice

- **A Glossary of Data Processing Terms**
- **Computer Forms and Printouts**
  - **Initial Registration Form**
  - **Encounter Form**
  - **Diagnostic Encounter Form**
  - **Family Visit Record**

Crosstabulation of Patients
Major Categories of Disease
Frequency List of Problems
Problem Encounters Listed by Diagnosis Class

A GLOSSARY OF DATA PROCESSING TERMS

Access Time: The interval of time from the giving of an instruction for accessing data to when the data are available for processing.

Acoustic Coupler: A form of modem which permits attachment of an ordinary telephone handset so that a computer can communicate over any telephone. See *modem*.

Accumulator: A hardware component, generally a register, used to accumulate the sum of a minicomputer's operation.

Address: The identifier of the location in a minicomputer's memory in which a data element is stored.

American Standard Code For Information Interchange (ASCII): A code for data transfer between a computer and peripheral devices. The code uses seven bits to fully describe an alphanumeric symbol and has been adopted for use by the American Standards Association. All personal computers now use this standard.

Application Software: Programs designed to perform operations on data that are directly related to an application.

Application-Support Software: Programs designed to perform operations which interface application software with other software components in a computer system. Any application-support program can be used by an application program as general operations. (A database management system is an example of an application-support program.) See also *utility programs*.

Arithmetic Logic Unit (ALU): The electronic circuitry of the central processing unit, used for performing all arithmetic and logical operations on data.

Assemble: An operation by which symbolic program statements are converted into machine language instructions.

Backup: Stand-by hardware and software which can take over processing in the event of failure of part of or all the components in a minicomputer system.

Basic: A quaint little language used by humans to tell computers what they are supposed to do. *BASIC* is an acronym for *b*eginners *a*ll-*p*urpose *s*ymbolic *in*struction *c*ode. It can be used with almost all personal computers and is extremely popular. BASIC should always be written in capital letters.

Batch: A group of programs stacked for individual execution by a minicomputer system. Each program runs to completion before the next one begins execution.

Baud Rate: A unit of measure indicating the speed at which data are transmitted over a communications link. *Baud* is used interchangeably with bits per second (bps); for example, 1,200 baud equals 1,200 bps.

Binary-Coded Decimal (BCD): An early code used for data transmission. The code uses four bits to represent each of the ten decimal digits, that is, 0000 = 0; 0001 = 1; 1000 = 8.

BIT: The fundamental unit of binary data—the smallest amount of information that can be known. A single bit can specify either of two alternatives. In computers, *bit* usually refers to the concept behind the words from which it was invented: *bi*nary digi*t*, meaning either a 1 or a 0. A bit can be thought of as representing a simple yes/no choice, the distinction between true and false, whether a circuit is on or off, or any other two-way choice.

Buffer: An allocation of storage used to temporarily hold data that are being transferred between two components in a minicomputer for processing in a single transmission.

Byte: The fundamental unit of information; used in the transmission and processing of data. A byte is 8 bits long. In practice a byte is usually used to represent an alphanumeric character or a number in the range of 0 to 255.

Cathode Ray Tube (CRT): A video display terminal which uses a cathode ray tube as its display element.

Central Processing Unit (CPU): The lead component of a minicomputer system. It performs all arithmetic and logical operations requested by the system as well as controlling the flow of information throughout the system.

Characters Per Second (cps): Units of measure used to describe the speed at which information is transferred between a minicomputer and associated peripheral components. Since a character of information is completely described in a byte, characters per second is used interchangeably with bytes per second.

Chip: A small (typically less than half a centimeter on a side and quite thin) piece of material (usually silicon) into which have been formed from a few dozen to tens of thousands of circuit elements. This is done by etching the material, depositing microscopic metal conductors, and selectively impregnating the material with various elements that change its properties. See *integrated circuit*. Also used to describe the integrated circuit that houses a chip. This is a somewhat colloquial usage and should be avoided.

Command: A request to the computer that is executed as soon as it is received.

Communications: The exchange of information between a minicomputer and another minicomputer or a minicomputer and peripheral devices.

Communications Link: The physical path over which information is exchanged.

Compile: The process by which verbally descriptive symbolic statements are converted into a less complex code for execution by a programmed run-time system.

Compiler: A program used to perform the compilation process on a symbolic program. A program that translates one computer language into another. Most commonly the term refers to a program that translates a higher level language into the computer's machine language.

Cursor: A symbol placed on the screen to let you know where the next character you type will appear.

Data: Information of any kind processed or maintained by a computer system.

Database: An organization of data elements according to a predefined plan.

Database Management System (DBMS): Application-support software designed to maintain a database. Application programs can request that the DBMS store or retrieve data elements that are members of a database.

Debug: The process of testing and correcting new programs.

Debugger: A utility program designed to interact between a user and a program being tested to facilitate the debugging process.

Dedicated Line: Physical communications link between two points, rented for a monthly fee from a communications utility.

Dial-Up Line: A switched communications link between two points.

Directory: A catalog of data files that is readable by a minicomputer system and which is generally stored on the same device that contains the data files.

Disk Drive (disc drive): A mechanical device used to house a rotating, magnetic disk memory for operation.

Diskette: A flexible rotating medium used as low-capacity secondary memory. See *floppy disk*.

Dump: To copy all or a large part of a computer's memory.

Edit: The process by which a symbolic program is modified or extended. Make changes in program or data.

Editor: A program used to perform the edit process. Also known as the text editor.

Emulation: The duplication of another minicomputer's instruction set in the hardware of a minicomputer.

File: A logical organization of data elements related to a similar topic.

Firmware: Hardware programmed at the time of manufacture to display a specific set of characteristics.

Floppy Disk: The name given to a diskette because the medium is flexible. See *diskette*.

Graphics: The pictorial display of information. Minicomputer graphics range from simple bar graphs to minicomputer-generated films used in flight simulators.

Handshaking: The orderly exchange of signals between two devices, which results in coupling the devices for communications.

Hard Copy: Information printed on paper or other durable surface. This term is used to distinguish printed information from the temporary image presented on the computer's CRT screen.

Hardware: The electronic, magnetic, and electromechanical equipment that a computer system is comprised of. Physical parts.

In-House System: Computer facilities owned and operated by the user whose data are processed by them.

Input/Output (I/O): Movement of information to and from a minicomputer system.

Input/Output Control Unit (IOCU): The electronic circuitry of the central processing unit used for moving information in and out of the computer.

Instruction: A coded command interpreted and executed by a minicomputer to perform operations on data that are local to it.

Interactive System: A system that processes data based on the direction it receives from a user communicating with it.

Interface. (1) The electronics that allow two different devices to communicate with one another. (2) More generally, any situation where two different entities (eg, a person and a computer) communicate.

Key: A predefined identifier used by software to facilitate the access of data elements.

Leased Line: See *dedicated line*.

Library: A catalogued organization of programs. By referring to a library, a user can gain access to several programs with one request.

Load: The process by which a program enters main memory and is available for execution.

Machine Language: Binary representation of instructions which are executed by the hardware of a computer.

Memory: The internal storage capacity of a computer measured in kilobytes. The micro memories range from 4,000 bytes (4K) for the smaller units to 64K for larger business-oriented micros. Even larger memory units are becoming available with each new micro produced. The IBM micro memory ranges from 16K to a massive 256K, which is large enough to swallow the contents of a 50,000 word novel with room to spare.

Microcomputer: A computer based on a microprocessor.

Microprocessor: A fundamental subsystem of electronic circuitry capable of program control; the subsystem completely contained within one semiconductor component; an integrated circuit that performs the task of executing instructions. The presence of a microprocessor in a product does not make it into a computer.

Modem: An abbreviation of *mo*dulator-*dem*odulator: A device that allows a computer to communicate over the telephone lines (and other communication media) by changing the digital information into musical tones (modulating) and from musical tones to digital information (demodulating).

Monitor: (1) A television set, often one that is specially manufactured to be connected to a computer. (2) A program supplied by the manufacturer that allows the user to control the operation of a computer. With computers that operate directly in a higher level language such as BASIC, the monitor may often be built into the language. See also *operating system*.

Multiprogramming: An operating concept in which several programs compete for system resources according to predetermined priorities. These programs execute in parallel: as one program is suspended, another can execute. Only one program has control of the central processing unit at any given time, but other components in the system can respond to requests made by the other programs. Hence, multiple programs execute during an interval of time.

Network: An organization of two or more programmable components which communicate with each other.

Off-Line: The movement of information without program control by a central processing unit.

Off-Line Processing: Operations performed by auxiliary equipment on data prior to their entry into the central processing unit of the computer. Human intervention is usually required between data entry and ultimate processing. Compare with *on-line processing*.

On-Line Processing: The processing of data under the complete and absolute control of the central processor, eliminating the need for human intervention.

Operating System (OS): The software necessary to control the operation of computer system hardware, direct the flow of information throughout a computer system, and schedule work for the computer system to process. The operating software forms a total operating environment for application support and application software. Sometimes called a *monitor*.

Peripheral Device: Any component that is connected to the minicomputer, but which is not part of the minicomputer (that is, main memory is not considered a peripheral device, since it is an integral part of the minicomputer; a disk drive is a peripheral device.)

Printer: In computerese, a peripheral that makes hard copy of letters and numerals. A line printer prints a whole line of text at a time. A serial printer prints one character at a time.

Program: A logical organization of instructions designed to perform a function or set of functions within a computer system. A program must be written in a language the computer can understand.

Programming Language: A verbal means of interchange between humans and computers.

Prompt: A symbol that appears on your computer's display to let you know that it is ready to pay attention to your commands.

Protocol: A predefined exchange of control information which precedes and follows transmitted information in a network. A protocol is used to reduce the acceptance of erroneous information.

Random-Access Memory (RAM): A semiconductor memory module capable of random access.

Read-Only Memory (ROM): A semiconductor memory loaded in a program at the time of its manufacture, which is capable of permitting its storage locations only to be read and not written on.

Record: A group of related data elements accessed as a unit by application support and application software.

Recovery: Action taken by a computer system to compensate for a failure.

Redundancy: The duplication of components in a minicomputer system, for purposes of backup. See *backup*.

Response Time: The time spent between the acceptance of a request for processing and display of the results yielded by the processing.

Seek Time: The time spent positioning the head assembly of a moving-head disk.

Software: The programming necessary to direct the hardware of a computer system in performing the functions of a given application.

Special Character: A character that can be displayed by the computer, but is not a letter or numeral. Here are some special characters !"#$%&*−=(|/=;:?

Symbolic Code: The alphanumeric statements that represent a program.

System Software: See *operating system*.

Syntax: The rules that specify exactly how an instruction can be written.

Teleprocessing: Information processing in which communication facilities are used.

Terminal: A peripheral component used to transfer information between humans and computers.

Timesharing: The allocation for computer system resources to several users on a time partition basis.

Track: The area formed by two concentric boundaries to the circumference of a rotating medium. Specified area on a magnetic tape.

Transfer Rate: The speed at which information is exchanged between secondary memory and the computer.

Variable: A name for a quantity. A variable in a computer language can be thought of as a box into which a value may be stored.

Word: The unit of measure equivalent to the smallest number of bits necessary to represent a machine instruction. An arbitrary number of binary digits or bytes handled as a unit by the computer for the purposes of operation, transmission, and storage.

Utility Programs: Programs that provide the very basic facilities of a computer system, for example, copying one tape onto another, copying information from memory onto other media. See *application-support software*.

Family Practice Center

School of Medicine
University of North Carolina
Chapel Hill, North Carolina*

Initial Registration Form

PLEASE DO NOT WRITE IN THIS AREA

7.0

| MO | DA | YR | UNIT NUMBER | ACCT STATUS |

CURRENT DATE

TYPE ACCT   CODE   AMOUNT   EFFECTIVE DATE
ARRANGEMENTS

MAIL FLAG

1,0,0,1
GROUP CODE

Person to whom bills are to be sent (guarantor)   Circle Right Answer

DO NOT WRITE
IN THIS AREA

Name: _____ Telephone: _____
      Last   First   Middle

NCMH UNIT NO.

Address: _____ Occupation: _____
         Street

TYPE PAY   TEAM

_____ How many people in your family?_____
City   County   State   Zip Code

DOCTOR ASSIGNED

Sex: Male/Female Race: White/Black/Asian/Indian/Other Date of birth: ___/___/___ Yearly income: $0-6,000 $6,000-8,800

$8,800-12,400   over $12,400

MEMBER CODE

Marital status: Married/Single/Divorced/Widowed/Separated Social Security No.: ___/___/___

Other enrolling family members (you may use "same" where it applies)

DO NOT WRITE
IN THIS AREA

Name: _____ Occupation: _____
      Last   First   Middle

NCMH UNIT NO.

Address: _____ Social Security No. ___/___/___
         Street

TYPE PAY   TEAM

_____ Relationship to Guarantor: _____
City   County   State   Zip Code

DOCTOR ASSIGNED

Sex: Male/Female Race: White/Black/Asian/Indian/Other Date of birth: ___/___/___ Marital status: Married/Single/Divorced/Widowed/Separated

MEMBER CODE

DO NOT WRITE
IN THIS AREA

Name: _____ Occupation: _____
      Last   First   Middle

NCMH UNIT NO.

Address: _____ Social Security No. ___/___/___
         Street

TYPE PAY   TEAM

_____ Relationship to Guarantor: _____
City   County   State   Zip Code

DOCTOR ASSIGNED

Sex: Male/Female Race: White/Black/Asian/Indian/Other Date of birth: ___/___/___ Marital status: Married/Single/Divorced/Widowed/Separated

MEMBER CODE

DO NOT WRITE
IN THIS AREA

Name: _____ Occupation: _____
      Last   First   Middle

NCMH UNIT NO.

Address: _____ Social Security No. ___/___/___
         Street

TYPE PAY   TEAM

_____ Relationship to Guarantor: _____
City   County   State   Zip Code

DOCTOR ASSIGNED

Sex: Male/Female Race: White/Black/Asian/Indian/Other Date of birth: ___/___/___ Marital status: Married/Single/Divorced/Widowed/Separated

MEMBER CODE

Friend or relative to notify in case of emergency with phone number other than your own

Name: _____ Telephone: _____
      Last   First   Area Code   Telephone

Insurance Policy information for all members

Insurance Co. _____ Policy or certificate no. _____ Group No. _____ Coverage codes_____

Group name (employer)_____ Address claim to: _____

List first names of enrolled members covered: _____ Policy holder _____

Insurance Co. _____ Policy or certificate no. _____ Group No. _____ Coverage codes_____

Group name (employer)_____ Address claim to: _____

List first names of enrolled members covered: _____ Policy holder _____

Insurance Co. _____ Policy or certificate no. _____ Group No. _____ Coverage codes_____

Group name (employer)_____ Address claim to: _____

List first names of enrolled members covered: _____ Policy holder _____

*Courtesy of Department of Family Medicine, University of North Carolina.

ENCOUNTER FORM*

RECEIPT NUMBER		
12629	☐ N (New)	☐ R (Return)

MONTH	DAY	YEAR	.	ATTENDING	FPC DOCTOR	TEAM	CLINIC		Imprint
				3 1 5 2			1 0 0 1		

PAYOR	BALANCE FORWARD	TODAYS CHARGES	AMOUNT PAID TODAY	BALANCE REMAINING	REC'D BY	# CHARGES
4 0 2	▲	▲	▲	▲	▲	

DR. EDWARD SHAHADY AND ASSOC. **PHONE (919) 966-2491**
FAMILY PRACTICE CENTER
SCHOOL OF MEDICINE – UNIVERSITY OF NORTH CAROLINA
BOX 513 NCMH
CHAPEL HILL, NC 27514

CK.	DESCRIPTION	CODE	AMT.	CK.	DESCRIPTION	CODE	AMT.	CK.	DESCRIPTION	CODE	AMT.	CK.	DESCRIPTION	CODE	AMT.
	PATIENT ENCOUNTERS — 01				**OFFICE PROCEDURES — 04**				**INJECTION & IMMUNIZATION — 05**				**LABORATORY — NCMH — 07**		
	Initial O.V.	90015	30		Anoscopy	46600	10		Allergy	90785	2		Electrolyte Panel	80006	
	Extended O.V.	90070	20		Allergy Test	95001	10		DPT	90701	3		Enzyme Profile	80004	
	Routine O.V.	90060	12		BP Check	90030	N/C		DT	90702	3		Na	84295	
	Short O.V.	90040	5		Cast minor		25		Flu	90718	1		K	84140	
	Well Baby Visit	90090	10		Cast Intermediate		35		Heparin	90750	1		Cl	82435	
	Out of Hours	90560	15		Catheterization (T)	53670	15		MMR	90707	10		CO2	82374	
	House Visit	90160	25		Dressing (SR)	90060	12		Measles - Rubella	90708	3		BUN	84520	
	Ins. Form Sent	99080			ECG	93000	25		Mumps	90704	3		Creat	82565	
	Nurse Visit	90030			Ear Irrigation	69200	5		Penicillin	90780	2		T.P.	84155	
	Consultation	90620			Ear Piercing	69090	5		Polio (Oral)	90712	1		Alb.	82040	
	Nursing Home Visit	90460			Excision Minor		40		Tetanus Toxoid	90703	1		SGPT	84460	
					Excision Interm. (T)		50		Vitamin B-12	90750	1		Alk. P.	84075	
					Eye Exam	90089			Hydro + XYLO	90750	1		SGOT	84450	
					Hearing Test	92551	2		Small Pox	90711	1		CPK	82550	
	PHYSICAL EXAMS — 02				Fracture Care		3		Therapeutic	90750	1		LDH	83615	
	Comp Athletic	90081	15		Incision & Drain (T)	10060	30		Tine Test	86585	1		Acid P.	84060	
	College	90082	15		Laceration Minor		50		Gammaglobulin	90726			Bili D	82250	
	Adult Comp	90088	30		Laceration Major (T)		75		Miscellaneous	90749			Bili T	82250	
	Employment	90088	30		Lumbar Puncture (T)	62270	75						Ca	82325	
	Insurance	90088	30		Manipulation	22500	20						Chol	82465	
	Pre-school	90095	15		Rectal Exam	90060	12						Fe	83545	
					Sigmoidoscopy	45300	20						TIBC	83555	
					Spirometry	94010	5		**LABORATORY — CLINIC — 06**				PO4	84100	
	OB/GYN — 03				Splint Finger	26720	10		Cold Aggl (Beside)	86150	3		Trig	84475	
	Total OB Care				Suture Removal (SR)	90060	12		Diff	85040	3		Uric Acid	84555	
	& Delivery	59400	400		Tonometry	92100	5		Glucose	84330	3		IND (Full CBC)	85060	
	IUD Insertion	58300	35		UNA Boot	29580	5		HCT	85055	2		DIFF	85040	
	IUD Removal	58301	15		Vasectomy (T)	55250	135		Gramstain	87000	5		Retics.	85640	
	IUD Follow-up	90040	3		Wart Removal	17100	15		Preg. Test	83340	3		Platelets	85580	
	Pelvic Exam	57410	15		Wart Paring	11050	10		Sediment	81015	2		Protime	85610	
	Routine OB Visit	59420	N/C		Toe Nail Removal	11750	35		Sed Rate	85650	3		Group & Type	86087	
	D & C	58120	150		Circumcision	54161	50		Sickledex	85660	3		Coombs Prenatal	86250	
	PAP	88100	2		Rhythm Strip	93040			Smear Des	85040	2		STS	86410	
	Diaphragm	90060	12						Throat Culture	87090	4		VDRL	86410	
									Urine Complete	81000	5		Latex. Fix	86350	
									Urine Culture	87080	6		ASO Titer	86060	
									Urine Dip Stick	81002	1		Rubella	86394	
									Vag Drop	87010	3		O & P		
									WBC	85030	3				
	SPECIAL INSTRUCTIONS AND REFERRALS:								GC	87080	6				
									Mono Test	86300	3				
									HGB	83020	2				
									Occult Blood	82270	3				
									Sperm Count	89310	3		**OTHER — 08**		
													Supplies	99070	
													Suture removal set		
													Other (List)		
													TODAY'S CHARGES →		

RETURN APPOINTMENT

IF INJURY — GIVE LOCATION AND CAUSE:

WEEKS: 10 MIN. 20 MIN. 30 MIN. 40 MIN. _____ MIN.
MONTHS: 10 MIN. 20 MIN. 30 MIN. 40 MIN. _____ MIN.
NURSE VISIT: _____ REASON

ICDA	ICDA	ICDA	DATE OF ONSET

FPC - 020 REV. 3/78   PATIENT

*Courtesy of Department of Family Medicine, University of North Carolina.

DIAGNOSTIC ENCOUNTER FORM*

☐ N (New)
☐ R (Return)

RECEIPT NUMBER
12629

MONTH	DAY	YEAR	ATTENDING	FPC DOCTOR	TEAM	CLINIC	
			3 1 5 2			1 0 0 1	Imprint

FAMILY PRACTICE CENTER
SCHOOL OF MEDICINE
UNC CHAPEL HILL, NORTH CAROLINA

PRESENTING PROBLEM(S)

DIAGNOSES   Please Circle N or O for Each Entry

ENVIRONMENT
• ••

N O	Housing	0102
N O	Instit'ization	0104
N O	Insurance Coverage	0106
N O	Legal	0108
N O	Leisure Recreation	0110
N O	Misuse of Practice	0112
N O	Nursing/Home Care	0114
N O	Occupational	0116
N O	Poor Social Support	0118
N O	Unemployment	0120
N O	Welfare Dependent	0122
N O	_____	0198

PSYCHOSOCIAL

N O	Adjustment problem of childhood	0302
N O	Adjustment problem of adolescence	0304
N O	Adjustment problem of adult life	0306
N O	Adjustment problem of late life	0308
N O	Alcohol abuse	0310
N O	Affective Psychosis	0312
N O	Anxiety Neurosis	0314
N O	Depressive Neurosis	0316
N O	Drug Abuse	0318
N O	Employment problem	0320
N O	Financial problem	0322
N O	Hearing disability	0324
N O	Interpersonal/ Relational	0326
N O	Marital conflict	0328
N O	Mental retardation	0330
N O	Multi-problem family	0332
N O	Parent-child problem	0334
N O	Psychophysiological disorder	0336
N O	Schizophrenia	0338
N O	Sexual problem	0340
N O	Sleep disturbance	0342
N O	Speech disturbance	0344
N O	Smoking	0346
N O	Transient situational disturbance	0348
N O	_____	0398

SKIN

N O	Acne	0502
N O	Atopy/Eczema	0504
N O	Cellulitis	0506
N O	Dermatitis, Contact	0508
N O	Nail Disease	0510
N O	Pruritus	0512
N O	Rash	0514
N O	Seborrhea	0516
N O	Subcutaneous Infect	0518
N O	Sweat Glands	0520
N O	Tumor, Benign	0522
N O	Ulcer, Skin	0524
N O	Urticaria	0526
N O	Warts, Corns	0528
N O	_____	0598

EYES/EARS

N O	Cataract	0702
N O	Conjunctivitis	0704
N O	Foreign Body	0706
N O	Glaucoma	0708
N O	Otitis Externa	0710
N O	Otitis Media, Acute	0712
N O	Otitis Media, Chronic	0714
N O	Wax in Ear	0716
N O	_____	0798

CARDIAC

N O	Angina	0902
N O	Arrythmia	0904
N O	Chest Pain	0906
N O	Congestive Failure	0908
N O	Ischemic Heart Dis.	0910
N O	M. I.	0912
N O	Murmur	0914
N O	Palpitation	0916
N O	Rheumatic Heart	0918
N O	Syncope	0920
N O	_____	0998

VASCULAR

N O	Atherosclerosis	1102
N O	Edema	1104
N O	Hypertension	1106
N O	Peripheral B. V. S.	1108
N O	Phlebitis	1110
N O	Raised B.P.	1112
N O	Stroke	1114
N O	Varicose V.	1116
N O	_____	1198

RESPIRATORY

N O	Asthma	1302
N O	Bronchitis, Acute	1304
N O	Bronchitis, Chronic	1306
N O	C.O.P.D./Emphysema	1308
N O	Cough	1310
N O	Dyspnea	1312
N O	Epistaxis	1314
N O	Hay Fever	1316
N O	Laryngitis	1318
N O	Pleurisy	1320
N O	Pneumonia	1322
N O	Sinusitis	1324
N O	Tonsillitis	1326
N O	_____	1398

NEUROLOGIC

N O	Dizziness	1902
N O	Epilepsy/Seizures	1904
N O	Migraine	1906
N O	Multiple Sclerosis	1908
N O	Neuralgia	1910
N O	Organic Brain Syn	1912
N O	Parkinsonism	1914
N O	Tension Headache	1916
N O	T. I. Attack	1918
N O	Vertigo	1920
N O	_____	1998

NEOPLASM

N O	Benign Breast Tumor	1702
N O	Malignant	1704
N O	Not Yet Diag.	1706
N O	_____	1798

DIGESTIVE

N O	Abdominal Pain	1502
N O	Anal Fissure	1504
N O	Cirrhosis	1506
N O	Colon, Irritable	1508
N O	Constipation	1510
N O	Dental	1512
N O	Diverticular	1514
N O	Esophagus	1516
N O	Gall Bladder	1518
N O	Gastritis	1520
N O	Hemmorrhoids	1522
N O	Hernia, Inguinal	1524
N O	Hernia, Other	1526
N O	Mouth, Other Dis	1528
N O	Nausea/Vomit	1530
N O	Pancreas	1532
N O	Stomach Disorder	1534
N O	Ulcer, Duodenal	1536
N O	Ulcer, Peptic	1538
N O	_____	1598

BONES/JOINTS

N O	Arthralgia	2102
N O	Bursitis/Tenosynov.	2104
N O	Fibrositis	2106
N O	Joint Derangement	2108
N O	Osteoarthritis	2110
N O	Pain, Joint	2112
N O	Pain, Limb	2114
N O	Pain, Lower Back	2116
N O	Rheumatoid Arthritis	2118
N O	Spine, Cervical	2120
N O	Spine, Lumbar	2122
N O	_____	2198

GENITAL

N O	Abnormal Pap Smear	2302
N O	Breast Disease	2304
N O	Infertility	2306
N O	Male Genitalia	2308
N O	Menopause Symptoms	2310
N O	Menstrual Disorder	2312
N O	Ovarian Disease	2314
N O	P.I.D./Salpingitis	2316
N O	Urethritis	2318
N O	Vaginitis	2320
N O	_____	2398

URINARY

N O	B. P. H.	2502
N O	Cystitis	2504
N O	Enuresis	2506
N O	Hematuria	2508
N O	Kidney, Ureter, Bladder	2510
N O	Prostatitis	2512
N O	Pyelonephritis	2514
N O	_____	2598

BLOOD

N O	Anemia Macrocytic	2702
N O	Anemia Microcytic	2704
N O	Lymphadenitis	2706
N O	Sickle Cell	2708
N O	_____	2798

A·M·E·N

N O	Allergy	2902
N O	Collagen Dis	2904
N O	Diabetes	2906
N O	Gout	2908
N O	Hyper Throid	2910
N O	Hypo Thyroid	2912
N O	Lipid Disorder	2914
N O	Obesity	2916
N O	_____	2998

INFECTIVE

N O	Dermatophytosis	3102
N O	Enteritis	3104
N O	Fever (FUO)	3106
N O	Gonorrhea	3108
N O	Hepatitis	3110
N O	Herpes Simplex	3112
N O	Impetigo	3114
N O	Influenza	3116
N O	Mononucleosis	3118
N O	Pedicul/Scabies	3120
N O	Pharyngitis	3122
N O	Strep Throat	3124
N O	TB	3126
N O	Viral Rash	3128
N O	Viral Syndrome	3130
N O	Worms	3132
N O	_____	3198

CONGENITAL

N O	_____	3398

ACCIDENTS/POISON

N O	Contusion	3502
N O	Bites/Stings	3504
N O	Burn	3506
N O	Dislocation	3508
N O	Fracture	3510
N O	Laceration	3512
N O	Sprain/Strain	3514
N O	_____	3598

PERINATAL

N O	_____	3798

PREGNANCY

N O	Abortion	3902
N O	Delivery	3904
N O	Pregnancy	3906
N O	Prenatal Care	3908
N O	Postnatal Care	3910
N O	_____	3998

PROPHYLACTIC

N O	B. C. Pill	4102
N O	Contraception, Other	4104
N O	Immunication	4106
N O	I.U.D.	4108
N O	Medical Exam	4110
N O	Sterilization	4112
N O	Well Child	4114
N O	_____	4198

*New Problem
**Old or Continuing Problem

*Courtesy of Department of Family Medicine, University of North Carolina.

Family Practice Center of Akron City Hospital
Family Visit Record *
From 09/01/75 Thru 06/30/76

Date   08/13/76
MS1R0040-P0200

Family Number: 003732

Family Members on File

First	Last Name	Age	Suffix
Greg		25	A
Joanne		22	B
Sarah			C

Visit Record

Name	Suffix	Doctor	Site	Date	Diagnosis	Disp Status Recall
Greg	A	Nurse	3	12/22/75	Other Class 90	Old
Joanne	B	McGrady	3	01/07/76	Prenatal Care	Old
		Nurse	3	01/16/76	Other Class 90	Old
		McGrady	3	02/04/76	Pregnancy	Old
		McGrady	3	03/04/76	Prenatal Care	Old
		McGrady	3	04/01/76	Prenatal Care	Old
		Miller	3	04/12/76	Conjunctivitis	New
		McGrady	3	04/15/76	Prenatal Care	Old
		McGrady	3	04/29/76	Other Class 62	New
		McGrady	3	05/13/76	Prenatal Care	Old
		Black	3	05/20/76	Prenatal Care	Old
		Hershberger	3	05/27/76	Prenatal Care	Old
		McGrady	3	06/03/76	Prenatal Care	Old
		Black	3	06/04/76	Prenatal Care	Old
		McGrady	4	06/04/76	Delivery	New
		Black	3	11/05/75	Pregnancy	New
		Black	3	11/05/75	Pap	New
		Nurse	3	11/26/75	Other Class 90	Old
		McGrady	3	12/02/75	Pregnancy	New
Sarah	C	McGrady	3	06/17/76	Well Baby Care	New

*Courtesy of Family Practice Center, Akron City Hospital, Akron, Ohio.

Family Practice Center of Akron City Hospital
Family Visit Record *
From 09/01/75 Thru 06/30/76

Date   08/13/76
MS1R0040-P0200

Family Number: 003742

Family Members on File

First	Last Name	Age	Suffix
David		44	A
Catherin		51	B
Janice		17	C
Dolores			D
David		15	E
Catherin		6	F
Carolyn		15	G
Nancy		18	H

Visit Record

Name	Suffix	Doctor	Site	Date	Diagnosis	Disp Status Recall
Catherin	B	Hoff	3	05/18/76	Hypertension	Old
		Hoff	3	05/18/76	Bronchitis–Acute	New
Janice	C	Hoff	3	01/27/76	Sinusitis	New
		Hoff	3	01/27/76	Constipation	New
		Hoff	3	01/27/76	Sprain, Strain	New
		Hoff	3	09/02/75	Viral Syndrome	New
		Hoff	3	09/02/75	Gastritis	New
		Hoff	3	09/23/75	Abdominal Pain	Old
		Hoff	3	10/24/75	Other Class 50	Old
Dolores	D	Hoff	3	12/23/75	Pap	New
David	E	Black	3	01/05/76	Other Class 86	New
		Black	3	01/09/76	Other Class 90	New

*Courtesy of Family Practice Center, Akron City Hospital, Akron, Ohio.

Crosstabulation of Patients*
Tabulation by Age and Sex for Each Clinic
From 07/01/76 Thru 07/31/76

Date   09/01/76
MS1R0046

Age
Controlling For
Clinic   **Value**   **1 City**

	Count Row Pct. Col. Pct.	Sex Female	Male	Unknown	Row Total
Age	Tot. Pct.	1	2	3	
0 to 1	1	20 52.6 4.1 1.9	18 47.4 8.2 1.7	0 0.0 0.0 0.0	38 3.7
1 Thru 10	2	27 47.4 5.6 2.6	28 49.1 12.8 2.7	2 3.5 0.6 0.2	57 5.5
11 Thru 20	3	67 67.7 13.8 6.5	30 30.3 13.7 2.9	2 2.0 0.6 0.2	99 9.6
21 Thru 40	4	166 73.8 34.3 16.1	55 24.4 25.1 5.3	4 1.8 1.2 0.4	225 21.8
41 Thru 60	5	82 66.1 16.9 8.0	41 33.1 18.7 4.0	1 0.8 0.3 0.1	124 12.0
61 and up	6	106 76.8 21.9 10.3	32 23.2 14.6 3.1	0 0.0 0.0 0.0	138 13.4
Unknown	7	16 4.6 3.3 1.6	15 4.3 6.8 1.5	319 91.1 97.3 30.9	350 33.9
	Column Total	484 46.9	219 21.2	328 31.8	1031 100.0

*Courtesy of Family Practice Center, Akron City Hospital, Akron, Ohio.

Family Practice Center of Akron City Hospital
Problem Encounters Listed by Diagnosis Class for Each Doctor*
Based on Visits From 08/01/76 Thru 08/30/76

Date 09/22/76
MS1R0027-P0180
Doctor 002 Hoff

Major Categories of Disease

Medical Class Code	Description	Number of Problem Encounters	Percent of Doctor's Total Encounters
10	Infectious Disease	14	6.70
14	Neoplasm	1	.48
18	Allergy, Endo, Meta, Nu	21	10.05
22	Blood	2	.96
26	Mental	16	7.66
30	Neurological	1	.48
34	Eyes and Ears	7	3.35
38	Cardiac Problems	6	2.87
42	Vascular Problems	28	13.40
46	Respiratory Problems	6	2.87
50	Digestive Problems	9	4.31
54	Urinary	5	2.39
58	Genital	12	5.74
62	Pregnancy	6	2.87
66	Skin, Cellular Tissue	9	4.31
72	Bones and Joints	12	5.74
76	Congenital Anomoly	0	.00
80	Perinatal Conditions	0	.00
82	Signs and Symptoms	14	6.70
86	Accidents, Poisoning	6	2.87
90	Prophylactic Proceed	34	16.27
98	CMI	0	.00

Total Encounters for this Doctor   209

Total Encounters for this Center   1,955

*Courtesy of Family Practice Center, Akron City Hospital, Akron, Ohio.

Frequency List of Problems
Family Practice Center of St. Thomas Hospital
Problem Incidence Listed by Frequency for Each Doctor
Based on Visits From 05/01/76 Thru 05/31/76

Date 06/23/76
MS1R0048-P0170

Doctor 001   East

Medical Class Code		Description	Number of Patients With This Problem	Percent of Doctor's Total
42	401M	Hypertension	37	12.37
18	277–	Obesity	33	11.04
38	413Y	Chronic Ischemdis	25	8.36
26	3000	Anxiety	17	5.69
18	250–	Diabetes	16	5.35
72	713Y	Osteoarthritis	10	3.34
42	412X	Artherosclerosis	8	2.68
86	848Y	Sprain, Strain	8	2.68
42	443Y	Peripheral	7	2.34
46	519Y	Other Class 46	7	2.34
72	7179	Myosites	7	2.34
10	054–	Pharyngitis	6	2.01
26	3004	Depression	6	2.01
90	Y10M	Medical Exam	6	2.01
18	242–	Thyroid Disease	5	1.67
18	691–	Allergy	5	1.67
38	427M	Arrhythmia	5	1.67
54	595Y	Cystitis	5	1.67
90	Y10Z	Pap	5	1.67
86	929Y	Bruise, Contusion	4	1.34
18	279X	Lipid Abnorm	3	1.00
30	437Y	Cerebrovascular Dis	3	1.00
34	381Y	Otitis Med–Acute	3	1.00
38	427Z	Congestive Failure	3	1.00
42	454–	Varicosities	3	1.00
46	461Y	Sinusitis	3	1.00
66	709Y	Other Class 66	3	1.00
30	349Y	Other Class 30	2	.67
38	391Y	Rheumatic	2	.67
42	451Y	Phlebitis	2	.67
50	009Y	Gastroenterology	2	.67
54	599Y	Other Class 54	2	.67
58	627–	Menopausal	2	.67
62	Y60–	Prenatal Care	2	.67
66	680Y	Infectious	2	.67
66	692Y	Contact Derm	2	.67
72	729Y	Other Class 72	2	.67
86	829Y	Fracture	2	.67
90	Y434	Contraception	2	.67
10	0799	Viral Syndrome	1	.33
14	195Y	Malignant	1	.33
18	493–	Asthma	1	.33
22	285Y	Anemia	1	.33
22	289Y	Other Class 22	1	.33
26	Y137	Family Disruption	1	.33
26	306Y	Other Class 26	1	.33

Problem Encounters Listed by Diagnosis Class for All Clinics*
Based on Visits From 07/01/76 Thru 12/31/76

Date 01/26/77
MS1R0029-P0180

Medical Class Code		Description	Number of Problem Encounters	Percent of Clinics' Total Encounters
			21	.08
			21	.08
10	011Y	TB + Skin Test	10	.04
10	034Y	Strep Throat	90	.34
10	039Y	Other Infectious Dis	148	.56
10	054–	Pharyngitis	590	2.22
10	057–	Viral Exanthem	37	.14
10	070–	Hepatitis	21	.08
10	075–	Mononucleosis	53	.20
10	0791	Warts	112	.42
10	0799	Viral Syndrome	612	2.30
10	098–	Gonorrhea	32	.12
10	110Y	Dermatophytosis	40	.15
10	133–	Pinworms, Pedic, Scab	29	.11
10	470Y	Influenza	35	.13
10		Infectious Disease	1,809	6.80
14	195Y	Malignant	133	.50
14	228Y	Benign	22	.08
14	239Y	Other Neoplasm	11	.04
14		Neoplasm	166	.62
18	242–	Thyroid Disease	178	.67
18	250–	Diabetes	623	2.34
18	269X	Feeding Problems	7	.03
18	274–	Gout	39	.15
18	277–	Obesity	779	2.93
18	279X	Lipid Abnorm	116	.44
18	279Y	Other Allergic Endo	47	.18
18	392–	Collagen Disease	9	.03
18	493–	Asthma	83	.31
18	691–	Allergy	534	2.01
18		Allergy, Endo, Meta, Nu	2,415	9.08
22	282–	Sickle Cell Disease	3	.01
22	285Y	Anemia	109	.41
22	289M	Lymphadenitis	13	.05
22	289Y	Other Blood	31	.12
22		Blood	156	.59
26	Y131	Economic Problem	12	.05
26	Y137	Family Disruption	83	.31
26	Y138	Social, Family Prob	192	.72
26	Y139	Parent–Child Problem	43	.16
26	Y145	Occupational Problem	14	.05
26	291Y	Alcoholism	76	.29
26	299Y	Psychoses	36	.14
26	3000	Anxiety	515	1.94

*Courtesy of Family Practice Center, Akron City Hospital, Akron, Ohio.

Appendix 2
Professional Relations

- **A Glossary of Professional Liability Terms**

A GLOSSARY OF PROFESSIONAL LIABILITY TERMS

The following definitions are provided as a ready reference for future use. Because many of these terms are defined as they relate to medical professional liability only, these definitions may vary from the general insurance definitions.

Cancellation: Termination of the insurance policy before its natural expiration.

> **Pro Rata:** The percentage of earned premium that is applied when the policy is cancelled by the company. Premium returned to the insured is the full proportionate part due for the unexpired policy term.

> **Short Rate:** The percentage of earned premium that is applied when the policy is cancelled by the insured. The company pays a return premium less than the pro rata part that is still unearned. The short rate cancellation table is standard in the insurance industry.

Claim: In medical malpractice, an oral or written request by a patient or patient's representative for compensation. A demand or calling upon an insurance company by a policyholder for something that is due and supposed to be due under the terms of an insurance policy.

Classification (Specialty): The assigning of an applicant to a certain group of practitioners (according to specialty) for rating purposes.

Contingent Fees: An arrangement in which an attorney agrees to represent a plaintiff for a certain percentage of the final settlement awarded the plaintiff.

Corporate Liability: Any liability of a corporation of which the insured are owners or shareholders or in which they have a financial interest.

Endorsement: A form attached to the policy which modifies the basic contract.

Excess: A type of policy which provides higher limits of liability than the basic or primary policy.

Exclusion: A statement in the policy or an endorsement which outlines what is not covered by the insurance.

Experience: A measure of what has happened in the past, as in "loss experience."

Incident: A potential claim where the patient has not made an oral or written request for compensation. A happening which provides the physician some reason to believe that a claim may be made against him or her at some future date.

Incurred Losses: The amount of claims for which an insurance company is thought to be liable. This includes actual amounts for settled claims, as well as estimates for as yet unreported or unsettled claims.

Informed Consent: A state which exists when a physician has adequately informed a patient of the nature of the treatment proposed, of the risks inherent in the procedure, and of alternative treatments.

Insuring Agreement: The section of an insurance policy which defines the coverage and outlines in general the responsibilities of the insurance company in the event of a claim.

Limits of Liability: Dollar amounts that represent maximum liability of the insurance company, for example, $1,000,000 per occurrence, $1,000,000 annual aggregate.

> **Per Occurrence:** The maximum amount payable by the company as a result of a single occurrence or continuous or repeated exposure to substantially the same general conditions.

> **Annual Aggregate:** The maximum amount payable by the company during any one policy year.

Locum Tenens: In medicine, a physician who temporarily acts for another.

Medical Malpractice: Professional negligence which results in injury to the patient.

Mutual Insurance Company: A company which is owned by its policyholders. All risks and all profits are the property of the policyholders.

> **Assessable:** A mutual company which can require its policyholders to pay money in addition to premium in the event of insolvency of the company.

> **Nonassessable:** A mutual company which cannot "assess" its policyholders.

Negligence: Failure to use due care for the protection of another.

Policy Period: The period of time for which coverage is in force.

Premium: The sum of money paid by the insured in return for compensation in the event of loss covered by the policy.

Professional Liability: The state of being liable, as in the case of malpractice.

Professional Liability policies

> **Occurrence Policy:** A professional liability policy in which an event that takes place during the term of an occurrence policy and which later becomes the basis for a professional liability claim is covered even though the applicable policy is no longer in force. A number of years could elapse between the occurrence and the surfacing of a claim.

> **Claims-Made Policy:** A professional liability policy in which coverage is provided for only those claims that are presented during a specific policy period. Prior acts may be covered either by the policy itself or by endorsement. Also, an extended reporting period may be offered when the policy is terminated to allow for claims that may surface subsequent to the date of termination.

Punitive Damages: Damages awarded separately and in addition to compensatory damages, in the belief that the physician should be punished for gross, malicious, or wanton misconduct.

Re Ipsa Loquitur: "The thing speaks for itself"—a doctrine of law with reference to cases where mere proof that an occurrence took place is sufficient under the circumstances to throw the burden upon defendants to prove that it was not due to their negligence.

Reporting Endorsement: If the claims-made policy is cancelled or nonrenewed the insured can purchase an additional reporting period in which claims may be reported. This is also known as "tail coverage."

Risk Management: A process which emphasizes the prevention of medical incidents which might lead to claims.

Statute of Limitations: A statutory cut-off period which establishes the time limits for the beginning of a legal action.

Surcharge: An additional percentage applied to the premium because of previous claims or adverse risk history.

Umbrella: A type of policy which provides high limits of liability above those provided by the basic policy and which also extends the coverage to include certain other defined personal injury items.

Underwriting: The process of determining whether a risk will be accepted or rejected by an insurer. In medical professional liability, underwriting is sometimes done by peer review in which physicians review a physician's application to determine if he is an acceptable risk.

Vicarious Liability: Under the legal doctrine of respondent superior, people are responsible not only for their own acts, but also for the acts of their employees and other agents in the course of their employment. This is particularly true where discretion of their manner and method of work is exercised.

Appendix 3
Marketing

- **Letter to New Patients**
- **Patient Information Guide**
- **Family Practice News**
- **Printed Material for Patient Education**
- **Addresses for Ordering Patient Education Materials**
- **Patient Education Handouts**

Letter to New Patients

To Our Patients:

This letter is our first opportunity to explain the policies and features of our medical practice. Please keep this information in a convenient place as a reference for questions which may arise about our practice.

Appointments

Office visits are by appointment only. When you call for an appointment, our receptionist will ask a few questions regarding the nature and urgency of your problem or concern. For routine health care, please call several days in advance. Emergencies and problems requiring immediate physician attention will be given priority. Notify us before coming to the office or going to the emergency room.

Appointments are scheduled between 8:00 am and 4:30 pm, Monday through Friday. Saturday morning office hours are for urgent problems only. Nursing personnel are available for routine laboratory work and tests from 8:00 am to 9:00 am daily.

Fees

Medical costs are increasing at a rapid rate and we are making every effort to keep fees reasonable. Our facility, staff, equipment, and supplies are suited for your health care but they are costly. Please help us maintain costs by paying for your care at the time service is rendered. Billing statements and processing insurance claims are expensive and time consuming.

We will economize, as long as your medical care is not sacrificed. Laboratory studies, tests, and prescriptions will be utilized in the most cost-effective manner. If you have any suggestions which will conserve health care dollars, please let us know.

Telephone

We receive nearly 100 phone calls each day! Except for emergencies, we will respond to calls at regular times during the day, usually in the late morning or at the end of afternoon office hours. Please convey your questions and concerns clearly and allow a reasonable time for callback. Our nurses are trained to respond to the majority of phone messages and will always be acting under our direction. We will seldom prescribe medication over the phone, unless the patient has been seen within the past day or two. Long distance calls will be returned collect.

Emergencies

Please inform us of any emergency or family distress. We have facilities for minor surgical procedures and may save time and money by seeing some emergencies in the office. If the situation is obviously critical or life threatening, go directly to the hospital emergency room and we will be informed.

Health Maintenance

We offer all patients continuing and comprehensive health care. Regardless of age or sex we would like to encourage patients to prevent health problems and assist us in detection of disease at its earliest stages. This will require routine examinations and periodic visits. Your physician will discuss a personal health maintenance program, following initial visits and tests. This is a recommendation, *not* a requirement.

(continued)

Consultations

Occasionally during your care, we may wish to consult another physician. This may require you to be seen by this physician. If you are in agreement we will arrange the appointment and send information. When you conclude your treatment with our consulting physician we will have all necessary medical information in your records.

Coverage

During regular office hours our telephone will be answered by office personnel. After office hours and on weekends our answering service will receive calls and forward them to one of the physicians in our practice.

We are available for emergencies on a 24-hour basis. If it is *not* a serious problem or emergency, please wait until regular office hours to contact us.

The physicians and office personnel are trained to assist you in detection, treatment, and prevention of illness. We would like a long and meaningful relationship with you and encourage you to express concerns or problems regardless of the issue.

Patient Information Guide

Topical Outline

Introduction and Overview

physicians
type of practice
location
board certification
comprehensive and continuous care
doctor/patient and staff/patient relationships

Registration and Appointments

enrollment procedures
office hours
telephone protocol
scheduling visits
cancellations and missed appointments
physician assignments
forms and policies

Finances

services and charges
fee for service
office collections
billing and third party payments
delineation of charges—routine visits, laboratory, x-ray
special procedures
counseling
preparation of forms and reports
nursing home and hospital care

Emergencies

hospital emergency phone number
coverage during and after hours

Health Maintenance

physical and diagnostic examinations
health hazards
patient education
preventive medicine and early disease detection
periodic checkups

Specialized Care

pediatrics
obstetrics
geriatrics
house calls, etc.

Telephone

prescriptions and refills
routine phone messages
emergency calls
after hours coverage
reports of x-ray and laboratory tests
callback and call-in times

Consultation and Referral

specialists
written communications
follow-up

Health Care Records

individual and family care
privacy and confidentiality
transferring
legal documents

Hospital Care

which hospitals
types of care
admission and discharge routines
routine and emergency procedures

Insurance

medicare
medicaid
workman's compensation and disability
private carriers, outpatient and inpatient claims
patients' responsibilities to physician and contract with insurance company
super bill on universal form
processing policies
year-end statements

FAMILY PRACTICE NEWS *

FAMILY PRACTICE CENTER
VOLUME 2 NUMBER 1

NORTH CAROLINA MEMORIAL HOSPITAL
FEBRUARY 1986

WINTER HEALTH TIPS

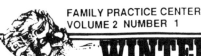

WHAT ARE THE SYMPTOMS OF COLDS OR FLU?

COLD:

- General discomfort
- Nasal stuffiness
- Sneezing
- Runny nose
- Watery eyes
- Mild sore throat
- Decreased appetite
- Small or absent fever

FLU:

- Headache
- General discomfort/ weakness
- Aches in muscles/joints
- Cough without phlegm
- Fever up to 102 degrees

SO WHAT CAN I DO ABOUT THIS?

Rest your body. Try to cut down or eliminate, for two or three days, anything that stresses your body.

- Get 8 hours of sleep a night.
- Drink a glass of water or non-caffeinated fluid every two hours (until three hours before bed) to keep the mucous membranes wet.
- Eat a balanced diet, that is, foods from all food groups (breads, poultry, vegetables/fruit and dairy products.
- Take your temperature. Although colds or flu can cause temperatures up to 102 degrees (particularly in children), they should not go higher. If you want to learn how to take your temperature, please ask the module nurse at the Family Practice Center. She will be happy to teach you.
- If you seem to have symptoms of the flu, call your doctor in the first 48 hours for his/her advice.
- Use a cool vaporizer in your bedroom at night. This will help you breath more easily and prevent a sore throat in the morning (a sore throat is usually the result of breathing through your mouth all night). Don't point the vaporizer directly at yourself.

- Use acetaminophen (Tylkenol, Datril, Panadol) as directed, for aches, pains and fevers. DO NOT USE ASPIRIN IN CHILDREN OR YOUNG PEOPLE UNDER 15 YEARS OF AGE. There has been some concern among doctors that taking aspirin could cause Reye's Syndrome if it is taken with the flu or taken following chicken pox. If you have any questions about Reye's Syndrome, please talk with your doctor.

- Decongestants (such as Sudafed, Novafed) help relieve stuffiness, but they can make you feel jittery. Antihistamines help dry up runny noses, but they can make you feel drowsy and should not be used if you are going to drive a car or operate machinery.

- Most cold preparations contain both a decongestant and an antihistamine (usually chlorpheniramine). If you use nasal spray antihistamines (such as Neo-Synephrine, Otrivin, Afrin), remember that they should be used for only three days. Stop using them for two days, and then resume use for three days. Using antihistamines for more than three consecutive days can produce congestion rather than relieve it!

WHEN SHOULD I CHECK WITH MY DOCTOR?

IF:

- Your temperature goes over 102 degrees for more than 24 hours.
- You have diarrhea or vomiting that is making you weaker.
- You start coughing up mucus that's thick and yellow or green.
- You seem to get better and then take a turn for the worse.
- You have a cough that doesn't let you sleep.

REMEMBER: COLDS and FLU are VIRUSES. They will NOT respond to antibiotics. The best we can do is to help ourselves through the illness and treat the symptoms. If you have any questions, please talk with your doctor.

* Courtesy of Department of Family Medicine, University of North Carolina.

TAKING CARE OF YOURSELF IN THE COLD

Getting caught unprepared for the winter weather can be dangerous. At the Family Practice Center we are concerned that you understand some basic facts about how to care for yourself and your loved ones in the cold weather. It is possible to enjoy the cold weather and be comfortable too.

A WORKING GUIDE TO DEALING WITH PROBLEMS IN THE COLD

MILD COLD
EXPOSURE

Signs and Symptoms | What to Do

- Hands and feet become numb.

- Ability to pick up or hold objects becomes more difficult.

- Occasional shiver or chill occurs.

- Put on mittens.

- Shoes should be loosely tied.

- Don't drink alcohol or caffine or smoke in the cold. These cause changes in the blood vessels that can cause heat loss and frostbite.

- Clothing should be loose, not tight, cotton or wool.

- WEAR A WARM HAT!

SEVERE COLD
EXPLOSURE

Signs and Symptoms | What to Do

- Shivering becomes uncontrollable, or muscle tightness occurs.

- Thinking becomes very dull.

- Ability to speak decreases, or person cannot respond.

- Behavior is irrational.

- Call an ambulance.

- Must get warm or may die.

- Take to warm area.

- Get out of cold clothes.

- Put warm items on skin-hot water bottles, warm body contact.

- If person cannot speak, do not give hot liquids. Otherwise, give hot liquids.

- Take to emergency room.

MODERATE
COLD EXPOSURE

Signs and Symptoms | What to Do

- Shivering becomes more intense.

- Attitude becomes more careless.

- Speech becomes more difficult.

- Hands/feet become very cold/numb.

- Leave. Go to a place that is warm—NOW.

- Take off cold clothes when you get inside.

- Drink hot liquids.

- If your feet hurt, get red or blister when rewarming, CALL THE DOCTOR.

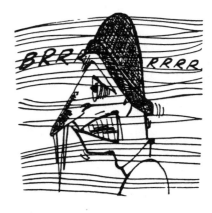

Printed Material for Patient Education

(Number in parentheses indicates address found on pp)

Circulatory System Diseases

Learning How to Live With Heart Trouble (12)
Watch Your High Blood Pressure, Pamphlet #483 (45)
Hypertension *Is* High Blood Pressure (30)

Contraception/Sterilization

Contraception with IUD's (54)
Women and the Pill (54)
Birth Control Handbook (33)
After Your Doctor Prescribes Ortho-Novum Tablets (40)
For the Patient: CU-7 (51)
Lippes Loop (40)
A Guide to the Use of Your Ortho Diaphragm (40)
Sterilization by Laparoscopy (3)
Elective Vasectomy (19)

Digestive System Diseases

How to Live with Your Ulcer (59)
Help for Your Hemorrhoids (59)
About Your Gas Crisis (53)
Understanding Your Irritable (Spastic) Colon (2)

Emotional Disorders

What to Do When a Member of Your Family is Depressed (16)
Stress (11)
Stress and Your Health (32)

Endocrine/Metabolic Disorders & Nutrition

You and Diabetes (57)
Toward Good Control: Guidebook for Diabetics (6)
Straight Talk About Diabetes: Guidebook for the Teenager and Young Adult Diabetic (6)
Diabetes in the News (a newspaper) (6)
Clinilog Diary (6)
Two Accepted Techniques for Self–Injection (8)
Feet First (for diabetics) (54)
Living with Diabetes (16)
Diabetes Diet Packet and Patient Instruction Guide (20)
Bland Diet Instructions (59)
Foods to Avoid on a Lipid–Lowering Regimen (8)
Pregnancy Diet (57)
Bulk Diet (57)
Residue–Restricted Diet (57)
Liquid Diet (57)
Low Fat Diet (57)
Bland Diet (57)
Geriatric Diet (57)

Convalescent Diet (57)
Hypochromic Anemia Diet (57)
Low-Sodium Diet (57)
Sodium-Restricted Diet (57)
Myths of Vitamins (54)
1000 Calories a Day (31)
Calorie Control for You (57)
Weight Control Plan Diet and Exercise (57)
Dietary Control of Cholesterol (21)
Hyperlipidemia—An American Epidemic (8)
Questions and Answers About Fats and Oils in Our Food (9)
Foods to Avoid on a Lipid-Lowering Regimen (8)
Good Eating for the Milk-Sensitive Person (50)

Genitourinary System Development & Diseases

Chronic Urethritis in the Female (19)
Chronic Prostatitis (19)
Feminine Hygiene (19)
Growing Up Young (23)
How Shall I Tell My Daughter (23)
The Miracle of You (23)
Very Personally Yours (22)
The Second 40 Years (8)

Infant & Child Care

Health and Immunization Record (20)
Facts About Breast Feeding (27)
Breast Feeding Your Baby (50)
The Phenomena of Early Development (50)
Caring for Your Baby (50)
Your Child's Appetite (50)
Your Baby Becomes a Toddler (50)
How Your Child Learns About Sex (50)
Developing Toilet Habits (50)
When Your Child is Contrary (50)
Your Children and Discipline (50)
Your Child's Fears (50)
When Your Child is Unruly (50)
Feeding Your Baby (50)
Mother and Baby Care at Home (Sp) (50)
Your Milk-Sensitive Infant (Sp) (50)
There Will Be a New Baby at Your House (Sp) (50)
Food for a Healthy Mother and Baby (Sp) (50)
Your Baby is Coming Soon (Sp) (50)
How to Fix Your Baby's Formula (Sp) (50)
Your Premature Infant (50)
Naming Your New Baby (50)
Your Child and Household Safety (15)
Your Child's Safety (32)
Your Child's Progress in School (50)
Memo to Parents About Immunization (32)
Baby's Day (23)
Your Growing Baby (50)
Children Learn What They Live (50)
The Sudden Infant Death Syndrome (54)

Infections/Parasitic Diseases

Questions and Answers About Head Lice (47)
Some Facts About Worms (also in Spanish) (40)
Treating Roundworm Infection (49)
Treating Pinworm (49)
"Flu" (1)
The Common Cold (41)
How to Treat the Common Cold (41)
Understanding Otitis Media (13)
How Fluids Help Your Cough or Cold (2)
Your Doctor Needs Your Help to Treat Your Urinary Tract Infection (48)
For Your Information . . . Vaginitis (40)
Understanding Your Vaginal Discharge (51)
A Woman Explains Vaginitis (31)
Facts You Should Know About V.D. (32)
V.D. Handbook (33)
V.D. — Epidemic Among Teenagers — Pamphlet #517 (45)

Miscellaneous

Getting Married (22)
The Years of Independence (22)
The Promise of the Mature Years (8)
Generation in the Middle (11)

Musculoskeletal System Diseases

Do the Following Exercises Twice a Day (for low back & abdomen) (2)
38 Pieces of Good Advice (for avoiding low back problems) (2)
How to Get Along With Your Back (26)
Arthritis: The Basic Facts (7)

Neoplasms

Cancer of the Colon and Rectum, HIS #124 (54)
How to Examine Your Breasts (4)
Cancer of the Breast, HIS #81 (54)
Breast Self Examination, NIH #74–649 (54)
Stay Healthy—Learn About Uterine Cancer (4)
Cancer of the Uterus, HIS #109 (54)
Cancer of the Bladder, HIS #149 (54)
Leukemias, Lymphomas, and Multiple Myeloma, HIS #144 (54)
Hodgkins Disease, NIH #72–172 (54)
Cancer of the Stomach, HIS #120 (54)
Cancer of the Mouth, HIS #132 (54)
Cancer of the Larynx, HIS #122 (54)
Cancer of the Prostate, HIS #127 (54)
Cancer of the Skin, HIS #75 (54)

Nervous System Diseases

What We Know About Headaches, Pamphlet #502 (45)
Migraine—Information for Patients (39)

Pregnancy, Postnatal Maternal Care

Becoming a Parent (50)
Be Good to Your Baby Before it is Born (25)
Birth Defects (22)
What to do about Minor Discomforts of Pregnancy (50)
Understanding Morning Sickness (31)
The Rh Negative Woman Asks About RhoGAM (40)
Facts About the Rh Factor (40)
Prenatal Care (43)
Before and After Having Your Baby (27)
Rapid Post Natal Figure Recovery (40)
Caring for Yourself After Your Baby is Born (50)
Abdominal Exercises (27)

Preventive Medicine

Adult Physical Fitness (54)
Youth Physical Fitness (54)
Beyond Diet: Exercise Your Way to Fitness and Heart Health (9)
Metropolitan Life's Exercise Guide (32)
Handle Yourself With Care (54)
Protecting Your Family From Accidental Poisoning (45)

Respiratory System Diseases, including Allergies

Cystic Fibrosis (17)
Emphysema and You (60)
Doctor, My Sinuses Are Killing Me (1)
Do's and Don'ts for Sinus Sufferers (2)
New Home Construction Suggestions for the Allergy Patient (2)
How to Reduce the "Allergic Load" for the Allergy-Prone Infant (2)
Taming the Outdoors for the Allergy Patient (2)
Ways to Help Allergy Patients Avoid "A Bad Day at the Office" (2)
Guide to "Desensitizing" a Room (2)

Smoking/Alcohol/Drug Abuse

Unless You Decide to Quit (54)
How to Talk to Your Teenager About Drinking and Driving (35)
Alcohol: A Family Affair (35)
Alcohol and Your Unborn Baby, # (ADM) 78-521 (54)
The Alcoholic American (11)
Alcoholic American (11)
Alcoholism (32)
Antabuse Therapy (8)
Druggism (32)

Addresses for Ordering Patient Education Materials

1. Abbott Laboratories
   North Chicago, Illinois 60064

2. A. H. Robbins Company
   Richmond, Virginia 23220

3. American College of Obstetricians and
      Gynecologists
   Suite 2700
   One East Wacker Drive
   Chicago, Illinois 60601

4. American Cancer Society
   Local Chapter or 777 3rd Avenue
   New York, New York 10017

5. American Heart Association
   44 East 23rd Street
   New York, New York 10010

6. Ames Company
   Division of Miles Laboratories, Inc.
   Elkhart, Indiana 46514

7. Arthritis Foundation
   National Office
   1212 the Avenue of the Americas
   New York, New York 10036

8. Ayerst Laboratories
   New York, New York 10017

9. Best Foods
   C.P.C. International, Inc.
   International Plaza
   Englewood Cliffs, New Jersey 07632

10. Blood Pressure Information Center
    120/80 National Institutes of Health
    Bethesda, Maryland 20014

11. Blueprint for Health
    Blue Cross Association
    840 N. Lakeshore Drive
    Chicago, Illinois 60611

12. Budlong Press Company
    5428 N. Virginia Avenue
    Chicago, Illinois 60625

13. Burroughs Wellcome Company
    Research Triangle Park
    North Carolina 27709

14. Cartoon Color Company
    9024 Lindblade Street
    Culver City, California 90230

15. Chemical Specialties Manufacturers
       Association
    Suite 1120
    1001 Connecticut Avenue, N.W.
    Washington, D.C. 20036

16. Ciba-Geigy Corporation
    Ardsley, New York 10502

17. Cystic Fibrosis Foundation
    3379 Peachtree Road, N.E.
    Atlanta, Georgia 30326

18. Dietor Systems
    P.O. Box 1501
    Ann Arbor, Michigan 48106

19. Eaton Labs
    Norwich, New York 13815

20. Eli Lilly & Company
    Indianapolis, Indiana 46206

21. Fleishman's Margarines
    625 Madison Avenue
    New York, New York 10022

22. Kimberly-Clark Corporation
    The Life Cycle Center
    Neenah, Wisconsin 54956

23. Kotex Products
    The Consumer Information Center
    Personal Products Company
    Milltown, New Jersey 08850

24. Lumex, Incorporated
    Bay Shore, New York 11706

25. March of Dimes National Foundation
    P.O. Box 2000
    White Plains, New York 10602

26. McNeill Labs, Inc.
    Fort Washington, Pennsylvania 19034
    Att: Sample Dept.

27. Meade–Johnson Company
    Evansville, Indiana 47721

28. Medical Focus, Incorporated
    142 Mineola Avenue
    Roslyn Heights, New York 11577

29. Medic Publishing Company
    P.O. Box 1636
    Bellevue, Washington 98009

30. Merck, Sharp, & Dohme
    West Point, Pennsylvania 19486

31. Merrill–National Laboratories
    Division of Richardson–Merrill, Inc.
    Cincinnati, Ohio 45215

32. Metropolitan Life Insurance Company
    1 Madison Avenue
    New York, New York 10010

33. Montreal Health Press
    P.O. Box 1000, Station G
    Montreal,Quebec, Canada

34. National Audio–Visual Center
    National Archives & Records Service
    Washington, D.C. 20409

35. National Clearinghouse for Alcohol
    Information
    P.O. Box 2345
    Rockville, Maryland 20852

36. Norwich Products, Inc.
    Norwich, New York 13815

37. Office of Communication
    U.S. Department of Agriculture
    Washington, D.C. 20250

38. Office of Research Reporting
    National Institutes of Child Health &
    Human Development
    National Institutes of Health
    Bethesda, Maryland 20014

39. Organon, Incorporated
    West Orange, New Jersey 07052

40. Ortho Pharmaceutical Corporation
    Raritan, New Jersey 08869

41. Patient Education Center
    North Carolina Memorial Hospital
    Chapel Hill, North Carolina 27514

42. Phizer Laboratories Division
    New York, New York 10017

43. Pritchett & Hill Associates
    2996 Grandview Avenue, N.E.
    Atlanta, Georgia 30305

44. Professional Research, Incorporated
    PRI Building 461 N. La Brea
    Los Angeles, California 90036

45. Public Affairs Pamphlets
    381 Park Avenue, South
    New York, New York 10016

46. Questions and Answers About Fats & Oils
    Department QAO-X
    Box 307
    Coventry, Connecticut 06238

47. Reed and Carnrick
    Kennelworth, New Jersey 07033

48. Roche Laboratories
    Division of Hoffmann-La Roche, Inc.
    Nutley, New Jersey 07110

49. Roerig
    Division of Phizer Pharmaceuticals
    New York, New York 10017

50. Ross Laboratories
    Columbus, Ohio 43216

51. Searle & Company
    Chicago, Illinois 60680

52. Standard Brands, Incorporated
    625 Madison Avenue
    New York, New York 10022

53. Stuart Pharmaceuticals
    Division of ICI, U.S. Incorporated
    Wilmington, Delaware 19897

54. Superintendent of Documents
    U.S. Government Printing Office
    Washington, D.C. 20402

55. Train–Aid
    229 N. Central Avenue
    Glendale, California 91203

56. Trainex Corporation
    P.O. Box 116
    Garden Grove, California 92642

57. Upjohn
    7000 Portage Road
    Kalamazoo, Michigan 49001

58. U.S. Feed Pharmaceuticals Manufacturing
    Corporation
    Puerto Rico 00701

59. Warner Chilcott, Division of
    Warner-Lambert Company
    Morris Plains, New Jersey 07950

60. Winthrop Labs
    New York, New York 10016

Patient Education Handouts

How To Take A Temperature

Temperatures should be taken by mouth in older children and by rectum in babies as described below. It is important to shake down the mercury in the thermometer to below 98 so as to get an accurate reading. Oral thermometers can be used rectally and rectal thermometers can be used orally. Remember not to wash your thermometer in hot water as this may ruin it. A child should not drink hot or cold liquids for several minutes before their temperature is to be taken orally.

BY MOUTH	BY RECTUM

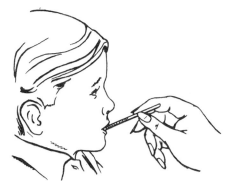

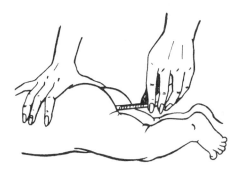

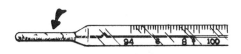

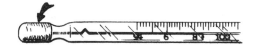

BY MOUTH	BY RECTUM
1. Shake down the thermometer.	1. Shake down the thermometer.
2. Place long, silver tip of thermometer under child's tongue.	2. Lubricate silver end of it.
3. Have child close lips gently, being careful not to bite thermometer.	3. Spread buttocks so that rectum can be easily seen.
4. Hold thermometer under tongue for two minutes.	4. Insert thermometer gently until silver tip can no longer be seen, then hold in place for two minutes.
5. Remove thermometer.	5. Remove thermometer.
6. Read degree of temperature (exactly where the mercury stops).	6. Read degree of temperature (exactly where the mercury stops).

House Dust Avoidance

As dust is one of the most common causes of allergic symptoms, it is very important to minimize exposure to it. The more completely you carry out the following recommendations, the more effective they will be. All the cleaning should be done in the allergic patient's absence and he or she should be kept out of the room for a few hours after the cleaning.

I. *The Patient's Bedroom*

    A. Remove all furniture, rugs, carpets, drapes and curtains.

    B. Clean the room from top to bottom with a cloth or mop dampened with water.

    C. Wax the floor.

    D. Scrub bed and springs (do this outside the bedroom).

    E. The mattress and box springs should have a dust (air) proof cover with a zipper fastener made of plastic or special material.

    F. All pillows in this room must be made of foam rubber or synthetic materials such as dacron and covered with plastic covers.

    G. Cotton mattress pads should not be used; however, a thin washed cotton sheet blanket can be used next to the mattress. Do not use comforters or quilts.

    H. A wooden chair which has been scrubbed may be used in this room.

    I. Rag rugs which must be washed once a week may be used on the floor.

    J. Plain light curtains which must be washed once a week may be used.

    K. If there is a hot air heating system in your house, shut off the duct to the patient's bedroom and cover the register with several layers of a cellophane wrap like Saran Wrap and seal it with tape.

    L. Clean this room thoroughly once a week with a damp cloth or water type vacuum cleaner. Keeping the room as bare as possible will simplify the weekly cleaning.

    M. Keep the windows in this room closed.

II. *Rest of the House*

    A. In cleaning the rest of the house, never use brooms or dusters. Use a water type vacuum or damp rags.

    B. Go over all overstuffed furniture and rugs with a water type vacuum cleaner often. Synthetic rug material is recommended. Use only rubberized rug pads.

    C. Remove all pets from the house.

    D. Use an exhaust fan in the kitchen while frying.

    E. Avoid keeping fruits or vegetables too long, as they may collect mold.

    F. Avoid damp, musty smelling places and if your basement is damp, use a dehumidifier in it.

    G. If air conditioners, dehumidifiers, or humidifiers are used, watch them closely for growth of mold and clean them frequently.

    H. Clean the furnace filter frequently.

    I. Blankets and clothing stored for a season should be cleaned thoroughly and aired before use.

Food Allergy in Children

I. *General Information*

The symptoms of food allergy in children may be clear cut or vague. They may include irritability, "colic", diarrhea, eczema, skin eruptions around the rectum, stuffy nose, vomiting and wheezing. Food allergy is more frequent in children from families in which other members have allergy problems.

The most common causes of food allergy are milk, eggs, wheat, corn, chocolate, peanuts, and orange juice. The best treatment is identification of the allergy-producing food and elimination of it from the diet of your child. The identification of the allergic food is done by elimination diet, then a challenge with the food.

II. *Directions for the Elimination Diet and Challenge Testing* (See attached sheets which show what foods contain milk, eggs, wheat, and corn)

A. Place the child on a diet consisting *only* of rice, lamb and water. This diet must be very strict to make the testing productive. You should stay on this diet for five (5) days. Note the effect this diet has on the suspected allergic symptoms in your child.

B. Next, add milk products in as high a concentration as your child will tolerate for five (5) days. Note whether there is a reappearance or increase in his or her allergic symptoms. If there is, notify us when this is noted. If not, proceed to "C".

C. Next, add eggs to the diet in as large amounts as your child will tolerate for the next five (5) days. Again, watch for reappearance or increase in allergic symptoms. If so, notify us; if not, proceed to "D".

D. Next, add wheat products to the diet in large amounts for five (5) days, watching for a reappearance or increase in allergic symptoms. If so, notify us; if not, proceed to "E".

E. Next, add corn products to the diet in large amounts for five (5) days, watching for the allergic symptoms to increase or reappear. If they do, notify us; if not, we will discuss further testing with other foods with you on your return office visit.

Vomiting and Diarrhea in Children

I. *General Information*

Vomiting and diarrhea are two common problems in infants and children. These are symptoms and not a disease(s) themselves. Fortunately, they are usually self-limiting. Infectious organisms, both bacterial and viral, are the most frequent causes of acute vomiting and diarrhea. Except in epidemic situations, the causative organism is seldom identified before the condition is brought under control by the body's defenses and by effective treatment.

Infections of the upper respiratory tract, throat, middle ear, or urinary tract might be the cause of your child's vomiting and diarrhea. Fever is often present. Too much fat, carbohydrate, or fresh fruit in the diet can provoke an episode of loose stools requiring an adjustment in the diet.

II. *Treatment*

The main treatment of acute vomiting and/or diarrhea is to put the intestines to rest by not eating solid food while at the same time replacing fluid losses. The clear liquid diet is the best way to do this. Clear liquids include: water, sweetened tea, half-strength Jello water (do not use red Jello because the child's vomitus or stools may look as if there is blood in it), beef broth, Kool-Aid, diluted Coke or Pepsi, crushed ice chips or popsicles.

Specifically, no milk, ice cream, eggs, creamy soups, or fruit juices should be given.

If vomiting accompanies the diarrhea, give very small amounts of the liquids more often. In children with diarrhea who are not vomiting, it is sometimes helpful to give them larger volumes of oral fluids, but at less frequent intervals to avoid stimulation of the gastro-colic reflex. (This basic reflex occurs when there is something eaten and the urge to move the bowels follows.)

After the symptoms subside, the first solid food should be Jello and then bananas, applesauce, and dry (unbuttered) toast. If these are tolerated well, you may offer half-strength formula or dilute low-fat milk. If this works well for a couple of days, advance slowly to regular feedings. If it does not, drop back to clear liquids for a couple more days.

III. *Notify Us If Any Of The Following Occurs:*

A. Persistent vomiting on clear liquids.
B. Dry tongue—no saliva.
C. Urine not passed in an 8–12 hour period.
D. Extreme irritability or lethargy.
E. Eyes sunken and dry.

Sore Throat

I. *General Information*

Germs make throats sore. The kinds of germs that cause sore throats usually come from other people with sore throats. There are viral germs and bacterial germs. Most sore throats are caused by viral germs, but it is the bacterial germs that we are more concerned about. Most bacterial sore throats are caused by streptococci. We routinely culture all sore throats since no one can tell by looking at the throat whether it is bacterial or viral. In 24–28 hours we will know whether "strep" bacteria are present from the throat culture, in which case we will call you and start penicillin or another appropriate antibiotic. (Our office will call you *only* if streptococci are found on the throat culture.)

II. *Treatment*

A. *Antibiotics:* The main purpose of giving antibiotics is to prevent the complications of a "strep" infection such as rheumatic fever and glomerulo-nephritis (kidney disease). This will require *ten full days* of antibiotic therapy *no matter how well the patient feels.* The antibiotic will do little to cure the sore throat faster and a one- to two-day delay while waiting for the culture results will make no difference.

If we have not started antibiotics immediately or do not start you on them in two days this is because no strep was cultured and your sore throat is being caused by one of many viruses. Antibiotics, unfortunately, will do nothing for a virus and, in fact, may do harm. The following are reasons why antibiotics are not used routinely:

1. *No Value:* The first and main reason, as we mentioned, is that they will do absolutely no good for a virus infection. Present day antibiotics do not kill virus germs.

2. *Allergy:* A person at any time in his or her life may become allergic to antibiotics, no matter how many times he or she has had them before.

3. *Resistance:* When penicillin, for example, is used, most of the bacteria which are sensitive to this drug *throughout the body are killed*, leaving behind the bacteria resistant to penicillin. Therefore a later infection such as pneumonia, kidney infection, etc., may be resistant to treatment.

4. *Yeast Overgrowth:* We know that many different kinds of bacteria as well as yeast live usually in harmony in the large intestines, female organs, etc., and by indiscriminate use of antibiotics we kill out useful bacteria too, often allowing yeast and other resistant bacteria to overgrow and start another infection.

5. *Diarrhea:* As mentioned above, the antibiotic not only kills the bacteria that may be causing the "strep" throat, but also kills bacteria in the intestines which are necessary for digestion of foods, which may result in severe diarrhea.

B. *Symptomatic Relief:* For any type of sore throat, viral or streptococcal, warm salt water gargle or irrigation is of definite benefit to shorten the course and make the throat feel better. Chloroseptic throat spray may be purchased from the drug store. It is helpful in relieving some of the pain associated with a sore, raw throat. Other throat lozenges or disks may have a soothing effect. Extra fluids and aspirin or Tylenol for fever and pain also have benefit.

III. *Final Notes*

The usual course for a sore throat is two to five days. Even if antibiotics are used for a strep throat, it is not unusual to have a fever for two to three days. If the sore throat persists more than two weeks, we definitely should see you or your child again. Finally, when antibiotics are used, they must be continued for the *full ten days*. Even if you feel well after five days of antibiotics, you should continue taking the medicine until it is gone. It is important to kill completely all the streptococci to prevent recurrence and/or complications. Saving antibiotics for the next time is unwise.

Irritable Colon

I. *General Information*

Irritable colon is a common disorder of the large intestine with pain in the lower abdomen and irregular bowel habits—either diarrhea or constipation, or sometimes alternating diarrhea and constipation. Bowel movements often have mucus mixed with them.

The diagnosis of irritable colon is made by the above history and usually confirmed by physical examination, blood tests, bowel X rays and sigmoidoscopy. The treatment of irritable colon is important to relieve symptoms and to prevent the development of diverticulosis.

II. *Treatment*

A. General Measures

1. Activity: stay active. Get back into a state of good physical condition by daily increasing the amount of exercise. Make your exercise fun if possible, but exercise.
2. Diet: a diet high in residue is very important. You should start the day with a bowl of All Bran, Bran Buds or 100% Bran. If you are unable to eat these let us know. Other high residue foods include whole grain bread, *fresh* fruits and *fresh* vegetables. Canned or frozen fruits and vegetables as well as instant quick-cooking foods and convenience snack foods do not have the high residue you need. Drink an adequate amount of fluids each day.
3. Bowel movements: when you have the urge for a bowel movement take the time for it at that time. Do not strain. The best time for most people is soon after breakfast.

B. Medication:

Your medications must be fitted to your own particular needs. Do not take laxatives and other medications without discussing these with us. As you follow the above measures your symptoms will subside. However, early in therapy and for an occasional flare-up of symptoms, you may need a stool softener, a bowel relaxant, or an anti-diarrhea agent. We will instruct you on the use of any of these drugs if they are indicated in your case.

III. *Notify Us if Any of the Following Occur:*

A. Passage of black or bloody bowel movements.
B. Sudden, more several abdominal pain which is different from your usual symptoms.
C. Persistent diarrhea leading to severe weakness.
D. Persistent constipation leading to vomiting.

MIGRAINE
HEADACHES*

WHAT ARE THE COMMON SYMPTOMS?

One or a number of the following may appear:

an "aura" or sense a headache is starting
changes in vision (such as double vision, sensitivity to light, even partial
            blindness which resolves after the headache goes away.)
weakness in an arm or leg
dizziness or unsteadiness in walking
drowsiness and/or slight confusion in thinking
throbbing headache
headache is usually one-sided
nausea and/or vomiting
abdominal pain relieved by vomiting (more common in children)

WHAT CAUSES THESE SYMPTOMS?

There are many types and causes of headaches. Some of the symptoms above can
happen without it being a "migraine". It is advised that if you have more
than the common, one-in-a-while headaches that are relieved by a simple
tylenol or aspirin that you seek out your family physician.

A "true" migraine results from rapid changes in the size of some blood
vessels in the brain. First the blood vessels shrink or "constrict" in size,
then get larger or "dilate". It is during the shrinking stage that some
people feel the "aura" that something is going to happen. It is during the
enlargement stage that the headache symptoms start. Treatment is best when
it can be started during the first, or shrinking stage.

WHAT THINGS ARE KNOWN TO TRIGGER MIGRAINES?

Here is a list of things associated with the onset of migraines:

FOODS

aged cheeses
herring
monosodium glutamate (MSG, the
    Chinese restaurant syndrome),
    also in some meat
    tenderizers
cured cold cuts, hot dogs

fermented, pickled or marinated foods
peanut butter
canned figs
chicken livers
chocolate
vinegar
avocado, spinach and orange pulp

*Courtesy of Department of Family Medicine, University of North Carolina.

MEDICATIONS

- Reserpine
- Nitroglycerine

ENVIRONMENTAL CONDITIONS

- bright sunlight
- stuffy rooms
- rapid weather changes

PSYCHOLOGIC

- overstress ("distress") from
  many causes. The headache
  usually starts after the
  stressful events are over.
- depression at varying levels

BODY CONDITIONS

- rapid changes in blood sugar
  (such as fasting or overeating
  foods that are high in sugar)
- hormone changes
  (such as ovulation, pregnancy
  menstrual periods, birth control
  pills)
- oversleeping
- fever
- genetic causes
  (migraines occur mostly in women
  and 60–80% run in families)

WHAT CAN I DO?

Withough question, the best defense is a making a good attempt to finding out what causes them—and then how to prevent them from happening, if that's possible. WORK WITH YOUR DOCTOR ON A PLAN

1. If you have an idea of what causes one, restructure your life such that you can avoid the cause.

2. If you don't know what causes them, think about the items listed above. Eliminate as many of the possible causes as you can and then add them back one by one. If you get a headache, that may be a clue to what causes them.

3. Work with your Family Doctor on a plan of action since some medications are powerful, (even over-the-counter medicines!)

WHEN SHOULD I SEE MY DOCTOR?

- If after reading the above it appears that you have been having migraines, talk with your family doctor about them as soon as possible.

YOUR FAMILY DOCTOR'S NAME IS:

PATIENT'S NAME _____

SPRAINS*

WHAT IS A SPRAIN?

A sprain is a tear in a muscle or ligament
resulting from some kind of trauma. The tear
results when there's more pressure on the muscle
or ligament than the body can handle (usually a sudden
twisting motion).

ARE THEY SERIOUS?

Sprains can be serious. They can be mild or severe depending on the amount
of force that caused them to happen. What is most important is that you know
what to do about it right away, and when to call your doctor.

WHAT ARE THE SIGNS AND SYMPTOMS OF A SPRAIN?

• PAIN is probably the easiest symptom to recognize. Your body is
   trying to tell you that you should rest the part. Pain is caused
   by both the injury (tear) of the muscles/ligaments and also by
   swelling and bleeding that occurs after the injury.

• SWELLING AND BLEEDING will result if there has been enough force.

• WEAKNESS in the part affected

CAUTION: JUST BECAUSE YOU CAN MOVE IT DOESN'T MEAN IT'S NOT BROKEN!!!

HOW CAN I TAKE CARE OF MYSELF AT HOME?

REST is the most important thing. If you use the injured part, you
   may injure it even more. That will mean a longer healing period
   and the possibility that it may not regain its original strength.

You should immediately put COLD PACKS on the sprained part. Take some
   ice cubes out of the freezer, put them in a towel and then put the
   towel against the skin. It is important that you treat your injury with
   COLD packs for the first TWO DAYS. The COLD packs need to stay on the
   injury for at least 20 MINUTES, THREE TIMES A DAY for the first 2 days.

UNC FAMILY PRACTICE   966-2491

*Courtesy of Department of Family Medicine, University of North Carolina.

DO NOT PUT HEAT on the injury UNTIL the pain and swelling have stopped,

then use moist heat to speed the healing process. That might mean at least three or four days. Putting heat on the injury later than the third day will make the swelling and bleeding worse. If you re-injure yourself, immediately put COLD packs back on it (even if you injured it 5 days ago and have been using heat). FOR SWELLING AND PAIN USE COLD.

WRAP the injured part. If you can, in an elastic bandage (like an ACE) after

putting the ice on it. Put it on snugly, but not too tight. You should be able to put a finger under the bandage without difficulty. The fingers or toes that stick out beyond the bandage should stay warm to the touch and pink (not bluish!). If they get blue or lose feeling, immediately loosen the bandage. The bandage is intended to cut down on swelling and add some support- not cut off circulation.

ELEVATE the part up to the level of the heart or higher (such as on a stool

or several pillows) after putting the COLD packs and bandage on. This will aid the circulation and cut down on swelling.

TAKE TYLENOL (acetaminophen) for pain, NOT ASPIRIN. Aspirin may cause

bleeding to continue.

WHEN SHOULD I CONTACT MY DOCTOR?

Since sprains can often be serious, we suggest you call the Family Practice Center doctor on-call (or your own primary doctor during the weekday) if:

1. the swelling starts immediately after the injury

2. there is bleeding

3. there is any loss of feeling

4. there is a deformity

5. you cannot move the part

6. your sprain continues to get worse, despite REST, COLD PACKS, ACE WRAP, ELEVATION

HOW LONG WILL IT TAKE THIS TO HEAL?

That will depend on the amount of damage that was done. Mild sprains may take only a week, severe sprains will take longer. Some may take 6 weeks or more to heal.

It's important that you pay attention to your pain and swelling. That's your

best guide to healing. If you use the injured part and it hurts—stop using it. If the injured part starts to swell—stop using it and apply cold

packs. Use the crutches or supportive devices your doctor gives you. Eat a balanced diet and get a good night's sleep. The more you care for yourself, the faster it will heal with the minimum damage.

MY FAMILY DOCTOR'S NAME IS:

966-2491

WATCHING SUGARS IN YOUR FOODS*

- Look at the ingredients on the label
- If any of the following words appear in the first 3 ingredients, DON'T eat that product...

- glucose
- dextrose
- sucrose
- corn sweeteners

- molasses
- syrup
- honey
- sugars

UNC FAMILY PRACTICE   966-2491

*Courtesy of Department of Family Medicine, University of North Carolina.

Appendix 4
Office Systems and Communications

- Health Care Records

- Relative and Absolute Values for 24 Procedures

Fam. No _____

PLEASE FILL OUT THIS FORM COMPLETELY TO HELP US WITH YOUR MEDICAL CARE

Please Print

1. Patient Name _____ Age _____ Sex _____
     Last   First   Middle

2. Marital Status (Circle one)   M   S   W   D   Sep   3. Birth Date _____ / _____ / _____

4. Address _____
    Change: Street   City   State   Zip Code

5. Home phone: _____   Change:

6. Occupation _____   Social Security Number _____

7. Person responsible for account _____
    Relationship to patient _____   Social Security Number _____
    Address _____   Phone _____
         Street   City   State   Zip Code
    Employer _____   Address _____
    Occupation _____   Business phone _____
    Employment change: Business phone:

8. Family Members:

Name	Birth Date	Relationship	Address
_____	___ / ___	_____	_____
_____	___ / ___	_____	_____
_____	___ / ___	_____	_____
_____	___ / ___	_____	_____
_____	___ / ___	_____	_____
_____	___ / ___	_____	_____

9. Medical Insurance: Yes _____   No _____
    In whose name is the insurance policy? _____
    Insurance Company: 1. _____
                         2. _____
    Insurance Numbers: 1. _____
                        2. _____

10. Medicare/Medicaid/Welfare Numbers _____   _____   _____

11. I hereby authorize the office of Dr. Ronald A. Kellogg and Dr. J. Henry Burkholder to furnish medical information to insurance agencies as may be requested for any illness or injury. (Optional)

    Signature of responsible party _____   Date _____

12. Who referred you to our office? _____

INITIAL HISTORY:

1. Why are you coming to the doctor?

2. List any chronic diseases you have:

3. What medication are you now taking? For each one give:

    Name   Strength   How often taken   How long been on this medication?
    1. _____
    2. _____
    3. _____

4. Are you allergic to any medications? _____ If so, what ones and what reaction occurs?

    _____

5. Do you smoke now? _____ If so, how many cigarettes _____ cigars _____ or pipes _____
    per day.
    If you smoked in the past, when did you quit? _____

6. Do you drink alcoholic beverages? _____ If so, what ones and how much per day _____
    and week _____ ?

7. Have you ever had a tetnus shot? _____ If so, how many and when was the last? _____

8. Date of last: Chest x ray _____   TB skin test _____ Result _____
                   Blood Tests _____   Eye Exam _____
                   Electrocardiogram _____ Pap Smear (if female) _____

9. Your past Hospitalizations:

Medical Admissions:		Operations	
Date	Reason	Date	Reasons

10. Family History - Please check if a blood related member of your family has had any of the following:

    _____ TB   _____ Cancer   _____ Lung Disease   _____ Anemia
    _____ Rheumatic Fever   _____ Heart Disease   _____ Kidney Disease   _____ Arthritis
    _____ Diabetis   _____ High Blood Pressure _____ Stomach Problems   _____ Mental Disease
    _____ Thyroid Diseases   _____ Strokes   _____ Bleeding Tendency   _____ Glaucoma

    Other Diseases _____

		Age if Living	State of health. If not good, state reasons.	Age Deceased	Cause of Death
Mother					
Father					
Brothers	Number Alive _____ Dead _____				
Sisters	Number Alive _____ Dead _____				
Children	Number Alive _____ Dead _____				

11. Other things about your health you wish the doctor to know.

12. Signature of person completing this form _____

PROBLEM LIST

NAME _____

ALLERGIES: _____ CHART NO. _____

I. DATE ENTERED	CHRONIC PROBLEM:	PLAN:
1.		
2.		
3.		
4.		
5.		
6.		
7.		
8.		
9.		
10.		

II. PAST HOSPITALIZATIONS (nonsurgical)

	DATE	DIAGNOSIS OR REASON:	HOSPITAL & DOCTOR	YEAR
1.				
2.				
3.				
4.				

III. PAST SURGERY

	DATE	SURGERY OR REASON:	HOSPITAL & DOCTOR	YEAR
1.				
2.				
3.				
4.				

IV. ALLERGIES & REACTIONS

VI FAMILY HISTORY

RA		Thyroid	
DM		Kidney	
CA		Bleeding	
BP		Anemia	
CVA		Psy	
PUL		Arth	
GI		Glaucoma	

VII. RED FLAGS - FHx - ROS

Drinks / wk.

Packs / day

V. HEALTH MAINTENANCE:

Activity	Date of Last	Dates/Results:					
1. Pap/breast							
2. Rectal							
3. Hematest X 3							
4. EKG							
5. Hgb/Hct							
6. Urine							
7. Tonometry							
8. Chest X-ray							
9. Tetanus							
10.							
11.							
12.							
13.							

#20

Name _____

Birth
Date _____

Fam. No. _____

I. PROBLEM LIST:

1. _____
2. _____
3. _____
4. _____
5. _____
6. _____

III. ALLERGIES:

V. RED FLAGS:

VI. PAST HISTORY:

Hospitalizations   **Surgery**

Other serious illnesses: OM, UTI,
   Seizures, Anemia, TB, DM, MR,
   Pneumonia

Medications:

II. IMMUNIZATIONS:

Age				Date Given	
2 mos.	DPT - 1	TOP - 1			
4 mos.	DPT - 2	TOP - 2			
6 mos.	DPT - 3	TOP - 3			
10 mos.	Tine Test				
14 mos.	MMR				
18 mos.	DPT-Boost-1	TOP-Boost-1			
4-5 yrs.	Td/Tine	TOP-Boost-2			
15 yrs.	Td	Tine			

IV. PERSON RESPONSIBLE:

Name: _____

Address: _____

Social Security Number: _____

Employer: _____

Phone: Home _____

   Business _____

Insurance Company: _____

   Policy Number: _____

VII. BIRTH HISTORY:

Pregnancy: Medications _____   Illness _____   Complications _____

   Bleeding _____   Anemia _____   Infections _____

Labor—Length _____

Delivery—Type _____

Birth—Weight _____   Maturity _____   Apgars _____

   —Cyanosis _____   Jaundice _____

Congenital Defects _____

VIII. FAMILY HISTORY:

Name	Birth Date	Sex	Health
Mother			
Father			
Sibs - 1			
2			
3			
4			

____ Diabetes
____ Bleeding Disorders
____ Color Blindness
____ Deaths $<$ 50 y.o.
____ Birth Defects
____ Sickle Cell
____ Congenital Hip
____ Strabismus
____ Mental Retardation
____ Childhood Deaths
____ Cystic Fibrosis
____ Thyroid Disease
____ High BP
____ TB
____ Heart Disease
____ Epilepsy

COMMENTS:

CHART NO. _____

NAME _____

HEALTH QUESTIONNAIRE: DATE _____

Please check the items which have occurred recently or frequently in the past.

A.   General

Circle the highest year reached in school | 1 2 3 4 5 6 7 8 | 1 2 3 4 | 1 2 3 4 |
Grade School   High School   College

____ Recent family illness or death
____ Any recent change in weight
____ Recurrent fever or chills

B.   Head and Eyes

____ Headaches more often than once a week
____ Vision affected by headaches
____ Fainting spells
____ Injury to head
____ Dizziness
____ Double or blurred vision
____ Pain in eyes
____ Decreased vision
____ Blind spots or blindness
____ Seeing colored halo around lights

C.   Ears, Nose, and Throat

____ Recent change in hearing
____ Drainage from the ears
____ Ringing or buzzing in the ears
____ Head colds more often than twice a month
____ Nose bleeds for no reason
____ Nasal drip when no cold
____ Sinus problem
____ Hoarseness without a cold
____ Lumps or swelling in the neck
____ Trouble swallowing
____ Change in voice
____ Thyroid enlargement - goiter

D.   Respiratory (Lungs)

____ Frequent cough
____ Cough up thick sputum
  (color _____ amount per day _____)
____ Cough up blood
____ Chest colds more often than twice a winter
____ Short of breath after walking ___ flights of stairs
____ Asthma
____ Night sweats
____ TB exposure or past history of TB
____ Hay fever

E.   Cardiac (heart)

____ Sleep with more than one pillow
____ Chest pain
____ Swelling of the ankles
____ Fast or irregular beating heart
____ Previous medication for heart trouble
____ Past heart murmur
____ Past heart attack
____ Pains in the legs with walking
____ High or low blood pressure

F.   Gastrointestinal (stomach)

____ Indigestion or heart burn
____ Stomach pains
____ Vomiting blood
____ Difficulty swallowing
____ Black or bloody bowel movements
____ Recent change in bowel movements
____ Frequent constipation
____ Rectal pain or bleeding
____ Intolerant of fried or fatty foods
____ Hepatitis
____ Jaundice or yellowing of the skin
____ History of ulcer disease

G.   Urinary

____ Urinate often at night
____ Pain or burning with urination
____ Blood in the urine
____ Loss of bladder control
____ Urinate frequently during the day
  (more than 5 - 6 times)
____ History of kidney stones

H.   Skin

____ Boils
____ Black and blue spots without injury
____ Cuts hard to heal
____ Colored moles that have recently changed
____ Persistent rash

I. **Endocrine (glands)**

___ Weight loss despite good appetite
___ Unusual loss of hair
___ Constantly thirsty
___ Recent weight gain
___ Craving sweets
___ Hot or cold room intolerance

J. **Musculoskeletal**

___ Gout
___ Stiffness or pain of joints
___ Arthritis
___ Paralysis or weakness
___ Back pain
___ Any body disability or deformity

K. **Neuropsychiatric**

___ Change in speech
___ Lost track of thoughts
___ Unable to express thoughts or feelings
___ Persistent numbness or tingling
___ Trouble coordinating
___ Loss of memory
___ Difficulty with words
___ Frequently ill
___ Afraid to be alone
___ Finds decisions difficult
___ Previously had a nervous breakdown
___ Loss of appetite
___ Unhappy with job
___ Cry frequently
___ Difficulty falling asleep
___ Often get spells of complete exhaustion
___ Often tired or exhausted in the morning
___ Severe aches or pains make it impossible
      for you to work
___ Feel unhappy and depressed
___ Life looks entirely hopeless
___ Wish that you were dead and away from it all
___ Tremors or convulsions
___ Loss of sex interest
___ Presently under tension
___ Loss of interest in home and family
___ Have you ever had counseling or psychiatric care?

L. **Women Only**

Number of pregnancies _____ , stillbirths _____
    miscarriages ___ , premature babies _____
___ On birth control pills or hormones
___ Problems with pregnancy
      What _____
___ Babies over nine pounds
___ Spotting between periods or after sex
___ Not having periods now. Date of last
      period _____
___ Excessive vaginal discharge
___ Lump or pain in breasts
___ Severe pain with periods

M. **Men Only**

___ Trouble starting stream
___ Reduced urinary stream
___ Cancer or tumor of the prostate
___ Lumps or sores on the penis or
      discharge from the penis
___ Loss of sex ability or nature
___ Rupture
___ Enlarged, swollen, tender or hard testicles
___ Doctor said prostate was enlarged

**List other things about your health you wish the
doctor to know**

_____

_____

_____

_____

_____

_____

Signature of person completing form _____

DATE	PROBLEM	GEN	EENT	HEART LUNGS	G. I.	G. U.	ORTHO	N./P.	CHART # _____
		1	2	3	4	5	6	7	PLAN

PROBLEMS 1. _____ 3. _____ CHART NO. _____

2. _____ 4. _____ NAME _____

GRAPHIC FLOW CHART			DATE OF VISIT 19												
		Wt. P O BP X													
		250													
		240													
		230													
		220													
		210													
		200													
		190													
		180													
		170													
		160													
		150													
		140													
		130													
		120													
		110													
		100													
		90													
		80													
		70													
		60													
Symptoms															
Medications / Compliance															
Examination															
Laboratory															
Next Appointment															

PEDS. FLOW SHEET   Allergies _____   Name _____

_____   Chart # _____

PROBLEM LIST   PLAN   Past Illnesses _____

1. _____   _____

2. _____   Surgery _____

3. _____

4. _____   Other Hosp. _____

5. _____   _____

____ Yo $\begin{smallmatrix}c\\n&m\\&f\\o\end{smallmatrix}$ born __/__/__ weighed _____ lbs ____ oz after ____ mo of pregnancy that was

complicated by: _____

delivered by Dr. _____ , labor of _____ hours, complications: _____

perinatal problems: _____

	NAME	BORN	SEX	HEALTH	OTHERS AT HOME
Father	_____	__/__	m	_____	_____
Mother	_____	__/__	f	_____	_____
Sib. 1	_____	__/__ m	f	_____	_____
Sib. 2	_____	__/__ m	f	_____	_____

Wt.* lbs.	Ht.* in.	H. C.* cm	Talk + Diet #	Age	Date	Immunizations (Initial)		Lab	C/o	Exam	Devel.
				1 m							
				2 m		DPT	TOP				
				4 m		DPT	TOP				
				6 m		DPT	TOP				
				9 m				Tine			
				12 m				hct			
				15 m		MMR					
				18 m		DPT	TOP				
				2 y.							
				3 y.				C & S Urine		Hearing	
				5 y.		Dt	TOP	Hearing & Vision Tine		BP _____	
				10 y.				Rubella titer (F) Tine		BP _____	
				15 y		Td		Vision Tine		BP _____	

* PLEASE CHART

Pregnancy Complications:

Medicines _____

Drugs _____

Alcohol _____

Infections _____

Bleeding _____

Anemia _____

Infections _____

Pregnancy _____

Family History: (fetal, child or early deaths - - 50)

DM _____

C.F. _____

TB _____

HBP _____

Bleeding problems _____

Sickle cell _____

Strabismus _____

Epilepsy _____

Thyroid problems _____

Other _____

Birth defects (hip, stature, heart, MR, other)

Deaths < 50 yo _____

Cholesterol / Triglycerides _____

Past Medical History:

UTI _____

DM _____

TB _____

Anemia _____

Seizures _____

Pneumonia _____

Ear infections _____

Skin infections _____

Other _____

Birthmarks and defects _____

Medicines past _____

Medicines present _____

Surgery (who/what/where/when) _____

_____

_____

_____

Other hospitalizations (who/why/where/when) _____

_____

_____

_____

Allergies (type of reaction/drug, allergens) _____

_____

_____

_____

COMMENTS: _____

DEVELOPMENTAL MILESTONES	Normal	Actual
WATCHES FACE	1 Mo.	
COOS, FOLLOWS MOVING OBJECTS	2 Mo.	
LAUGHS	3 Mo.	
HOLDS HEAD ERECT	4 Mo.	
PUTS THINGS IN MOUTH	4½ Mo.	
ROLLS OVER	5 Mo.	
REACHES FOR OBJECTS	6 Mo.	
SITS WITHOUT SUPPORT	8 Mo.	
PLAYS PEEK-A-BOO, CRAWLS	9 Mo.	
TRANSFERS	9 Mo.	
PULLS UP TO STANDING	10 Mo.	
TRIES TO EAT WITH FINGERS	11 Mo.	
WALKS	12 Mo.	
MA MA, DA DA	12 Mo.	
THUMB-FINGER GRASP	12 Mo.	
WALKS WITHOUT SUPPORT	14 Mo.	
CLIMBS ON FURNITURE	15 Mo.	
TRIES TO USE CUP AND SPOON	18 Mo.	
SPEAKS A FEW WORDS	18 Mo.	
WALKS UP AND DOWN STAIRS	22 Mo.	
THREE WORD SENTENCES	24 Mo.	
PLAYS ALONE; 'HELPS' CLEAN HOUSE	24 Mo.	
DRAWS O	24 Mo.	
KNOWS SOME BODY PARTS	3 Yr.	
PEDALS TRICYCLE	3 Yr.	
DRAWS + X	4 Yr.	
ASKS "WHY"	4 Yr.	
USES FULL SENTENCES	4 Yr.	
PLAYS COOPERATIVELY	4 Yr.	
DEVELOPS BLADDER & BOWEL CONTROL	4 Yr.	
KNOWS FIRST & LAST NAME	4 Yr.	
DRESSES SELF	5 Yr.	
KNOWS COLORS	5 Yr.	
DRAWS □ △	5 Yr.	
DROPS INFANTILE SPEECH PATTERNS	5 Yrs.	
DRAWS ◇	6 Yrs.	

OB FLOW SHEET   ALLERGIES: _____   NAME _____

_____   CHART NUMBER _____

_____ y.o. $\begin{matrix} S & C \\ M & N \\ D & O \end{matrix}$ g____ p _____Ab ____ LNMP _____ EDC* _____ largest _____ lb. ____ oz.

longest labor ____ hrs., shortest ____ hrs., height _____ diagonal conjugate _____

bispinous _____ arch _____ weight before pregnant _____ lbs.

Complications:

PMH:

ABO_____ Rh ____($\begin{smallmatrix}20, 24, 28, \\ 32, 34, 36.\end{smallmatrix}$) rubella _____ (12 week)

LBS.	Sug/Ptn	BP	FHT	FUNDUS	TALK^0	DATE	WKS.	LAB	C/O$^+$	EXAM
					Bleed		6	Preg. Prof.		
					$		8			
					Preg.		12			
					Labs		16			
					Sibs		20	hct %		
					Limits		24			
					Hid Anes		28	BP$_l$ BP$_s$		
					Class		32	U/C		
					Baby		34	hct %		
					Labor		36	BP$_l$ BP$_s$		
					Hosp		37	gc RPR		
					Family		38			
					Mood		39			
					GM$_0$		40			
							41			
							42			

Delivery date _____ Weight _____ Sex_____ Complications: _____

Baby Name _____

*enter on OB calendar $^0\checkmark$ each talk when given   +each visit ask about bleeding, calf pain, N/V, UTI, edema, h/A

#16

Pregnant?

Menarche _____ yrs. old	Form of birth control _____
Periods regular _____	Morning sickness _____
Usual cycle _____ days	Breast change _____
Flow _____ days	Skin changes _____
LNMP _____	(-3/+7/+1) EDC _____
Prior MP _____	Father _____
Any spotting since _____	Feelings (self) _____
Quickening date _____	_____
Do you feel pregnant? _____	Feelings (other) _____
	_____

Other pregnancies (include miscarriages and Ab's)

	Birth Date	Sex	Weight	Mom+	Children ever have*
1.					
2.					
3.					
4.					
5.					

+ any problems of HBP, toxemia, preeclampsia, seizures, Rh, sugar, diabetes, bleeding, transfusions, anemia, jaundice, over 5 days in hospital, C-sections, breech, UTI

* jaundice, premature, birth defects, infections, surgery, hospitalizations, poor growth, other.

PMH Meds   Allergies

Surgery   Transfusions

Illnesses: Tb, hepatitis, phlebitis, anemia, thyroid, sugar, kidney, GC, VD, epilepsy, heart disease, rheumatic fever

FHx Above illnesses
or
C. F., sickle cell, birth defects, child deaths, premature, bleeding problems, mental retardation, twins

EXPOSURES:

Diet _____	Meds _____	X rays _____
Cigarettes _____	Employment _____	Cats _____
Alcohol _____	Hobbies _____	Farm animals _____
Drugs _____	Rubella _____	Other _____

Well Child Care

Name —   Fam. No. —

		1 mo.	2	4	6	10	14	18	2 yo.	3	5	8	12	15		
Date																Date
Age																Age
Immunizations																Immunizations
DPT			○	○	○			○								DPT
TOP			○	○	○			○			○					TOP
Td											○			○		Td
Tine-PPD						○					○			○		Tine-PPD
MMR							○									MMR
Lab																Lab
Hgb/Hct			○				○			○	○	○		○		Hgb/Hct
U/A								○				○				U/A
UC										○	○	○				UC
BP										○	○	○	○	○		BP
Vision											○		○	○		Vision
Hearing										○	○	○				Hearing

		1	2	4	6	10	14	18	2	3	5	8	12	15		
Physical Exam.																Physical Exam.
Fontanels																Fontanels
Hershberg-Cover																Hershberg-Cover
Ear-Drum																Ear-Drum
Hearing																Hearing
Nose																Nose
Throat																Throat
Mouth																Mouth
Teeth																Teeth
Cervical Glands																Cervical Glands
Thyroid																Thyroid
Lungs																Lungs
Heart																Heart
Abd. Mass L/S																Abd. Mass L/S
Hernia																Hernia
Femoral Pulse																Femoral Pulse
Genitalia																Genitalia
Testis ↓↓																Testis ↓↓
Rectum																Rectum
Hips-Barlow																Hips-Barlow
Legs																Legs
Feet																Feet
Walking																Walking
Scoliosis-Kyphosis																Scoliosis-Kyphosis
Moro/T G																Moro/T G
		1 mo.	2	4	6	10	14	18	2 yo	3	5	8	12	15		

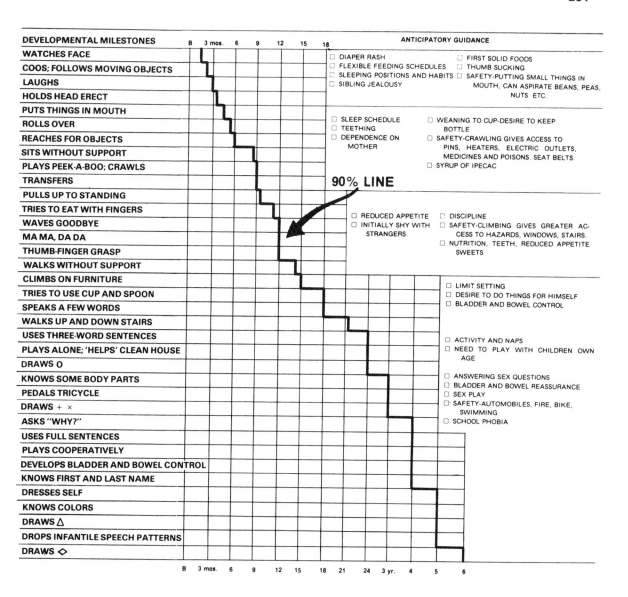

DEVELOPMENTAL MILESTONES	B	3 mos.	6	9	12	15	18	ANTICIPATORY GUIDANCE
WATCHES FACE								☐ DIAPER RASH ☐ FIRST SOLID FOODS
COOS; FOLLOWS MOVING OBJECTS								☐ FLEXIBLE FEEDING SCHEDULES ☐ THUMB SUCKING
LAUGHS								☐ SLEEPING POSITIONS AND HABITS ☐ SAFETY-PUTTING SMALL THINGS IN
HOLDS HEAD ERECT								☐ SIBLING JEALOUSY MOUTH, CAN ASPIRATE BEANS, PEAS, NUTS ETC.
PUTS THINGS IN MOUTH								
ROLLS OVER								☐ SLEEP SCHEDULE ☐ WEANING TO CUP-DESIRE TO KEEP
REACHES FOR OBJECTS								☐ TEETHING BOTTLE
SITS WITHOUT SUPPORT								☐ DEPENDENCE ON ☐ SAFETY-CRAWLING GIVES ACCESS TO
PLAYS PEEK-A-BOO; CRAWLS								MOTHER PINS, HEATERS, ELECTRIC OUTLETS, MEDICINES AND POISONS. SEAT BELTS.
TRANSFERS								☐ SYRUP OF IPECAC
PULLS UP TO STANDING								**90% LINE**
TRIES TO EAT WITH FINGERS								
WAVES GOODBYE								☐ REDUCED APPETITE ☐ DISCIPLINE
MA MA, DA DA								☐ INITIALLY SHY WITH ☐ SAFETY-CLIMBING GIVES GREATER AC-
THUMB-FINGER GRASP								STRANGERS CESS TO HAZARDS, WINDOWS, STAIRS. ☐ NUTRITION, TEETH, REDUCED APPETITE
WALKS WITHOUT SUPPORT								SWEETS
CLIMBS ON FURNITURE								☐ LIMIT SETTING
TRIES TO USE CUP AND SPOON								☐ DESIRE TO DO THINGS FOR HIMSELF
SPEAKS A FEW WORDS								☐ BLADDER AND BOWEL CONTROL
WALKS UP AND DOWN STAIRS								
USES THREE-WORD SENTENCES								☐ ACTIVITY AND NAPS
PLAYS ALONE; 'HELPS' CLEAN HOUSE								☐ NEED TO PLAY WITH CHILDREN OWN AGE
DRAWS O								
KNOWS SOME BODY PARTS								☐ ANSWERING SEX QUESTIONS
PEDALS TRICYCLE								☐ BLADDER AND BOWEL REASSURANCE
DRAWS + ×								☐ SEX PLAY
ASKS "WHY?"								☐ SAFETY-AUTOMOBILES, FIRE, BIKE, SWIMMING
USES FULL SENTENCES								☐ SCHOOL PHOBIA
PLAYS COOPERATIVELY								
DEVELOPS BLADDER AND BOWEL CONTROL								
KNOWS FIRST AND LAST NAME								
DRESSES SELF								
KNOWS COLORS								
DRAWS △								
DROPS INFANTILE SPEECH PATTERNS								
DRAWS ◇								

	B	3 mos.	6	9	12	15	18	21	24	3 yr.	4	5	6

PHYSICAL EXAM

	NAME							CHART NO.				
	DATE											
		R	L	R	L	R	L	R	L	R	L	
	Weight Ideal											
	Height Pulse											
	B P Sitting											
	Supine											
ENT	T M's											
	Nose											
	Lips Tongue											
	Gums Teeth											
	Throat Voice											
	Hearing											
EYES	Pupils											
	E O M											
	Fundi											
	Fields											
	Tonometry											
NECK	Trachea											
	Thyroid											
	Cervical Nodes											
	Carotid Pulse											
	Bruits											
	Supra Clavicular											
	JVD HJR											
BREASTS	Masses											
	Nipple											
	Axilla											
CHEST & LUNGS	Percussion											
	Auscultation											
	FEV, FVC											
CV	Thrust Thrill											
	Murmur											
	Gallop											
ABDOMEN	Shape											
	Bowel Sounds											
	Tenderness											
	Liver Spleen											
	Masses Bruit											
	Femoral Pulse											
	Inguinal Nodes											
SKIN	Texture											
	Nodules											
	Eruptions											
	Scars											

#27

	Date	R	L	R	L	R	L	R	L	R	L
Pelvic	Hernia										
Rectal	Ext. Genitalia										
	Rectal										
	Guine Prostate										
	Vagina PAP										
	Cervix										
	Uterus										
	Adnexa										
Ext.	Clubbing Cyanosis										
	Edema										
	Radial Pulse										
	DP Pulse										
	PT Pulse										
	Joints										
Neuro.	Cranial										
	Nerves										
	Motor										
	Sensory										
	DTR's Triceps										
	Biceps										
	Knee										
	Ankle										
R L	Babinski										
	Vibration										
	Position										
	F→N H→S										
	Romberg										
	Gait										
	Affect										

Date

Date

Date

Date

Date

Date

Relative and Absolute Values for 24 Procedures Common to Both the Time-Based and Charge-Based Relative Value Scales.

Procedure (CPT-4 Code)	Time-Based[1]			Charge-Based[2]		
	Relative Value	Scale Rank	Absolute Value	Relative Value	Scale Rank	Absolute Value
Brief hospital visit established patient (90240)	0.68	(1.00)	8.04	0.96	(3.00)	$15.52
Minimal office visit, established patient (90030)	0.72	(2.00)	8.61	0.51	(1.00)	8.26
Brief office visit, established patient (90040)	0.77	(3.00)	9.13	0.85	(2.00)	13.72
Brief office visit, new patient (90000)	0.85	(4.00)	10.08	1.32	(8.00)	21.34
Limited hospital visit, established patient (90250)	0.96	(5.00)	11.44	1.25	(5.00)	20.11
Limited office visit, established patient (90050)	1.00	(6.00)	11.87	1.00	(4.00)	16.10
Brief hospital visit, new patient (90200)	1.11	(7.00)	13.13	2.46	(15.00)	39.69
Chemotherapy (96030)	1.17	(8.00)	13.88	1.30	(6.00)	20.91
Limited office visit, new patient (90010)	1.23	(9.00)	14.63	1.70	(12.00)	27.38
Electrocardiogram (93000)	1.36	(10.00)	16.19	1.71	(13.00)	27.68
Extended hospital visit, established patient (90270)	1.40	(11.00)	16.67	2.12	(14.00)	34.18
Extended office visit, established patient (90070)	1.50	(12.00)	17.85	1.65	(11.00)	26.71
Brief home visit, established patient (90140)	1.52	(13.00)	18.08	1.30	(7.00)	20.92
Limited home visit, established patient (90150)	1.69	(14.00)	20.04	1.52	(9.00)	24.54
Arthrocentesis (20610)	2.03	(15.00)	24.12	1.59	(10.00)	25.62
Comprehensive office visit, new patient (90220)	2.16	(16.00)	25.68	3.14	(18.00)	50.71
Comprehensive office visit, established patient (90080)	2.27	(17.00)	26.98	2.68	(16.00)	43.25
Comprehensive hospital visit, new patient (90220)	3.14	(18.00)	37.30	3.73	(19.00)	60.18
Herniorrhaphy (49505)	3.52	(19.00)	41.82	27.2	(20.00)	439.38
Thoracentesis (32000)	3.71	(20.00)	44.11	3.08	(17.00)	49.75
Hysterectomy (58265)	4.73	(21.00)	56.13	53.3	(23.00)	861.21
Cholecystectomy (47600)	5.02	(22.00)	59.62	43.7	(22.00)	705.65
Colon resection (44140)	8.27	(23.00)	98.25	60.20	(24.00)	972.29
Heart catherization (93527)	10.20	(24.00)	120.92	33.00	(21.00)	532.28

[1] Mean time per procedure are in minutes.

[2] Mean Health Care Financing Administration (unindexed) prevailing charges are in dollars.

NOTES: The time-based and charge-based means for all procedures are 2.54 and 10.47, respectively. The time-based and charge-based standard deviations for all procedures are 2.37 and 17.85, respectively. The Pearson and Spearman correlations between the two scales are 0.8 and 0.90, respectively. (Reprinted with permission from Juba D and Hadley J (1985). Relative value scales for physicians services. Health Care Financing Review 6(4). Health Care Financing Administration, US Dept of Health and Human Services.)

Appendix 5
Practice Site

- Floor Plans
- Preliminary Architectural Program: Sample Data Retrieval Sheet
- Corporation Benefits Available to the Physician-Executive
- Physician Agreement Summary

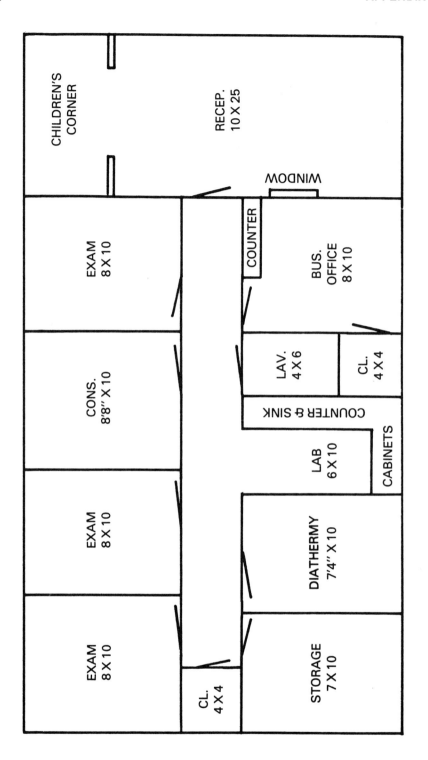

Solo Doctor—Simple Basic Design
Dimensions: 25′ × 44′ = 1,100 Square Feet
Scale: 1/6″ = 1′
Expansible

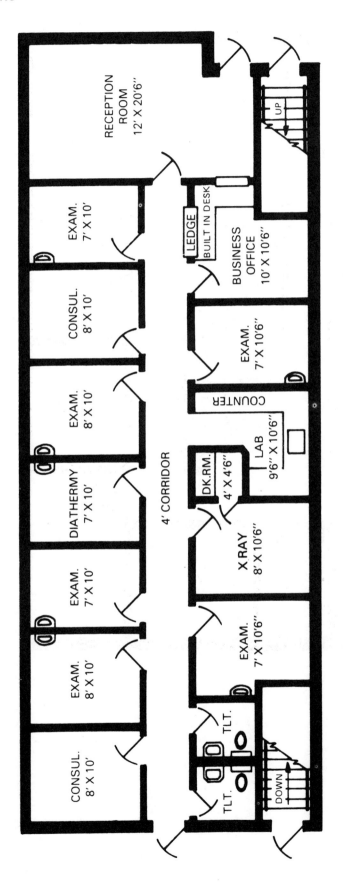

Two Doctors—Single Corridor
Good Design Feature: Business office counters and windows to reception room and corridor
Dimensions: 25′ × 68′ = 1,700 Square Feet
Scale: 1/8″ = 1′

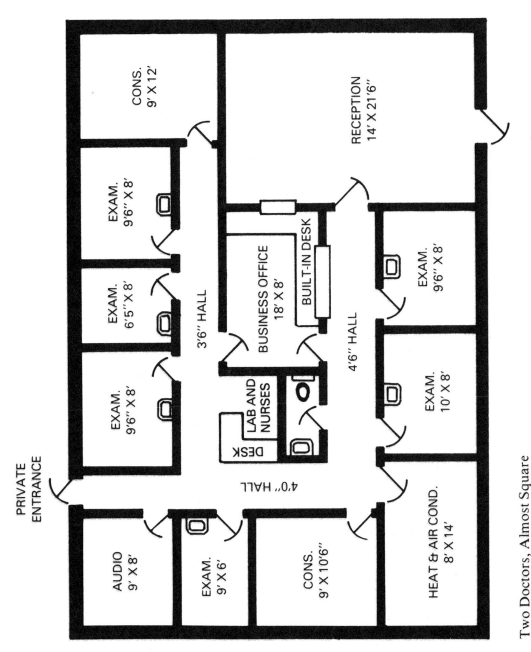

Two Doctors, Almost Square
Good Design Features: Built-in desk in business office, windows and nurses station
Dimensions: 36' × 51' = 1,836 Square Feet
Scale: 1/8" = 1'
Expansible

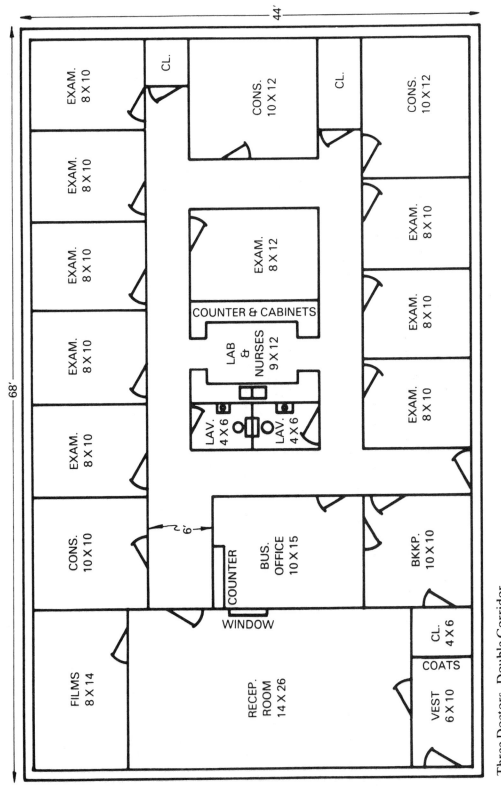

Three Doctors, Double Corridor
Good Design Features: Separate bookkeeping office, combined lab–nurses station
Dimensions: 44′ × 68′ = 2,992 Square Feet
Scale: 1/8″ = 1′
Expansible two directions

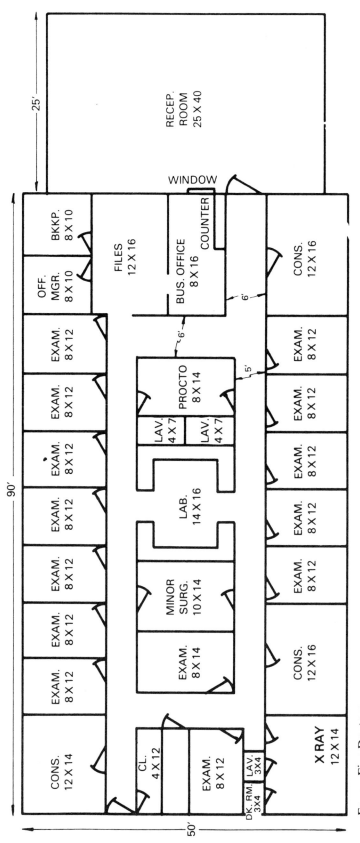

Four—Five Doctors
Good Design Feature: Multiple business offices, shared consultation offices
Dimensions: 50′ × 90′ main building plus reception
Area: 5,500 Square Feet
Scale: 1/12″ = 1′
Expansible

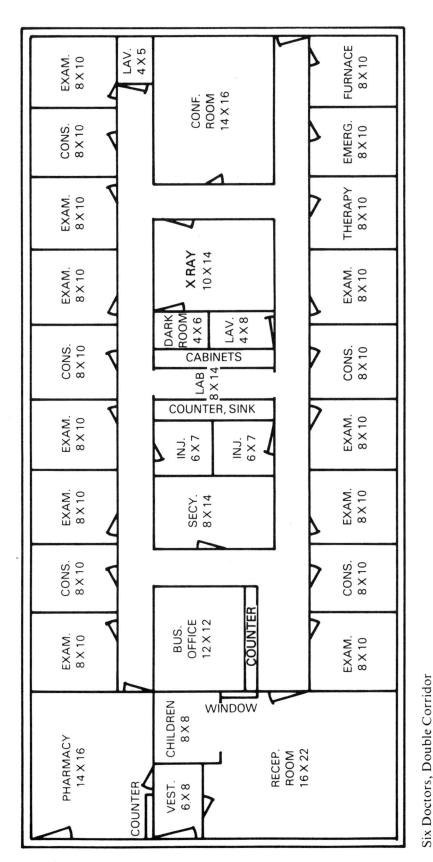

Six Doctors, Double Corridor
Good Design Features: Injection rooms, pharmacy, conference room (can also be staff lounge), children's reception area

Dimensions: 45′ × 93′ = 4,185 Square Feet
Scale: 1″ = 10′
Expansible

Preliminary Architectural Program*
Sample Data Retrieval Sheet

I. Initial Goals and Scope of the Project

II. Services to be Provided on Site

It has been proposed that the following services be provided:

A. Complete history and physical examination with appropriate laboratory tests as indicated or desired.

B. Management of stabilized chronic disorders under physician supervision.

C. Management of uncomplicated pre and postnatal states under physician supervision.

D. Provision of well–child care.

E. Family planning as requested by the patients.

F. Counseling as appropriate within the limitations and abilities of the staff.

G. In addition, certain specimens such as pap smears or blood for chemical analysis may be obtained at the health center and transported to the appropriate laboratory.

H. Provision on site of select testing and screening procedures as appropriate:

_____ Anthropometry: measure height and weight

_____ Vital Signs: determine blood pressure, pulse, temperature, respiratory rate

_____ Tonometry: glaucoma screening

_____ Audiometry: determine hearing capacity (referred to local health department)

_____ Spirometry: lung capacity screening

_____ Vision Testing: check seeing ability for color, perception, etc. (nonverbal test)

_____ Electrocardiogram: measure electrical activity of heart (referred to area hospital)

_____ Phonocardiogram: detect and measure heart sounds and murmurs (referred to area hospital)

_____ Pap Smear: detect cervical cancer

_____ Proctosigmoidoscopy: detect polyps or cancer in the lower colon (referred to back-up physician)

_____ Glucose Ingestion: detect diabetes

_____ Tine Skin Test: detect tuberculosis

_____ Pregnancy Test

_____ Mononucleosis Test

_____ Sickle Cell Anemia Test

_____ Parasite Detection

_____ Throat & Urine Cultures: detect types of infections

_____ Urinalysis: specific gravity, pH, sugar, albumin, acetone, bacteria

_____ Blood Chemistry: white blood count, blood sugar, hematocrits/hemoglobins

*From Alford's FACILITY PLANNING, DESIGN AND CONSTRUCTION OF RURAL HEALTH CENTERS, Copyright 1979 by University of North Carolina at Chapel Hill. Reprinted with permission from Ballinger Publishing Company.

_____   EENT Screening: instrument–assisted visual survey of eyes, ears, nose, and throat

_____   Skinfold: determine degree of obesity

_____   Dental & Soft Tissue Exam: oral survey with no fillings or cleaning

_____   Visual & Tactile Physical Exam

_____   Psychological Questionnaire

_____   Medical History Interview

_____   Other: Future addition of simple x ray for chest and extremities

III. Staffing Program

     RNs
     LPNs
     Clinical Aides
     Physicians
       backup
       visiting specialist
     Receptionist/Secretary
     Administrative Aides
     Business Administration (consulting accountant)
     Maintenance
     Outreach:
       visiting public health staff
     Other

IV. Anticipated Patient Load

V. Anticipated number of examination/treatment rooms

VI. Anticipated maximum number of patient associates occupying waiting area at any given time

VII. Patient Types

     A. Well–child (newborn through adolescence)

       _____   Routine preventive treatment

       _____   Physical examinations

       _____   Monitoring of total state of health

     B. Adult Screening (adolescence through geriatric)

       _____   Routine preventive treatment

       _____   Physical examinations

       _____   Monitoring of total state of health

     C. Chronic disease (all ages)

       _____   Prolonged monitoring, repeated treatments, and consultation as required

     D. Minor Illness (all ages)

       _____   Diagnosis, treatment, and consultation

     E. Minor Trauma (all ages)

       _____   Render treatment as required by specific nature of the injury

F. Emergency (all ages)

_____   Take action to sustain life for patients in critical condition until they can reach a major medical facility

G. OB/GYN (women, adolescence through geriatric)

_____   Routine pre and postnatal medical supervision

_____   Routine gynecological monitoring

VIII. Anticipated activity settings and requirements

Phase I:

A. Entrances

_____   Patient and visitors

_____   Staff and emergency

B. Reception and Clerical

_____   Monitor waiting area

_____   Patient data

_____   Financial interview

_____   Scheduling

_____   General business and administrative activities

C. General Waiting

_____   Lounge area

_____   Community notice area

_____   Health education information

_____   Coat storage

_____   Public toilets

D. Staff Office(s)

_____   Reference reading material

_____   Consultation and patient interview

_____   Charting

_____   Dictation/dictaphone

_____   Family Nurse Practice (FNP)

_____   Visiting physician and specialists

E. Clinical Control

_____   Medications

_____   Testing

_____   Clinical Control

_____   Vital Signs

F. Laboratory

    _____ Patient toilet (handicapped)

    _____ Testing

    _____ Sample taking

    _____ Analysis

    _____ Charting

G. Examination/Treatment

    _____ Pediatric exam

    _____ Minor trauma area

    _____ Testing

    _____ Examination

    _____ Consultation

    _____ Undressing/dressing

    _____ Treatment

H. General Storage

    _____ Supplies (clinical, business, health education)

    _____ Medication (locked storage)

    _____ Personal effects

I. Utility

J. Mechanical

K. The Site: provide parking for a minimum of 18 vehicles

CORPORATION BENEFITS AVAILABLE TO
THE PHYSICIAN-EXECUTIVE

1. Face amount of group life insurance.
   a. While actively in practice _____
   b. After retirement _____

2. Hospitalization benefits for self and family. (Describe) _____
   _____

3. Major Medical Benefits.
   a. Deductible _____
   b. Top limits _____

4. Availability of medical and dental reimbursement program.
   Top limit _____

5. Wage continuation program, if disabled. (Describe) _____
   _____

6. Disability insurance benefits.   Amount _____
                                     Paid personally _____
                                     Paid by corporation _____

7. Automobile reimbursement
   a. Auto _____
   b. Repairs _____
   d. Gas _____

8. Reimbursement on dues and subscriptions: _____

9. Reimbursement for attending conferences: _____

10. Vacation policy.
    a. How vacation times are determined _____
    b. Amount of time available _____
    c. Compensation arrangements if more time is taken _____

11. Pension/profit sharing plan—find out details of each.
    a. Where are the funds invested? _____
    b. What is the formula? _____
    c. What is the vesting schedule? _____
    d. What are the eligibility requirements? _____
    e. What does the most recent actuarial valuation show past service liability to be? _____
    f. Availability of voluntary contribution under the plan? _____

12. Procedure by which a new physician becomes a stockholder.
    a. Waiting time _____
    b. Terms of the purchase _____
    c. What assets are included _____
    d. At what point an equal stockholder _____

13. How accounts receivable are handled.
    a. In buying in _____
    b. Paying off an existing stockholder _____

14. How termination benefits are handled.
    a. Stock interest _____
    b. Receivables _____

15. Does the firm's attorney do the estate planning for the new physician? _____
    Who pays the fee, the group or the new physician? _____

16. Does the firm's accountant do the tax return of the new physician? _____
    Who pays the fee, the group or the new physician? _____

17. Does the firm arrange for a line of credit for the new physician? _____

18. Does the practice own its own building? _____

19. Are there provisions for the new physician to eventually buy into that building? _____
    a. Share of interest _____
    b. Terms of buy-in _____

20. Policy for time off to prepare for Boards. _____

21. Who pays for malpractice insurance? _____ Umbrella? _____
    a. Amounts of coverage _____
    b. Claims made or occurrence policy? _____

22. Are there any privileges restricted to senior physicians? _____
    _____

23. Are there any extra duties expected of the new physician that are not performed by the established physician? _____
    a. Evening calls _____
    b. Weekend calls _____

24. Is the new physician invited to all corporation meetings and discussions with professional advisors? _____
    a. At the time he associates with the practice? _____
    b. When he becomes a stockholder? _____

25. A copy of the Employment Contract governing each of these items? _____
    Will it be available for signature prior to employment? _____

PHYSICIAN AGREEMENT SUMMARY

Physician Participation. As a private practice physician you have the opportunity to participate in the HealthAmerica prepaid plan as a supplement to your existing practice. Your patients choose the prepaid plan and remain your patient with no disruption of your practice. The excellent benefits offered by HealthAmerica and high quality care provided by participating physicians has resulted in rapid growth, making HealthAmerica the largest HMO in North Carolina.

Enrollment. HealthAmerica is offered to employers with fifteen or more employees. The employee/subscriber has a choice to remain in their traditional insurance plan or to join HealthAmerica by selecting one of the Health-America participating physicians. The physician/group so chosen must accept the member and the responsibility of providing or supervising all care. However, physicians may limit the number of members that will be accepted into their practice.

If the physician-patient relationship becomes unacceptable either the physician or the patient may request, in writing, a transfer to another practice. Physicians may not request to transfer patients because of high utilization resulting from the patient's medical condition.

Payment for Services. The HealthAmerica Plan covers virtually all medically necessary care with a few limitations which are outlined in the Agreement. The participating physician is responsible to provide primary care services and manage necessary consultant and hospital care required by members. HealthAmerica divides the health care dollar used to pay for these services into four funds as described below:

Primary Physician Capitation: **Features:** Capitation dollars are paid to the Primary Physician on a monthly basis for each member in the practice on an age and sex adjusted basis. Age and sex adjustment is utilized to reflect the differing amounts of care normally required by women and men within specific age groups and to insure adequate reimbursement for the members in each practice. HealthAmerica pays

100% of the capitation dollars to the practice at the beginning of each month with no amount withheld as is common in other HMO's. All prepaid plans have an element of risk for the Primary Physician, but HealthAmerica has limited this risk to a maximum of up to 10% of the Primary Physician Capitation if deficits occur in the Individual Referral Services Fund, the Shared Risk Fund for Referral Services or the Hospital Services Fund and the Financial Review Committee determines that care provided or authorized was not medically appropriate. **Covers:** Primary care services, outpatient laboratory and immunizations and injections and routine radiology performed by the Primary Physician in the office.

Individual Referral Services Fund: **Features:** HealthAmerica pays for services covered by the Individual Referral Fund approved and authorized for payment by the Primary Physician. This fund is practice specific with allocations made monthly for each member in the practice on an age and sex adjusted basis. The fund is protected by a single stop-loss of $1200 per member per calendar year for all consultant costs and effective management of services. Physicians receive quarterly fund reports and any deficit is automatically reviewed by the Financial Review Committee. **Covers:** All consultant services and outpatient radiology provided outside the primary physician's office.

Shared Risk Fund for Referral Services: **Features:** A practice specific allocation is made monthly for each member in the practice on an age and sex adjusted basis. These practice specific funds are then pooled with all other participating practices' shared risk funds. 100% of any surplus in the fund is distributed annually to the Primary Physician according to the practices' pro rata contribution to the fund surplus and any deficit is automatically reviewed by the Financial Review Committee. Physicians receive quarterly fund reports. **Covers:** All charges greater than the $1200 stop-loss amount in the Individual Referral Services Fund and all charges greater than the total funds available in the Individual Referral Services Fund.

Hospital Services Fund: **Features:** A practice specific allocation is made monthly for each member in the practice on an age, sex and regionally adjusted basis. Practice specific funds are then pooled and all hospital costs below the corporate reinsurance level are paid out of the pooled Hospital Services Fund. A $10,000 per member per calendar year stop-loss limits the amount of hospital costs allocated against the practice specific Hospital Services Fund when the status of that fund is being calculated. 50% of any surplus in the pooled fund is distributed annually to individual practices based on the practices' pro rata contribution to the surplus. Physicians receive quarterly fund reports. **Covers:** Hospital room, board and ancillary services; radiology, pathology and ekg interpretation; emergency and ambulance services; inpatient mental health. Hospital and outpatient chemotherapy, radiation therapy and dialysis.

Special Financial Considerations. Experience indicates that the age and sex adjusted capitation will provide participating physicians with an equitable compensation for providing and managing care in a cost conscious manner. However, adverse experience can have a negative impact on the adequacy of the capitation for an individual practice. Consequently, HealthAmerica will make a retrospective review of a participating physician's financial experience to assure equitable reimbursement for providing members appropriate medical care and management of covered services. All physician/practices are evaluated during their first year of participation. If HealthAmerica determines that the physician is practicing in a cost conscious manner, the contract will be renewed with the assurance that during the second and subsequent years a minimum of 90% of the fee for service equivalent will be achieved for pro-

viding medically appropriate care and conscientious management of services required by HealthAmerica members. Determination of the fee for service equivalent is based on the HealthAmerica reasonable fee schedule for services reported on HealthAmerica encounter forms.

Financial Review Committee. The Financial Review Committee includes participating family physicians, pediatricians and internists from each region of North Carolina. The Committee automatically reviews all practices that have deficits. Practices with fund deficits may be required to reimburse HealthAmerica up to 10% of their capitation if the Committee determines that inappropriate management of care was provided. Practices will not be held at risk when adverse selection or catastrophic illness has affected their financial experience. The Committee examines the financial experience of any practice that requests a review and makes recommendations regarding practices which may be eligible for special financial consideration. The 90% assurance provided for practices after the first year of evaluation will not apply if the Committee determines that the practice did not provide appropriate care and management.

Quality Assurance. HealthAmerica is committed to providing high quality, cost effective care. Physicians agree to participate in the HealthAmerica Advisory Medical Council which meets regularly to adopt quality of care guidelines and conduct quality assurance reviews. Physicians also agree to maintain up to date medical records in accordance with accepted professional standards and to allow inspection of records and facilities as required by HealthAmerica.

Appendix 6
Financial Management

A SELECTED GLOSSARY OF FINANCIAL MANAGEMENT

Accrual Accounting: A basis of accounting that identifies revenue with the period in which service is provided and expenses with the period in which resources are consumed. Because revenues and expenses are easier to predict on an accrual basis, accrual accounting is normally used to prepare operating budgets.

Assets: The organization's resources which will benefit the future.

Balance: The difference between the sum of debit entries minus the sum of credit entries in an account. If positive, the difference is called a *debit* balance; if negative, a *credit* balance.

Balance Sheet: A summarized statement as of a given date of the financial position of a group showing assets, liabilities, and equity.

Benefit-Cost Analysis: An evaluation of the relationship between the benefits expressed in dollars and the dollar costs of a particular project or activity.

Capital Expenditure Budget: The portion of the group's comprehensive budget that relates to the

procurement or disposition of long-lived productive resources.

Cash Basis: The basis of accounting under which revenues are recorded only when cash is received and expenses are recorded when cash is paid.

Cash Budget: A portion of the comprehensive budget that relates to the plan of expected cash inflows, outflows, and balances.

Cash-Flow Statement: A form of the statement of changes in financial position where the cash inflows and outflows for a group are explained.

Chart of Accounts: A list of accounts systematically arranged, applicable to a specific group, giving account names and numbers.

Cost Accounting: The body of accounting which provides for the assembling and recording of all the elements of cost incurred to accomplish a purpose, to carry on an activity or operation, or to complete a unit of work or a specific job.

Cost Center: An organizational segment of a group that is separately recognized in the group's records, accounts, and reports. Program-oriented budgeting, accounting, and reporting aspects of an information system are usually built upon the identification and use of a set of cost centers.

Current Liabilities: Liabilities that will mature and require payment from current assets within the coming year.

Database: Information available to group practice management for planning, decision making, and control functions.

Debt Service: Expenditures for the retirement of noncurrent or long-term debt, including principal and interest on such debt.

Direct Costs: Costs that are directly attributable to a specific cost objective, such as cost center, and are traceable to that cost objective.

Encumbrances: In fund accounting, purchase orders, contracts, and/or other commitments which are chargable to an appropriation and for which a part of the appropriation is reserved. They cease to be encumbrances when paid or cancelled or when actual liability is established.

Expenditures: In fund accounting, the incurrence of a cost either through the commitment of credit or the disbursement of cash. In other accounting systems, only the disbursement of cash is considered an expenditure.

Expenses: In the accrual basis of accounting, resources consumed in the process of generating revenue, regardless of when the payment for the source is made.

Expired Costs: In the cash basis of accounting, the amount of cash expended in the process of generating revenue.

Financial Management: The process of dealing with problems of cost effectiveness, control of expenditures, use of financial data, preparation of budgets, concepts of cash flow, cost accounting, resource allocations, investments, capital financing, etc.

Financial Statements: The general purpose reports on the stewardship of the group prepared for management and external purposes. They include the statement of financial position, income statement, statement of retained earnings, and the statements of changes in financial position.

Fiscal Period: Any period of time at which a group determines its financial position and the results of its operations, and closes its books. It is usually a year, though not necessarily a calendar year. The most common fiscal period for groups is January 1 through December 31.

Fixed Costs: Costs which are incurred regardless of the volume of encounters and do not vary with utilization rates; as distinct from variable costs.

Fund Balance: In fund accounting, the excess of the assets of a fund over its liabilities and reserves, except in the case of funds subject to budgetary accounting where, prior to the end of a fiscal period, it represents the excess of the fund's assets and estimated revenues for the period over its liabilities, reserves, and appropriations for the period.

Goal: A broad statement of the direction toward which all decisions and activities of a clinic are focused.

Gross Income: Revenues before deducting any expenses; an expression employed in the accounting process for individuals, financial institutions, and the like.

Income: Excess of revenues earned over the expenses incurred in carrying on the group's operations. It should not be used without an appropriate modifier such as operating, nonoperating, or net. Note that the term *income* should not be used in lieu of revenue.

Income Statement: A statement that evaluates operating performance by comparing revenues with expired costs.

Indirect Expenses: Those elements of cost necessary in the provision of a service which are of such a nature that they cannot be readily or accurately identified with or traced to the specific service.

Ledger: A group of accounts in which are recorded the financial transactions of a group.

Liabilities: Incurred expenses for which payment has not yet been made. An obligation arising out of past events or transactions payable in cash or other resources, usually at some specified or determinable date in the future.

Management Information System: A network of communication channels that acquires, retrieves, and redistributes data used in managing the group and in supporting the individual and collective decision-making process.

Objectives: Specific quantitive and time-performance targets to achieve a firm's goals.

Overhead: Those elements of cost necessary in the performance of a service which do not become an integral part of the service, such as rent, heat, light, supplies, supervision, management.

Planning: The selection or identification of the overall, long-range goals, priorities, and objectives of the organization, and the formulation of various courses of action in terms of identification of needs and relative costs or benefits for the purposes of deciding on courses of action to be followed in working toward achieving those goals, priorities, and objectives.

Proforma: Budgeted financial statements developed from certain specified planning assumptions.

Program Budgeting: A budgetary system used in the public sector that relates resources used to the output of the organization, rather than on specific inputs.

Receipts, Revenues: Additions to assets which do not incur an obligation that must be met at some future date and do not represent exchanges of property for money.

Variable Costs: Costs that vary in total dollar amount in direct proportion to the changes in activity. The cost per unit of output is assumed to be constant over the relevant range of activity.

Variance: The difference between actual results and planned results.

Working Capital: The excess of current assets over current liabilities.

Zero-Based Budget: A budget process which assumes that all programs or line-item categories should be reassessed each budget period to see if the program or category should be continued. If it cannot be justified, it is dropped or not funded.

Index